Proactive Support of Labor

The Challenge of Normal Childbirth

Second edition

Proactive Support of Labor

The Challenge of Normal Childbirth

Second edition

Paul Reuwer
Consultant Obstetrician-Gynecologist and Master of the Labor and Delivery Unit at the St. Elisabeth Hospital, Tilburg, The Netherlands

Hein Bruinse
Professor Emeritus of Obstetrics at the University Medical Centre Utrecht, The Netherlands

Arie Franx
Professor of Obstetrics and Chair of Division Woman and Baby, University Medical Centre Utrecht, The Netherlands

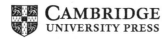
CAMBRIDGE
UNIVERSITY PRESS

CAMBRIDGE
UNIVERSITY PRESS

University Printing House, Cambridge CB2 8BS, United Kingdom

One Liberty Plaza, 20th Floor, New York, NY 10006, USA

477 Williamstown Road, Port Melbourne, VIC 3207, Australia

314-321, 3rd Floor, Plot 3, Splendor Forum, Jasola District Centre, New Delhi - 110025, India

79 Anson Road, #06-04/06, Singapore 079906

Cambridge University Press is part of the University of Cambridge.

It furthers the University's mission by disseminating knowledge in the pursuit of education, learning and research at the highest international levels of excellence.

www.cambridge.org
Information on this title: www.cambridge.org/9781107426580

© Paul Reuwer, Hein Bruinse, and Arie Franx (2009) 2015

First published 2009
Second edition 2015

A catalogue record for this publication is available from the British Library

Library of Congress Cataloging in Publication data
Reuwer, Paul, author.
Proactive support of labor : the challenge of normal childbirth / Paul Reuwer, Hein Bruinse, Arie Franx. – Second edition.
    p. ; cm.
Includes index.
ISBN 978-1-107-42658-0
I. Bruinse, Hein, author.   II. Franx, Arie, author.   III. Title.
[DNLM: 1. Maternal Health Services.   2. Delivery, Obstetric – methods.
3. Natural Childbirth.   4. Obstetric Labor Complications – prevention & control.
5. Pregnancy Outcome. WA 310.1] RG524
618.2–dc23

2015007322

ISBN 978-1-107-42658-0 Paperback

....

Every effort has been made in preparing this book to provide accurate and up-to-date information which is in accord with accepted standards and practice at the time of publication. Although case histories are drawn from actual cases, every effort has been made to disguise the identities of the individuals involved. Nevertheless, the authors, editors and publishers can make no warranties that the information contained herein is totally free from error, not least because clinical standards are constantly changing through research and regulation. The authors, editors and publishers therefore disclaim all liability for direct or consequential damages resulting from the use of material contained in this book. Readers are strongly advised to pay careful attention to information provided by the manufacturer of any drugs or equipment that they plan to use.

This book is dedicated to Kieran O'Driscoll, great obstetrician and distinguished teacher, pioneer in the development and evaluation of conceptual birth care. His fundamental insight and inspiring work provided the starting point of this treatise.

Contents

Section III – Proactive support of labor

Foreword to the first edition

Improvements in the care of the pregnant woman and fetal patient during the birthing process have been a success story for modern obstetrics. Less than a century ago, maternal mortality during labor was commonplace in most developed countries, and fetal mortality and morbidity were even more common. The keystone of modern obstetrics was the introduction of hospital and safe cesarean deliveries in the early twentieth century. However, too much of a good thing can sometimes lead to other problems.

In their book *Proactive Support of Labor*, Drs Reuwer, Bruinse, and Franx make an important contribution to modern obstetrics by providing a critical counterbalance to technologic interference in labor and delivery. The authors introduce the concept of "proactive support of labor" as an acceptable alternative to traditional labor and delivery management in order to shorten labor and ultimately ensure a safer delivery. They propose that results of improved labor and delivery management should be evaluated not only in physical terms (e.g., reduced morbidity and mortality) but also in terms of emotion and patient satisfaction. This concept is designed to improve not only the overall outcome but also patient satisfaction.

We agree that the perspective provided in this book should be carefully considered by all providers of healthcare to women in labor. The call for humanistic and evidence-based obstetric care in labor and delivery by including the emotional needs of women in labor should be embraced throughout the world.

Amos Grunebaum
Director of Obstetrics, New York Weill Cornell
Medical College, New York Presbyterian Hospital

Frank A. Chervenak
Chairman of Obstetrics and Gynecology,
New York Weill Cornell Medical College,
New York Presbyterian Hospital

Preface

The central message remains unchanged in the updated Second Edition of this book and continues to emphasize the need for fundamental reforms in the world of obstetrics and midwifery. The policy proposals – aimed at enhancement of women's satisfaction with the childbirth experience and a safe reduction of the cesarean birth rate – stay the same.

New is the deeply researched treatise on the worrying misapplication of evidence-based medicine, leading to false evidence claiming a tempering effect of labor inductions on cesarean rates. Many other prevalent misinterpretations of the literature are exhibited, and several new examples of disturbing misguidance from official guidelines are exposed.

The chapters on audit and quality control have been rewritten. The clinical procedures and outcomes are now analyzed according to the Robson ten-group classification system, providing the best evidence of the effectiveness and safety of the combined policies and the overall strategy of *proactive support of labor*.

The authors wish to express their special gratitude to the nurses and midwives in the integrated birth center Livive, in recognition of their unfailing cooperation at all times. We highly appreciated the criticism, advice, and support we received from esteemed and befriended colleagues, in particular Marc Keirse and Michael Nicholl from Australia and Michael Robson from Ireland. The authors owe many thanks to Simone Valk, Dutch midwife to her bone marrow, for her comments on manuscript drafts and her promotional activities. She developed the interactive partogram-app and the website on keeping birth normal, both based on this book.

Web-links

Readers are encouraged to share their opinions and comments in the interactive web-forum: www.proactivesupportoflabor.com

A book-related partogram app can be downloaded at www.apparentapps.com. This interactive app is available to both professionals and clients/patients, and gives advices for the timely correction of abnormal labor, based on the policies explained in this book.

Clear information and guidance for pregnant women and partners to meet the challenge of normal birth can be found in plain lay-language at www.keepingbirthnormal.com.

General introduction

The natural process of birth increasingly involves medical intervention, but the benefits of this trend are questionable at best. The inexorable growth in cesarean delivery rates is not validated by tangible improvements in perinatal outcomes. Rather, short- and long-term maternal morbidity has risen significantly.

Apart from the physical impact, giving birth is one of the most profound emotional experiences in a woman's life, but women's satisfaction with childbirth remains a cause for common concern. Despite all good intentions, modern maternity care is often perceived as professional but impersonal, and labor is not infrequently described as a traumatic or even "dehumanizing" life-event. This must be changed.

1.1 Purpose

The aim of this book is to present a simple, cohesive, and evidence-based plan for the care of the normal, healthy woman in labor, designed to restore the balance between natural birth and medical intervention. The main target is to improve professional labor and delivery skills in order to promote spontaneous delivery and enhance women's satisfaction with childbirth. *Proactive support of labor* is a carefully orchestrated and audited expert team approach involving the laboring woman, nurse, midwife, and obstetrician, committed to a safe and good birth experience for both mother and baby. Emphasis is placed as much on the physical challenge as on the emotional impact of childbirth. The principles and practices are universally applicable.

> The objective is to enhance women's childbirth experience by improving professional labor and delivery skills and the overall quality of routine intrapartum care.

1.2 Target readership

This book is directed to:

- All professionals who are primarily responsible for the quality of childbirth: obstetricians, midwives, and labor room nurses. Obstetricians are in the prime position to enhance all standards of care by creating the conditions for nurses and midwives to execute their labor support tasks properly;
- Medical students and student-midwives engaging in their first practical contacts with childbirth;
- All other healthcare providers involved in birth care such as family practitioners, childbirth educators, doulas, physiotherapists, sonographers, anesthesiologists, and home health nurses;
- Hospital administrators, healthcare policymakers and health insurers, since high-quality care in labor requires a sound organization, which should coincide with sound economics;
- Last but not least pregnant women and other interested laypersons. No experience with childbirth is needed to understand the relevance and significance of this book. Mothers-to-be have the most to gain from supportive care during their labor and delivery effectively preventing everyday labor disorders and promoting a safe and rewarding delivery. Although professional language is used, the text should be readily understandable to an educated lay audience.

1.3 Presentation

This book is divided into three sections. The first section is a mirror for reflection, unveiling the mechanisms in everyday childbirth that explain excessive operative delivery rates and avoidable discontent of many women with their labor experience. The second section goes back to the basics and reviews the physiological prerequisites for a rewarding and safe birth that are all too often neglected in common childbirth practice. The third section proposes structural measures to solve most problems by introducing the simple principles and safe practice of *proactive support of labor*. Special attention should be paid to the subsection and paragraph headings as many address topics of critical relevance that are seldom, if ever, discussed in standard textbooks.

Section 1 A wake-up call

To solve a problem, one must first admit that the problem exists and identify its causes. Inconsistencies in care, controversial midwifery and medical services, and unfounded concepts and dogmas on both sides of the aisle will be identified and discussed in detail, as well as the self-sustaining mechanisms and stubborn nuisance values hampering structural improvements. Deeply researched analysis of "evidence-based" guidelines will identify many pitfalls and flaws, and will debunk detrimental misguidance from several poorly designed randomized controlled trials and uncritical meta-analyses.

Many elements of care during pregnancy and childbirth can facilitate or jeopardize the successful accomplishment of this natural process.

The preventable or overtly iatrogenic (provider-caused) nature of many birth disorders in mainstream practices will be exposed, and the numerous examples of avoidable harm to women and babies will confront childbirth professionals, and may even shock lay readers. The defiant and provocative tone we adopt is by no means intended to question the integrity and devotion of birth care providers, or to belittle their efforts, but to promote debate and to guide structural and real evidence-based reforms. We wrote this section to serve as a mirror and an eye-opener, laying bare the fundamental problems plaguing current childbirth practices all over the world.

Section 2 Back to basics

Leading ideas about labor and delivery have been relayed from teacher to student and from textbook to textbook without any serious attempt at verification until they have become the main impediments to improvements in everyday care. Recognition of the latent phase of labor is one of the prime examples. The critical reappraisals in this section will show that many accepted and guiding concepts in the world of childbirth are scientifically unfounded, mutually in conflict, and sometimes even plain fallacies.

It is all too frequent in medicine to find ignorance about the most common events.

The chapters in this section offer a fundamental reinterpretation of the basic biophysics dominating the natural process of birth. The basic biology is organized in a coherent manner, giving structure and direction to a scientifically based policy for the supervision of labor. We will emphasize the differences between nulliparous and multiparous labors and challenge the classic understanding of the onset of labor and the course of normal cervical dilatation. It is not the mechanics of delivery, but primarily the dynamics of first-stage labor that provide the optimal chance for a successful, safe, and rewarding birth. Furthermore, a basic knowledge of the biophysical changes in the uterus prior to labor is essential for an accurate understanding of the initiation of the birth process and the negative impact of labor induction. Equally important is knowledge of the physics of uterine contractions, dilatation, and expulsion. Crucial to expert care of labor is recognition of the parasympathetic condition controlling birth and the negative impact that anxiety and stress have on the effectiveness and safety of labor. These fundamental, universally valid aspects of childbirth are of such importance that each must be examined in considerable detail before genuine progress in labor supervision can be made.

Section 3 Proactive support of labor

The emphasis of this book is to organize basic scientific understanding of parturition and hard clinical evidence into an integrated, all-embracing birth-plan. This section provides a step-by-step exposition of the policy framework designed to prevent common labor disorders and to detect and treat problems at an early stage before they are compounded. Safety is crucial, and simplicity is the key. This science- and evidence-based policy offers providers a foothold in negotiating the complexity of daily practice and guards them against clinical stalemates, inconsistent (non-) policies of care, and mismanagement of labor with self-created birth complications. If caregivers follow the strategy promoted in this book, all elements of high-quality birth care will fall into place including honoring women's needs and desires, fetal and maternal monitoring, pain relief, and the prevention and timely correction of everyday labor complications.

> **Proactive support of labor**
>
> *A simple and evidence-based approach specifically designed to promote safe and rewarding labor and delivery. It should appeal to both obstetricians and midwives.*

The key points include a clear diagnosis of the onset of labor, early recognition and correction of dysfunctional labor, consistent conduct, personal attention and commitment, and continuous supportive care on a one-on-one basis extended to all women in labor.

Proactive support of labor encourages an active interest in the supervision of first-stage labor by all members of the delivery team and facilitates constant support and good communication in labor. The central birth-plan promotes the development of team spirit between doctors, midwives and nurses, and dictates good labor ward organization that will improve labor care immensely. This well-defined policy at last makes possible a meaningful daily audit of all procedures in the supervision of childbirth, promoting and ensuring safe, high-quality care. This approach effectively restricts operative delivery rates without any detrimental effects to the infants. Most importantly, this integrated women-centered care system invariably improves mothers' satisfaction with their childbirth experience.

1.4 Advice for readers

Although childbirth is the same physiological process worldwide, childbirth services – even if confined to western countries – have proved to be strongly influenced by cultural differences, medico-legal issues, social pressures, and politics. Therefore, transcultural diversities in birth philosophies, childbirth practices, and care organizations should not be ignored and will be addressed throughout this book. Time and again, *proactive support of labor* will be contrasted with ubiquitous but controversial approaches – ranging from "all natural" midwifery care to high-tech, fully medicalized childbirth – in order to illustrate the need for structural reforms in each type of care. Typical American or European issues should not distract

from the universally valid observations, statements, and evidence-based policy proposals on the supervision of labor made here.

This book describes a cohesive and consistent concept of birth care universally applicable to all societal contexts. All aspects of childbirth will be discussed, but the emphasis is placed on redefining basic birth parameters, reinterpretation of physiological data, hard clinical evidence, emotional support, and strict adherence to logic. For this reason, we recommend reading the chapters in the order in which they are presented. The numbers in brackets represent cross-references within the text.

> *The authors recommend reading the chapters in the order in which they are presented.*

1.4.1 Classification of birth professionals

Terminology with regard to childbirth professionals may be quite confusing as many doctors of unequal educational status are involved, ranging from junior residents to senior consultants. Likewise, the titles "nurse," "nurse-midwife," and "midwife" may cover dissimilar and often overlapping content, substance, and responsibilities. Sensitivity to status and emotion are involved here, and a few terms as used in this book may therefore benefit from definition:

Obstetricians hold a specialist qualification in obstetrics and gynecology. They bear the ultimate responsibility for the medical well-being of their patients. They may also be called "consultants."

Midwives. The general term "midwife," as used in this book, is a state-registered caregiver who has completed four years of vocational education at one of the official midwifery schools, including practice training programs in accredited hospitals and home birth practices. They are regarded as specialists in the supervision of normal pregnancy and delivery. Midwives provide antenatal and postnatal care and supervise normal deliveries independently in primary birth centers or at the woman's home. They are trained in risk assessment and the detection of disease, at which point they will or should seek consultation and transfer the patient. A "clinical midwife" is a postgraduate with two years' additional education and medical training, often to the academic level of a master degree in "advanced midwifery" working exclusively in the hospital.

Labor room nurses are general nurses with two years' additional training in maternity care. They support women in labor and assist midwives and doctors. Labor room nurses do not perform vaginal examinations or deliveries. Whenever the term "nurse" is used in this book, labor room nurses are meant unless indicated otherwise.

Residents are doctors in training to become a medical specialist. Senior residents are in their final years of training and largely function at a level equal to obstetricians after formal authorization.

Interns are undergraduate medical students performing their clinical rotations.

"Laborist" or "OB-hospitalist" is a new breed of caregiver still in its infancy but spreading fast. The titles refer to medical officers who work exclusively in the hospital, keeping watch over women in labor and performing deliveries. Their role should be compared with that of other and more familiar hospital-based doctors such as emergency room physicians. Confusingly, education and responsibilities vary widely ranging from the level of junior residents to fully certified obstetricians. The titles are, therefore, avoided except in Chapter 25 on professional working relations and organization. It is for laborists/OB-hospitalists to decide how to recognize themselves in this book: either as residents or fully qualified obstetricians.

Family practitioners. Some primary care physicians (general practitioners) still attend births, mainly in the woman's home. Their childbirth services resemble those of community-based midwives. Although they are not specifically mentioned throughout this book for reasons of readability, this group of primary care providers is not forgotten: whenever independent midwives are mentioned, readers may include family practitioners as well.

2

Medical excess in normal childbirth

"Not everything that is faced can be changed, but nothing can be changed until it is faced."
–James Arthur Baldwin

The purpose of professional care during labor and delivery is to ensure that every child is born as healthy as possible while causing the least possible damage to the mother. For the most part, this dual goal was realized during the twentieth century as demonstrated by the sharp reduction of maternal and perinatal mortality. In the past three decades, however, obstetrics has failed to maintain its objectives. The once-declining rate of maternal morbidity and mortality is now on the increase, primarily because of the ever-increasing cesarean birth rate in low-risk pregnancies.[1-5] This is a trend that must be changed.

2.1 The cesarean pandemic

The ideal overall cesarean rate is not known, but on the basis of available databases no noticeable improvement in fetal outcome is observed once cesarean rates rise above 10–15%.[6] By now, however, the cesarean birth rate in all developed countries far exceeds these target figures.[7] In the USA, for instance, one in three babies is currently delivered by cesarean section, but the US rates of cerebral palsy and perinatal mortality have remained steady over the past decades.[8-10] The "cesarean problem" that first seemed to be an American affliction is now international. In the last two decades, there has been a 100% increase in cesarean births in England, and the cesarean birth rate continues to climb.[11] The cesarean rates in urban Brazil and China even rocketed to 47% and 60%.[7]

The increase in cesarean delivery-related maternal morbidity and mortality rates, without any evidence of improvement in overall fetal outcomes, is indicative of the failure of current childbirth methods.

Liability concerns regarding uterine rupture have effectively sliced VBAC-rates (Vaginal Birth After Cesarean) worldwide, and the old adage "once a cesarean, always a cesarean" again prevails in many nations.[12] Relatively low overall cesarean rates in the Netherlands and the Scandinavian countries are largely explained by relatively high VBAC rates whereas, there too, about one in four first pregnancies ends with a cesarean delivery.[13]

2.1.1 Operative solutions for failed labors

The cesarean pandemic is not the result of standard elective surgery for indications such as breech presentations, multiple pregnancies, or severely compromised pregnancies, since they represent only a small minority of all births. Neither do emergency interventions, to rescue babies from neurological damage or death, explain the rising cesarean rates. The overall US cesarean rate for "fetal distress" has remained stable between 3.8% and 4.2%.[14,15] The alarming observation is that the vast majority of cesarean deliveries today are performed as the easy-exit strategy for disorders in the first (dilatation) stage of labors in healthy women with a single term fetus in the cephalic presentation – the precise group presumed to be low risk. Predictably, fetal outcome in this group has not improved at all during the past three decades despite this trend.[1-7]

There is a growing tendency to resolve the problems of first-stage labor by surgical intervention.

The American College of Obstetricians and Gynecologists (ACOG) identified dystocia or failure to progress as the primary impetus for the startling expansion of cesarean deliveries, in particular in first labors.[16] These failed labors and related repeat operations in next pregnancies account for two-thirds of all cesarean deliveries in the USA.[8,16] National statistics

5

from all other countries with accurate obstetric records confirm similar trends worldwide. Faced with decreasing VBAC rates, a reduction in the primary cesarean section rate should have a significant effect on the need for subsequent surgical delivery and, therefore, a large impact on the overall cesarean delivery rate.[8] Clearly, when trying to reduce undue cesarean rates one should focus on the supervision of low-risk first labors. That is precisely the emphasis of this book (Sections 2 and 3).

> Failure to progress accounts for the majority of cesarean deliveries in first labors and, by inference, for the largest proportion of repeat procedures.

A detailed discussion regarding the recent trend of elective (planned) cesareans for no reason other than the patient's request falls outside the scope of this book. Nonetheless, such requests must be considered in the overall context of current practice in which the woman – upon denial of her request – has a very high chance of a cesarean or an instrument-assisted vaginal delivery anyhow. In fact, most demands for elective cesarean relate to a previous traumatic labor experience or discouraging horror stories from others. Indeed, the overall cesarean rate is effectively determined – directly and indirectly – by the women-friendly conduct and care of first labors.

> Cesarean delivery reduction programs, to be effective and safe, should primarily focus on the conduct and care of low-risk first labors.

2.2   Instrumental delivery rates

With rising cesarean rates, fewer women reach the second (expulsion) stage of labor, and the rates of instrumental vaginal deliveries should, therefore, decline. However, this has not always happened. Many hospitals with high cesarean rates also have high operative vaginal delivery rates.[17,18] The main indication is second-stage arrest. A forceps or vacuum delivery is not a trivial intervention either as it is particularly damaging to a woman's pelvic floor, potentially risky, and certainly painful for her child.[19] Instrumental vaginal delivery is worryingly associated with serious perinatal birth injuries.[19-21]

First-time mothers-to-be (nulliparas) face the highest risks of operative delivery. Even if a nullipara manages to escape the major surgery of a cesarean, she still has a 25% chance of an instrument-assisted vaginal delivery, in most cases for failure to progress.[19-21] Of course, these are average figures as the rates vary greatly among hospitals and even among practitioners in the same institution. Overall, however, less than half of all women in western countries deliver their first babies spontaneously by the normal route nowadays. There are only two possible explanations: either modern women are no longer capable of normal childbirth or modern childbirth services fail.

> Currently, less than half of all first-time mothers in western countries give birth via the normal route without surgical or instrumental intervention.

2.3   Conceptual flaws

High intervention rates in childbirth are often attributed to the supposedly changing needs of childbearing women and their babies. Some authors suggest a causal association between increasing maternal age and weight and dysfunctional labor.[22-30] In reality, however, the predominant contributors to excessive operative delivery rates more likely relate directly to the caregivers and reflect birth philosophies, culture, organization, the degree to which doctors are paid on a "piecework" basis, their propensity for convenience and control, the extent to which malpractice litigation is feared, and so forth. It is impossible to express the relative impact of each of these factors in absolute numbers, but they all contribute to current obstetric performance. The literature addressing these topics is extensive but mostly vague, and it generally misses the point: the spiraling operative delivery rates actually reflect a progressive lack of understanding of the labor process and, consequently, declining labor and delivery skills of today's birth professionals.

> The majority of problems surrounding childbirth can be attributed to the widespread lack of a consistent and cohesive policy framework for the supervision of normal labor.

2.3.1   Professional controversies

Professional birth care should be based on an astute comprehension of the fundamental processes of parturition such as the cervical and myometrial changes in late pregnancy, the onset of labor, the pattern of normal dilatation, and the length of normal labor. Although nature designed a biological blueprint for labor and delivery – fine-tuned over millions of years of evolution – knowledge and appreciation of the basic biophysical processes controlling birth vary significantly among care providers. As a result, professional views range from understanding childbirth as a natural process, best supervised with the least possible interference, to the emphasis being placed on risks – leading to highly medicalized "management" of labor. This diversity in birth philosophies and practices echoes differences in opinion or lack of scientific knowledge, and the inexorable rise in failed labors seriously calls into question whether midwives and obstetricians still operate from valid concepts of childbirth, if from any concept at all.

Professional conduct and care of labor and delivery should be based on solid, scientific knowledge of the physiology of parturition.

2.4 Counting the costs

The high failure rate of normal labor and delivery is more detrimental than meets the eye and includes severe psychological and physical harm to women, and adverse neonatal outcomes, as well as serious economic and social damage.

2.4.1 Psychological harm

Ideally, women experience childbirth as an empowering and ultimately gratifying event in which the care providers are allowed to partake. Unfortunately, practice shows that many women do not achieve this rewarding scenario, in particular not for their first labor. Apart from the physical burden of a stalled labor that ends in a forceps, vacuum, or cesarean delivery, the woman may sustain substantial emotional damage owing to a feeling of frustration and failure. An operative delivery denies her the unique experience of giving birth to her child by her own efforts as well as the sense of accomplishment from which she could gain further self-esteem and self-confidence. The harsh reality of daily practice is that current birth care turns many a birth into an ordeal.

In the worst-case scenario, the parturient ends up in a deplorable condition; after a whole day or more of exhausting labor, she undergoes abdominal surgery or a difficult instrumental extraction. The psychological

damage from such a poorly managed labor can be worse than the emotional impact of an emergency cesarean for acute fetal distress: a lasting aversion to all things related to birth maintained by recurring nightmares and complicated by feelings of inadequacy and even conscious or subconscious feelings of hostility toward her child.

The emotional impact of women's labor experience remains a matter of common but underrated concern.

The prevalence and severity of these life-lasting effects are strongly underestimated as they mainly develop outside the field of vision of childbirth professionals. Too many women, estimated between 9 and 20%, experience labor and delivery as a genuinely traumatic event.[31–37] Approximately 3% of all women develop a full-blown chronic post-traumatic stress disorder (PTSD) following childbirth, and an additional 22 to 40% experience some post-traumatic stress symptoms.[31–37] About half the women with childbirth-related PTSD also suffer postpartum depression.[33,36,38,39] Importantly, the prevalence of PTSD (symptoms) is reportedly much higher after intrapartum cesarean section and instrumental delivery.[34,38] Usually, PTSD following childbirth is not self-limiting and impairs mother–child bonding, affects the intimate partner relationship, and gives rise to severe fear of childbirth in a subsequent pregnancy, all too often leading to a request for an elective cesarean section.[35,39–44]

Childbirth-related depression and PTSD are chronic conditions permeating throughout a woman's lifetime.

2.4.2 Direct physical harm

Although cesarean section is safer than ever before, it remains major abdominal surgery, and the direct risks are far from negligible. The short-term complications, such as excessive blood loss, infectious morbidity, thromboembolic complications, longer recovery time, extended hospital stay, and the chance of rehospitalization are all too well understood.[2,16,45–50] Moreover, the baseline morbidity associated with cesarean section rockets in obese women, and obesity is another epidemic disease of modern times.[51]

Less well known is that the overall maternal mortality rate for cesarean section is nearly five times greater than that for planned vaginal birth (relative risk [RR] = 4.9; 95% confidence interval [CI] = 3.0–8.0), and the maternal death rate has been slowly but steadily increasing in western countries since the 1980s.[47] The need for emergency hysterectomies has also increased: in about 1 per 200 cesarean deliveries as compared with 1 per 1000 vaginal deliveries.[48,49,52,53] More than 40% of postpartum hysterectomies for massive hemorrhaging follow cesarean delivery.

Spiraling cesarean delivery rates hugely increase severe maternal morbidity.

2.4.3 Long-term medical harm

The negative implications of a cesarean section for future childbirth are the most alarming although generally underrated. Firstly, the risk of unexplained stillbirth in women with a cesarean scar is doubled,[54] and secondly, up to 90% of American pregnant women with a previous cesarean undergo a repeat operation for fear of uterine rupture.[10] Many US hospitals have banned VBACs. Inevitably, the more first cesarean deliveries performed today, the more repeat cesareans will be necessary tomorrow.

The most distressing are the uterine scar-related complications as a result of placental implantation in the lower uterine segment with placenta previa, accreta, or even percreta, leading to massive hemorrhaging. In effect, 2–3% of pregnant women with a cesarean scar – regardless of whether they are scheduled for elective cesarean or a vaginal birth – require massive blood transfusions, embolization therapy, or extensive surgery including emergency hysterectomies and post-treatment intensive care as a result of life-threatening uterine rupture or massive bleeding from the placental implantation site.[2,55–60] Too many women suffer severe harm or even die because of these catastrophic complications in pregnancies that follow an unnecessary primary (first-time) cesarean delivery. These secondary harms are, in fact, primarily iatrogenic.

The initial cesarean delivery is associated with increasing maternal morbidity and mortality, but the downstream effects are even greater because of the relatively higher risks from repeat cesareans in future pregnancies.

Other unforeseen harm includes lifelong discomfort and pain from adhesions, scar endometriosis, or nerve entrapment in the abdominal wall. The amount of attention given to these late complications is inversely proportional to the gravity of long-term patient burden. The same holds for adhesions related difficulties in abdominal surgery many years later. In survey-studies on cesarean-related morbidity, these late sequelae are usually underreported or undetected altogether.

2.4.4 Increased neonatal mortality

In the past, it was assumed that babies were delivered by cesarean because they were medically at risk, thereby explaining the higher infant and neonatal mortality rates typically associated with cesarean births. However, research of the US Centers for Disease Control and Prevention, analyzing over 5.7 million live births and nearly 12 000 infant deaths over a four-year period in the USA, suggested that the mechanism of cesarean birth itself poses a risk of neonatal mortality.[61] The study showed that for mothers at low risk, neonatal mortality rates are nearly three times higher among infants delivered by cesarean (1.77 per 1000 live births) than for those delivered vaginally (0.62 per 1000 live births). The increased risk for neonatal mortality related to cesarean delivery persisted even after adjustment for sociodemographic and medical risk factors. The authors concluded: "Timely cesareans in response to medical conditions have proved to be life-saving for countless babies. At present, we are witnessing a different phenomenon: a nearly threefold increased risk for neonatal mortality in low-risk infants following cesarean birth with no formal medical indication." The overall rate of babies delivered by cesarean among women with no indication save women's request more than doubled in the USA and UK in the last decade. Although neonatal mortality rate for this low-risk group remains low – regardless of delivery method – unnecessary cesarean births might inadvertently put more babies at risk for neonatal morbidity and mortality.

Unbridled expansion of cesarean births in low-risk infants inadvertently increases neonatal morbidity and mortality.

2.4.5 Neonatal and long-term morbidity

No single scientific report indicates that newborns profit from cesarean delivery after an uneventful pregnancy. On the contrary, planned cesarean in uncomplicated pregnancies is associated with a three-fold increase of short-term neonatal respiratory morbidity – necessitating admission to advanced care nurseries – compared with a trial of labor (RR 3.58, 95% CI 3.35–3.58).[62] Levine *et al.* also found a fivefold greater risk of persistent pulmonary hypertension for elective cesarean than for vaginal deliveries.[63] Older literature suggested that neonatal pulmonary hypertension, respiratory distress, and transient tachypnea in elective cesarean deliveries are the exclusive result of iatrogenic prematurity.[64] However, the evidence from well-dated pregnancies shows otherwise.[62] Labor itself benefits the newborn owing to less respiratory morbidity and mortality. Labor induces the release of fetal catecholamines and prostaglandins that promote lung surfactant secretion. In addition, epinephrine (adrenaline) release during labor and the physical compression of the fetal thorax help to remove fetal lung fluid and facilitate postnatal lung adaptation.[65] Moreover, babies born spontaneously are spared the potentially harmful effects of maternal anesthetic medication, such as analgesics and vasopressors, and of standard prophylactic antibiotics.

A beneficial effect of vaginal birth might also hold true for other aspects of later health, as birth by cesarean is associated with a higher incidence of allergic diseases, obesity, and diabetes, possibly or probably related to an altered neonatal bacterial colonization of the skin and gut influencing the immune system.[66–72] Even an association between cesarean birth and the chance of developing psychosis in later life has been suggested, possibly due to an altered perinatal adjustment of the dopamine metabolism.[73]

> There is no evidence whatsoever to indicate that elective cesarean after an uncomplicated pregnancy is of any benefit for babies. Rather, the reverse is true.

2.4.6 Economic damage

Cesarean section has now achieved the dubious distinction of being the most frequently performed inpatient operation of any category. In the USA alone, more than 1.2 million cesareans are performed each year, relegating hysterectomy – not without a tinge of irony – into a lower place in the surgical league tables.[74,75] A systematic review of health economic studies demonstrated that cesarean delivery costs a health service at least 3 to 5 times more than vaginal delivery.[76] This accounts for the direct expenses only, not those resulting from related repeat procedures and complications in subsequent pregnancies. Nearly a quarter of all US hospital stays are related to pregnancy and childbirth, but most people do not realize what a big chunk of hospital care that is: it involves approximately 4 million women and their babies each year in the USA alone. Cesarean deliveries cost more than $16 billion in the USA alone each year. Consumer watchdog group Public Citizen estimated that at least half of these are unnecessary and result in 1.1 million extra hospital days. Soon the costs of the cesarean pandemic will become unsustainable. Clearly, uncritical use of cesarean deliveries is a huge waste of resources, both financial and professional, and to the detriment of those who really need medical attention.

> The billions of dollars spent worldwide on "unnecesareans" are an inexcusable assault on increasingly limited healthcare budgets.

2.4.7 Prejudice of future reproduction

Cesarean section undermines fertility.[77] A Scottish study followed over 25 000 women who had their first single child – multiple births were excluded. Women who had delivered their firstborn by cesarean were 9% less likely to conceive again compared with those who had a spontaneous natural delivery (66.9% versus 73.9%).[78] It was concluded either that women were avoiding second pregnancy because of the negative experience of cesarean delivery or that the surgery itself directly affected fertility. The latter surely plays a role because women who have undergone cesarean section are more likely to suffer an ectopic pregnancy, with 9.5 occurring per 1000 pregnancies compared with women after spontaneous delivery, who suffer 5.7 per 1000 pregnancies.

2.4.8 Social damage

The social effects of obstetric excess are also disturbing. WHO consultant and male feminist Marsden Wagner, an influential and outspoken critic of medicalized childbirth, was intentionally provocative but essentially correct when he wrote: "[A] woman giving birth is a human being, not a machine and just a container for making babies. Showing women – half of all people – that they are inferior and inadequate by taking away their power to give birth is a tragedy for all society." He concluded: "Respecting the woman as an important and valuable human being and making certain that the woman's experience while giving birth is fulfilling and empowering is not just a nice extra, it is absolutely essential as it makes the woman strong and therefore makes society strong."[79]

2.4.9 Dangerous export

Perhaps the most tragic result of the trend toward surgery-oriented obstetrics is its widespread export to underdeveloped countries from which so many graduates are trained in American and European institutes. In the developing world, a uterine scar is a far more dangerous condition than in the western world, and extremely limited healthcare resources could be utilized far more wisely.

2.4.10 Declining overall quality of childbirth

Since most surgical interventions are performed to resolve problems of labor in low-risk pregnancies, spontaneous delivery rates are currently the most realistic objective measure of professional labor and delivery skills. By this criterion, the overall standard of maternity care has declined markedly over the last decades. Considering the impressive list of harms inflicted on mothers and the lack of evidence of any benefits for the newborns – rather the opposite is the case – the obstetrical establishment has some pertinent questions to answer about the explosive growth of operative deliveries in low-risk pregnancies and the dissatisfaction of women subjected to their care.

> *Spontaneous delivery rates in low-risk pregnancies are the most realistic measure of the standard of care afforded to mothers.*

References

1. Clark SL, Belfort MA, Dildy GA, *et al.* Maternal death in the 21st century: causes, prevention, and relationship to cesarean delivery. Am J Obstet Gynecol 2008;**199**:36. e1–36.e5; discussion 91–2

2. Liu S, Liston RM, Joseph KS, *et al.* Maternal mortality and severe morbidity associated with low-risk planned cesarean delivery versus planned vaginal delivery at term. Maternal Health Study Group of the Canadian Perinatal Surveillance System. CMAJ 2007;**176**:455–60

3. Glantz J. Obstetric variation, intervention, and outcomes: doing more but accomplishing less. Birth 2012;**39**:286–90

4. Gregory KD, Jackson S, Korst L, Fridman M. Cesarean versus vaginal delivery: whose risks? Whose benefits? Am J Perinatol 2012;**29**:7–18

5. Hamilton BE, Hoyert DL, Martin JA, Strobino DM, Guyer B. Annual summary of vital statistics: 2010–2011. Pediatrics 2013;**131**:548–58

6. World Health Organisation. Appropriate technology for birth. Lancet 1985;**2**:436–7

7. Gibbons L, Belizán JM, Lauer, JA, *et al.* The global numbers and costs of additionally needed and unnecessary caesarean sections performed per year: Overuse as a barrier to universal coverage. *World Health Report* 2010; Background Paper 30

8. American College of Obstetricians and Gynecologists. Obstetric Care Consensus No. 1: Safe prevention of the primary cesarean delivery. Obstet Gynecol 2014;**123**:693–711

9. Nelson KB. Can we prevent cerebral palsy? N Engl J Med 2003;**349**:1765–9

10. Hankins GD, Speer M. Defining the pathogenesis and pathophysiology of neonatal encephalopathy and cerebral palsy. Obstet Gynecol 2003;**102**:628–36

11. NHS Institute for Innovation and Improvement. Focus on: Caesarean section 2012. http://www.institute.nhs.uk

12. Guise JM, Eden K, Emeis C, *et al.* Vaginal Birth After Cesarean: New Insights. Evidence Report/Technology Assessment No. 191. AHRQ Publication No. 10–E003. Rockville (MD): Agency for Healthcare Research and Quality; 2010

13. Perinatal Registration The Netherlands 2013.www.per inatreg.nl

14. Barber EL, Lundsberg LS, Belanger K, *et al.* Indications contributing to the increasing cesarean delivery rate. Obstet Gynecol 2011;**118**:29–38

15. Hendrix NW, Chaucan SP. Cesarean delivery for nonreassuring fetal heart rate tracing. Obstet Gynecol N Am 2005;**32**:273–86

16. ACOG. *Task Force on Cesarean Delivery Rates: Evaluation of Cesarean Delivery.* American College of Obstetricians and Gynecologists; 2000

17. RCOG. *Operative Vaginal Delivery.* Green-top Guideline No. 26. London: Royal College of Obstetricians and Gynaecologists; 2011

18. Stephenson PA, Bakoula C, Hemminki E, *et al.* Patterns of use of obstetrical interventions in 12 countries. Paediatr Perinat Epidemiol 1993;**7**:45–54

19. Keriakos R, Sugumar S, Hilal N. Instrumental vaginal delivery – back to basics. J Obstet Gynaecol 2013;**33**:781–86

20. O'Mahony F, Settatree R, Platt C, Johanson R. Review of singleton fetal and neonatal deaths associated with cranial trauma and cephalic delivery during a national intrapartum-related confidential enquiry. Br J Obstet Gynaecol 2005;**112**:619–26

21. Wegner EK, Bernstein IM. Operative vaginal delivery. UpToDate. Accessed November 2014; www.uptodate.com

22. Main DM, Main EK, Moore DH 2nd. The relationship between maternal age and uterine dysfunction as a continuous effect throughout reproductive life. Am J Obstet Gynecol 2000;**182**:258–9

23. Liu S, Rusen ID, Joseph KS, *et al*. Recent trends in caesarean delivery rates and indications for caesarean delivery in Canada. J Obstet Gynaecol Can 2004;**26**:735–42

24. Ecker JL, Chen KT, Cohen AP, Riley LE, Lieberman ES. Increased risk of cesarean delivery with advancing age: indications and associated factors in nulliparous women. Am J Obstet Gynecol 2001;**185**:883–7

25. Jensen H, Agger AO, Rasmussen KL. The influence of prepregnancy body mass index on labor complications. Acta Obstet Gynecol Scand 1999;**78**:799–802

26. Usha Kiran TS, Hemmadi S, Bethel J, Evans J. Outcome of pregnancy in a woman with an increased body mass index. Br J Obstet Gynaecol 2005;**112**:768–72

27. Cedergren MI. Maternal morbid obesity and the risk of adverse pregnancy outcome. Obstet Gynecol 2004;**103**:219–24

28. Declercq E, Menacker F, MacDorman M. Maternal risk profiles and the primary cesarean rate in the United States, 1991–2002. Am J Public Health 2006;**96**:867–72

29. Declercq E, Menacker F, MacDorman M. Rise in "no indicated risk" primary caesareans in the United States, 1991–2001: cross sectional analysis. Br Med J 2005;**330**:71–2

30. Heffner LJ, Elkin E, Fretts RC. Impact of labor induction, gestational age and maternal age on cesarean delivery rates. Obstet Gynecol 2003;**102**:287–93

31. Stramrood CA, Paarlberg KM, Huis In 't Veld EM, *et al*. Posttraumatic stress following childbirth in homelike- and hospital settings. J Psychosom Obstet Gynaecol 2011;**32**:88–97

32. Boorman RJ. Childbirth and criteria for traumatic events. Midwifery 2014;**30**:255–61

33. Alcorn KL, O'Donovan A, Patrick JC, Creedy D, Devilly GJ. A prospective longitudinal study of the prevalence of post-traumatic stress disorder resulting from childbirth events. Psychol Med 2010;**40**:1849–59

34. Soderquist J, Wijma B, Thorbert G, Wijma K. Risk factors in pregnancy for post-traumatic stress and depression after childbirth. BJOG 2009;**116**:672–80

35. White T, Matthey S, Boyd K, Barnett B. Postnatal depression and post-traumatic stress after childbirth: Prevalence, course and co-occurrence. J Reprod Infant Psychol 2006;**24**:107–20

36. Ayers S, Joseph S, Kenzie-McHarg K, Slade P, Wijma K. Post-traumatic stress disorder following childbirth: current issues and recommendations for future research. J Psychosom Obstet Gynaecol 2008;**29**:240–50

37. Wijma K, Soderquist J, Wijma B. Posttraumatic stress disorder after childbirth: a cross sectional study. J Anxiety Disord 1997;**11**:587–97

38. Ryding EL, Wijma K, Wijma B. Psychological impact of emergency cesarean section in comparison with elective cesarean section, instrumental and normal vaginal delivery. J Psychosom Obstet Gynaecol 1998;**19**:135–44

39. Stramrood CA, Wessel I, Doornbos B, *et al*. Posttraumatic stress disorder following preeclampsia and PPROM: a prospective study with 15 months follow-up. Reprod Sci 2011;**18**:645–53

40. Soderquist J, Wijma B, Wijma K. The longitudinal course of post-traumatic stress after childbirth. J Psychosom Obstet Gynaecol 2006;**27**:113–19

41. Parfitt YM, Ayers S. The effect of post-natal symptoms of post-traumatic stress and depression on the couple's relationship and parent–baby bond. J Reprod Infant Psychol 2009;**27**:127–42

42. Rouhe H, Salmela-Aro K, Halmesmaki E, Saisto T. Fear of childbirth according to parity, gestational age, and obstetric history. BJOG 2009;**116**:67–73

43. Gottvall K, Waldenstrom U. Does a traumatic birth experience have an impact on future reproduction? BJOG 2002;**109**:254–60

44. Fuglenes D, Aas E, Botten G, Oian P, Kristiansen IS. Why do some pregnant women prefer cesarean? The influence of parity, delivery experiences, and fear. Am J Obstet Gynecol 2011;**205**:45–9

45. National Collaborating Centre for Women's and Children's Health. Caesarean Section: Clinical Guideline. RCOG Press, 2004

46. Hall MH, Bewley S. Maternal mortality and mode of delivery. Lancet 1999;**354**:776

47. Harper MA, Byington RP, Espeland MA, *et al*. Pregnancy-related death and health care services. Obstet Gynecol 2003;**102**:273

48. Shellhaas for the NICHD MFMU Network. The MFMU cesarean registry: Cesarean hysterectomy – its indications, morbidities, and mortality. Am J Obstet Gynecol 2001;**185**:S123

49. Kastner ES, Figueroa R, Garry D, *et al.* Emergency peripartum hysterectomy: experience at a community teaching hospital. Obstet Gynecol 2002;**99**:971

50. Knight M, Kurinczuk JJ, Spark P, Brocklehurst P. United Kingdom Obstetric Surveillance System Steering Committee. Cesarean delivery and peripartum hysterectomy. Obstet Gynecol 2008;**111**:97–105

51. Myles TD, Gooch J, Santolaya J. Obesity as an independent risk factor for infectious morbidity in patients who undergo cesarean delivery. Obstet Gynecol 2002;**100**:959

52. Marshall NE, Fu R, Guise JM. Impact of multiple cesarean deliveries on maternal morbidity: a systematic review. Am J Obstet Gynecol 2011;**205**:262. e1–8

53. Kwee A, Bots ML, Visser GH, Bruinse HW. Emergency peripartum hysterectomy. A prospective study in the Netherlands. Eur J Obstet Gynecol Reprod Biol 2006;**124**:187–92

54. Smith GC, Pell JP, Dobbie R. Caesarean section and risk of unexplained stillbirth in subsequent pregnancy. Lancet 2003;**362**:1779–84

55. Silver RM, Landon MB, Rouse DJ, *et al.* National Institute of Child Health and Human Development Maternal-Fetal Medicine Units Network. Maternal morbidity associated with multiple repeat cesarean deliveries. Obstet Gynecol 2006;**107**:1226–32

56. Solheim KN, Esakoff TF, Little SE, *et al.* The effect of cesarean delivery rates on the future incidence of placenta previa, placenta accreta, and maternal mortality. J Matern Fetal Neonatal Med 2011;**24**:1341–6

57. Green R, Gardeil F, Turner MJ. Long-term effects of cesarean sections. Am J Obstet Gynecol 1996;**176**:254–5

58. Kwee A, Bots ML, Visser GH, Bruinse HW. Obstetric management and outcome of pregnancy in women with a history of caesarean section in The Netherlands. Eur J Obstet Gynecol Reprod Biol 2007;**132**:171–6

59. Kwee A, Bots ML, Visser GH, Bruinse HW. Uterine rupture and its complications in the Netherlands: a prospective study. Eur J Obstet Gynecol Reprod Biol 2006;**128**:257–61

60. Guise JM, McDonagh MS, Osterwell P, *et al.* Systematic review of the incidence and consequences of uterine rupture in women with a previous cesarean section. Br Med J 2004;**329**:1–7

61. MacDorman MF, Declercq E, Menacker F, Malloy MH. Infant and neonatal mortality for primary cesarean and vaginal births to women with "no indicated risk," United States, 1998–2001 birth cohorts. Birth 2006;**3**: 175–82

62. Fogelson NS, Menard MK, Hulsey T, Ebeling M. Neonatal impact of elective repeat cesarean delivery at term: A comment on patient choice cesarean delivery. Am J Obstet Gynecol 2005;**192**:1433–6

63. Levine EM, Ghai V, Barton JJ, Strom CM. Mode of delivery and risk of respiratory diseases in newborns. Obstet Gynecol 2001;**97**:439–42

64. Bowers SK. Prevention of iatrogenic respiratory distress syndrome: elective repeat section and spontaneous delivery. Am J Obstet Gynecol 1982;**143**:186–9

65. Doherty EG, Eichenwald EC. Cesarean delivery: emphasis on the neonate. Clin Obstet Gynecol 2004;**47**:332–41

66. Darmasseelane, K, Hyde MJ, Santhakumaran S, Gale C, Modi N. Mode of delivery and offspring body mass index, overweight and obesity in adult life: a systematic review and meta-analysis. PLoS One 2014;**9**: e87896

67. Hyde MJ, Mostyn A, Modi N, Kemp PR. The health implications of birth by caesarean section. Biol Rev Camb Philos Soc 2012;**87**:229–43

68. Laubereau B, Filipiak-Pittroff B, von Berg A, *et al.* Caesarean section and gastrointestinal symptoms, atopic dermatitis, and sensitisation during the first year of life. Arch Dis Child 2004;**89**:993–7

69. Ajslev TA, Andersen CS, Gamborg M *et al.* Childhood overweight after establishment of the gut microbiota: the role of delivery mode, pre-pregnancy weight and early administration of antibiotics. Int J Obes 2011;**35**:522–9

70. Dominguez-Bello MG, Costello EK, Contreras M *et al.* Delivery mode shapes the acquisition and structure of the initial microbiota across multiple body habitats in newborns. Proc Natl Acad Sci USA 2011;**107**:11971–5

71. Nue J, Rushing J. Cesarean versus vaginal delivery: long term infant outcomes and the hygiene hypothesis. Clin Perinatol 2011;**38**:321–31

72. Tollånes MC, Moster D, Daltveit AK, Irgens LM. Cesarean section and risk of severe childhood asthma: a population-based cohort study. J Pediatr 2008;**153**:112–16

73. Seeman P, Weinshenker D, Quirion R, *et al.* Dopamine supersensitivity correlates with D2High states, implying many paths to psychosis. Proc Natl Acad Sci USA 2005;**102**:3513–18

74. Ventura SJ, Martin JA, Curtin SC, Mathews TJ, Park MM. Births: Final data for 1998. Natl Vital Stat Rep 2000;**48**:1–10

75. Agency for Healthcare Research and Quality's Healthcare Cost and Utilization Project. Nationwide Inpatient Sample 2003. www.hcup.ahrq.gov/

76. Henderson J, McCandlish R, Kumiega L, Petrou S. Systematic review of economic aspects of alternative modes of delivery. Br J Obstet Gynaecol 2001;**108**:149–57

77. Murphy DJ, Stirrat GM, Heron J; ALSPAC Study Team. The relationship between Cesarean section and sub-fertility in a population-based sample of 14 541 pregnancies. Hum Reprod 2002;**17**:1914–17

78. Mollison J, Porter M, Campbell D, Bhattacharya S. Primary mode of delivery and subsequent pregnancy. Br J Obstet Gynaecol 2005;**112**: 1061–5

79. Wagner M. Fish can't see water: the need to humanize birth. Int J Gynaecol Obstet 2001;**75**: 25–37

3

Avoidable causes of failed labors

Dysfunctional labor is the primary indication for cesarean delivery in first pregnancies and, therefore, the indirect cause of most repeat operations (2.1.1). The terminology favored to describe the problem is "failure to progress," or "dystocia," from the Greek meaning abnormal labor as opposed to "eutocia" meaning normal labor. These medical terms, however, serve as a cloak to obscure a lack of true meaning because they relay little if any information about the underlying problems. Similarly, we can describe patients with thyroid disease as euthyroid or dysthyroid, but it gives no information whatsoever for the institution of treatment. Clearly, we cannot hope to tackle the problem of failed labors without resorting to cesarean delivery, unless we explore the pathophysiological heterogeneity of the condition and attempt to define causal diagnoses.

Dystocia, or failure to progress, is not a diagnosis but a common symptom of a variety of labor disorders.

3.1 Dynamic labor disorders

The ability of the fetus to negotiate the birth canal depends on *the powers, the passage*, and *the passenger*. This leaves, in essence, only two main explanations when labor stalls:

1. Mechanical obstruction, resulting from fetopelvic disproportion or fetal malposition.
2. Dynamic disorders in which the uterine force or the remaining strength of the birthing woman is insufficient: δυναμιζ (dynamis) is the Greek word for "power" or "force."

Faced with the virtual disappearance of pelvic anatomical deformities ("*the passage*") since the elimination of rickets a good century ago, and a stable mean birth weight ("*the passenger*"), the only possible explanation for the rise in operative deliveries for "dystocia" must be an increase in the incidence of dynamic labor disorders ("*the powers*") that arise in initially normal cases. If scrutinized, dynamic dystocia, in turn, consists of a broad spectrum of specific and identifiably distinct labor disorders (Sections 2 and 3), which too frequently pass unnoticed and are, therefore, treated after the fact with surgery. In many cases, dynamic labor disorders are even plainly iatrogenic from the outset, in particular when labor is induced.[1–15] These are harsh but at the same time hopeful conclusions, because they implicitly carry the real possibility of reducing operative delivery rates and enhancing women's labor experience by improving professional labor and delivery skills.

Fundamental problem 1

Traumatic childbirth experiences and high operative delivery rates predominantly result from growing rates of (iatrogenic) dynamic labor disorders.

3.1.1 Symptom-based interventions

Even dynamic dystocia is not a diagnosis but a syndrome of a variety of labor problems. A detailed causal diagnosis allows for other measures rather than the easiest way out using surgery or traction. Clearly, as long as the pathophysiology of the daily problems in the delivery room is not recognized and the various dynamic labor disorders are not properly defined and diagnosed, one cannot begin to formulate an effective policy to reduce undue operative delivery rates. Such detailed analyses will be provided in Sections 2 and 3.

Fundamental problem 2

Failure to submit "dystocia" to detailed analysis and diagnosis renders a structured policy for the reduction of operative delivery rates virtually impossible.

3.1.2 Lack of definitions

The widely differing criteria for dystocia manifest the lack of a scientific foundation for current childbirth practices. Scientific disciplines are based on universally valid definitions, but within obstetrics and midwifery one will search in vain for a common set of definitions, even for the most elementary parameters of birth. The onset of labor, the normal progression and duration of labor, and objective criteria distinguishing between a normal and an abnormal course of labor are poorly defined. The development and evaluation of a system of high-quality care is hampered by a pseudo-exact understanding of basic concepts such as the latent phase of labor compared with false labor, efficient compared with inefficient contractions, normal progression compared with prolonged labor, pelvic adequacy compared with fetopelvic disproportion, and fetal reserves compared with fetal distress. This imprecision instigates subjective and thus arbitrary care, based on beliefs and unfounded doctrines rather than solid evidence-based norms. Consequently, both the chance of intervention and the form it takes are determined more by the personal perspective of the caregiver than by the particular obstetric situation and reliable evidence.

Fundamental problem 3

The main obstacle for high-quality birth care is a lack of strict definitions and, consequently, absence of prospective criteria for the distinction between "normal" and "abnormal" labor.

3.2 Lack of an overall plan

The lack of commonly held definitions leads to a lack of consistent standards for the conduct and care of normal childbirth. Rates of induction, labor augmentation, and operative delivery vary enormously between hospitals in most countries, even after correcting for differences between populations.[16] The consequences of such arbitrariness are immense for the pregnant woman: in the US, for instance, she does not know that she is up to ten times more likely to have a cesarean or instrumental delivery in one hospital than in another, without a shred of evidence of any benefit to herself or her child.[17]

3.2.1 Non-management of first-stage labor

The authoritative textbook *Williams Obstetrics* argues: "It is generally agreed that dystocia leading to cesarean delivery is overdiagnosed in the USA and elsewhere. Factors leading to increased use of cesarean delivery for dystocia, however, are controversial. Those implicated have included incorrect diagnosis of dystocia, fear of litigation and even clinician convenience."[18] Although this holds true, it could be stated with even stronger arguments that dystocia is often underdiagnosed, that is to say, not recognized in good time, not causally specified, and not corrected in a due manner. These omissions leave surgery as the only solution after the fact. In other words:

High operative delivery rates result from the widespread disregard for a systematic policy aimed at short labor and a safe, spontaneous delivery.

3.2.2 Lack of professional interest

Unfortunately, many obstetricians worldwide show little interest in the prevention of first-stage labor disorders, which is surprising as labor is the final common pathway for all pregnancies entrusted to their care. In the private sector, the doctor is often not in the hospital and must be called in by the nurse when trouble develops. Or private doctors typically arrive just in time to cut the cord and write the bill. Women in public hospitals often do not see the specialist at all. The busy obstetrician/gynecologist has other things to do. Thus, nurses, midwives, and the least experienced interns and residents are the main attendants of the tedious hours of first-stage labor. If the labor becomes increasingly difficult, it is these attendants – not the specialist who is ultimately responsible and accountable – who must sell the decision of waiting to the helpless woman in distress and her desperate partner.

Obstetricians confidently approve epidural analgesia or large amounts of opioid drugs, far out of harm's way from behind a desk or from their beds over the telephone. Since a call schedule of two nights a week is the rule rather than the exception, many obstetricians try to lessen this nocturnal inconvenience by coming to the labor room only when strictly necessary. Their attitude to labor might very well be the reverse in the daytime, especially in busy maternity units, where there is constant pressure to keep patients moving through. In the late afternoon, obstetricians (on duty that night) may advise speeding up labor or considering a cesarean, often without having seen the patient at all.

In many childbirth settings, the care provided depends strongly on the time of day that labor happens to begin.

In many hospitals, the responsibility for the management of labor is passed on to nurse-midwives and residents, who are often allowed to act unsupervised after only a few weeks on the labor and delivery ward ("see one, do one, teach one"). Close supervision by an obstetrician is indeed available for acute problems or the actual (assisted) birth, but proactive supervision during the first stage of labor is non-existent. The lack of guidelines on how to proceed when a labor gets tough exposes the resident or midwife to the possibility of unfair criticism from either the patient or the distant supervisor or both. Such grievances contribute to the low morale and lack of team spirit that is characteristic of all too many delivery wards. "And whenever there is a lack of trust, decisions are avoided, care is not pursued effectively, and cesarean deliveries are performed unnecessarily because surgery provides a soft option for those anxious to avoid blame."[19]

Lack of team spirit in the labor ward is detrimental to the quality of birth care.

Most gynecologists enter the delivery room only when they are needed to solve problems, honing their skills in the "tricks of the trade": vacuum, forceps, and cesarean. They are often involved in other subspecialties and regard obstetrics as a simple but burdensome part of a much broader profession (obstetrics and gynecology). That is why most consultants typically seek intellectual fulfillment outside the labor room. As a result, birth attendance and care are left in the hands of lower-qualified personnel, and when there is a problem the specialist quickly performs an operative delivery in the midst of all his or her other work obligations. These common practices emphasize the need for a new, inspiring childbirth system that encourages an active interest in first-stage labor by all professional staff, including the consultants. Obstetricians need to return to the labor ward – both intellectually and physically – and take on the many challenges it presents (Section 3).

Fundamental problem 4

Lack of direct involvement at consultant level in first-stage labor is indicative of the state of apathy within the obstetric establishment regarding the supervision of labor.

3.2.3   Discontinuous care

As a result of the 8-hour work shifts, women commonly have several caregivers over the length of their labor. This discontinuity is compounded by poor handover practices that have been demonstrated to be a significant contributing factor in medical errors and inadvertent harm.[20–22] Furthermore, the turnover in personnel makes it difficult to maintain consistent and high-standard birth care, if a central care policy is not formulated and implemented. What one attendant regards as normal another finds abnormal and vice versa. This variance results in inconsistencies in guidance and a lack of clarity at the bedside. Additional disagreement regarding criteria for normal progress of labor results in heated, endless discussions between nurse-midwives and obstetricians, and, most importantly, it stands in the way of effective cooperation.

Fundamental problem 5

Impersonal and discontinuous care is caused by the lack of a central birth-plan.

In some western countries, community-based midwives still attend births at the woman's home or in primary birth centers, claiming to provide more personal care. But the famous Dutch example shows that it is typical for many self-employed midwives to remain with a parturient only when approaching full dilatation. In the long first stage of labor, it is presumed that intermittent care with periodic visits at three-hourly intervals will suffice (Chapter 5). As a result, many Dutch women giving birth at home go through the greatest part of their dilatation stage unattended and unsupported by professional help.

3.2.4   Tolerance of long labors

The traditional midwifery approach to labor is to wait for the natural process to unfold. This method originates in the fundamental philosophy that the natural process of birth neither can be improved nor needs improvement. As a result, they see no alternative to waiting, even when labor takes a very long time. In this tradition of care, which is passed on from generation to generation without question, the main task of the midwife is to ensure that no direct problem arises to make intervention necessary. If Mother Nature fails, there is always the obstetrician as back-up, solving the problem after the fact. It should be noted, however, that midwives are not alone in defending this passive wait-and-see attitude; it is one that is conveniently shared by many obstetricians.

> *Tolerance of long labors increases surgical intervention rates and undermines women's satisfaction with the labor experience.*

Despite claims of providing "holistic" care, too little attention is given to the relationship between the length of labor and the woman's exhaustion. When the patience of birth attendants exceeds the stamina of a laboring woman, a cascade of unmanageable complications may be the result. After an unnecessarily long first stage, most women can no longer push, no longer want to push, or may not even reach the point of pushing. Thus, the decision to intervene is belatedly motivated by compassion. This passive approach toward first-stage labor, together with women's increasing unwillingness to tolerate protracted pain and stress, is accountable for the greater proportion of cesarean births. These operations are, in fact, emergency solutions that could have been prevented by much earlier and far less invasive measures (Section 3).

> *After an unnecessarily long dilatation time, women can no longer push, no longer want to push, or may even not reach the point of pushing.*

The patience exhibited by caregivers during labor contrasts sharply with clinicians' impatience during late pregnancy. About 25% of all pregnant women in western countries give birth after having their labor induced.[23–26] Labor may be induced because of a supposed medical indication or for opportunistic reasons on the part of the obstetrician – those who deliver during the day are not, after all, delivering at night – or at the request of the pregnant woman herself. An induced uterus is not yet ready for labor and so must be coerced into contractions. It is for this reason that a woman's labor, when induced, is often much less effective than if one had waited for the spontaneous onset to occur (Chapter 8). Induction increases the chance of a long labor due to inefficient and thus ineffective contractions and seriously increases the risk of cesarean delivery because of non-progressing dilatation (Chapter 23). Induction also increases the likelihood of a forceps or vacuum delivery owing to the woman's

exhaustion and heightens the risk of fetal distress as a result of overstimulation.[27–29]

> **Fundamental problem 6**
>
> *Induction is one of the leading causes of iatrogenic labor disorders.*

3.2.5 The paradox

In the final analysis, avoidable operative deliveries result from two common policies that are strangely practiced side by side: the interventional approach with excessive use of inductions leading to long and troublesome labor, and the passive approach in spontaneous labor in which a protracted first stage is not recognized and treated in a timely manner, so that it is only possible to attend to the problems after the fact.

> *Both overuse of induction and underuse of acceleration after spontaneous labor onset mark the professional indifference to long labors.*

The fundamental explanation of this paradox is the still widely dominating mechanistic view of birth oriented toward the mechanics of birth and manual skill, rather than the dynamics of first-stage labor.

3.3 Mechanics-oriented view of childbirth

To reiterate, the mechanism of labor is basically simple and dependent on the interaction of three factors:

- *The passenger*, meaning the dimensions and attitude of the fetus's head
- *The passage*, meaning the shape and size of the woman's pelvis
- *The powers*, meaning the efficacy of uterine contractions

The first two represent the mechanical or anatomical condition, and the third variable represents the dynamic prerequisite for a successful birth. By and large, the impact of the mechanical factors is grossly overrated while the true dominance of the dynamic factor is often unrecognized or severely underestimated.

3.3.1 Historical background

Tolerance of long labor goes back to ancient history. After all, women have been giving birth since the beginning of humanity, sometimes after two or three days of agony. Until about a century ago, attendance of childbirth was the exclusive domain of midwives, and nothing could be done to resolve the problem of overly long labors without introducing extreme hazards. Surgery was almost invariably lethal and not an option. Hence, the course and outcome of birth was a trial by ordeal and believed to be God's will.

By default, midwifery care was limited to moral support – an emotionally heavy and sometimes even superhuman task. This might explain why alcohol consumption among midwives was a popular topic described with disdain in the classic world literature from the Victorian era. Whether the unborn child was still alive was mostly unknown. When the woman finally reached full dilatation, she might be nearly dead from exhaustion. In privileged circles, the "master" would then arrive and solve the problem with his "iron hands" (forceps). Otherwise, arrested birth meant death for both mother and child. Delivery literally meant mechanical deliverance – a skilled trade.

Empiricism helped in the further evolution of this handcraft in the twentieth century. The master became the obstetrician, and medical advances in antiseptics, blood typing, and anesthesiology made it much safer to operate in the event of arrested labor. The perception of the natural birth process, however, remained predominantly mechanistic. Women in labor are still reaping the sorry harvest, as the passive attitude in first-stage labor still prevails to this day in many birth settings.

Fundamental problem 7

Traditionally, obstetrics has been strongly oriented toward the mechanics of birth and manual skill. The importance of optimal dynamics is still highly underestimated.

3.3.2 The mechanistic paradox

The mechanistic approach explains the language of obstetrics and midwifery, in which the doctor or midwife "delivers" the baby or "does" the delivery instead of the mother herself. The word "midwife" literally means "standing with/by women." But if labor is slow and increasingly difficult, the orthodox midwife then typically feels there is nothing she can do – beyond tender loving care – to resolve this predicament without the introduction of presumed extraneous hazards

to mother or child. From her mechanistic point of view, the midwife is patiently waiting for … full dilatation.

In hospitals, long and difficult labor is regarded as a burden, but one that is acceptable and can be relieved by an epidural or large amounts of opioid drugs. Acceleration of labor is not considered before at least 3 cm dilatation has been reached ("active labor established") or, even worse, until a woman shows the first signs of exhaustion. What is more, in many hospitals, oxytocin treatment is an option during business hours only. For a woman whose cervix dilates unsatisfactorily late at night, sedation is typically the course of action. And in the morning, the sleepless and distressing night is followed by the "total package" of an epidural, electronic fetal monitoring, an intrauterine pressure catheter, and an oxytocin drip. At this point, meconium is present in the amniotic fluid, and the uterus is by now beyond stimulation. Morale crumbled hours before, and the now emotionally drained patient shuts herself off from her attendants, in whom she has progressively lost all trust. All the same, orthodox care providers eagerly await and expect the achievement of the ultimate goal: full dilatation.

Fundamental problem 8

The dilatation stage of labor comprises more than 90% of the total time of birth, but it is insufficiently recognized that the majority of birth disorders arise or are created during exactly this first stage.

As soon as the cervix no longer presents an obstacle, the attitude of the providers undergoes a change as sudden as it is radical. They use a strict time limit on pushing, and nearly every invasive intervention seems permissible to force a vaginal birth. These care providers do not seem to realize that if a baby can safely be pulled through the birth canal by forceps or vacuum extractor then delivery should, in principle, have been possible by the expulsive force of the woman herself – provided she has enough strength remaining. Obstetricians spend a great deal of their training in learning manual and operative skills to solve an arrested birth while little or no attention is given to the possibility of preventing the situation.

The sudden transition from an extremely expectant approach during the first stage to an equally aggressive approach in the second stage epitomizes the still widely prevalent mechanistic view of birth.

Characteristic of the passive attitude toward the first stage of labor – known in French as *la période du désespoir* or the period of despair and hopelessness – is the manner in which patience has been elevated to the level of a professional ethic in midwifery and conventional obstetrics alike. Orthodox publications discuss the idea of "masterly expectancy" and claim "patience is not a weakness but a controlled force" and "the clock is the midwife's enemy." Each of these contentions highlights the focus on "the main event," the expulsion of the fetus, while the importance of a smooth first stage of labor is neglected. This oversight is the core of a multitude of problems that will be addressed in detail in the next chapters. In reality, physical and emotional exhaustion is the most frequent and most underrated complication of birth nowadays, and attention to the prevention of long labor is far more worthwhile than the attention that is usually devoted to its operative resolution.

> *Physical and emotional exhaustion is the most frequent and most underrated complication of first labors. The central problem of unduly long labors can be solved by much simpler methods than resorting to cesarean delivery.*

References

1. Johnson AM, Bellerose L, Billstrom R, Deckers E, Beller P. Evaluating outcomes of labor inductions beyond 39 weeks of gestation. Obstet Gynecol 2014;**123** Suppl 1:58S

2. Seyb ST, Berka RJ, Socol ML, Doodley SL. Risk of cesarean delivery with elective induction of labor at term in nulliparous women. *Obstet Gynecol* 1999;**94**:600–7

3. Macer JA, Macer CL, Chan LS. Elective induction versus spontaneous labor: a retrospective study of complications and outcome. *Am J Obstet Gynecol* 1992;**166**:1690–6

4. Cammu H, Marten G, Ruyssinck G, Amy JJ. Outcome after elective induction in nulliparous women: a matched cohort study. *Am J Obstet Gynecol* 2002;**186**:240–4

5. Luthy DA, Malmgren JA, Zingheim RW. Increased Cesarean section rates associated with elective induction in nulliparous women; the physician effect. *Am J Obstet Gynecol* 2004;**191**:1511–15

6. Dublin S, Lydon-Rochelle M, Kaplan RC, Watts DH, Critchlow CW. Maternal and fetal outcomes after induction without an identified indication. *Am J Obstet Gynecol* 2000;**18**:986–94

7. Van Gemund N, Hardeman A, Scherjon SA, Kanhai HH. Intervention rates after elective induction of labor compared to labor with a spontaneous onset: a matched cohort study. *Gynecol Obstet Invest* 2003;**56**:133–8

8. Maslow AS, Sweeny AL. Elective induction of labor as a risk factor for cesarean delivery among low-risk women at term. *Obstet Gynecol* 2000;**95**:917–22

9. Smith KM, Hoffman MK, Scicione A. Elective induction of labor in nulliparous women increases the risk of cesarean section. Obstet Gynecol 2003;**101**:S45

10. Kauffman K, Bailit J, Grobman W. Elective induction: an analysis of economic and health consequences. *Am J Obstet Gynecol* 2001;**185**:209

11. Vahratian A, Zhang J, Troendle JF, *et al.* Labor progression and risk of cesarean delivery in electively induced nulliparas. *Obstet Gynecol* 2005;**105**:698–704

12. Hamar B, Mann S, Greenberg P, *et al.* Low-risk inductions of labor and cesarean delivery for nulliparous and parous women at term. Am J Obstet Gynecol 2001;**185**:215

13. Yeast JD, Jones A, Poskin M. Induction of labor and the relationship to cesarean delivery; a review of 7001 consecutive inductions. *Am J Obstet Gynecol* 1999;**180**:628–33

14. Johnson DP, Davis NR, Brown AJ. Risk of cesarean delivery after induction at term in nulliparous women with an unfavorable cervix. Am J Obstet Gynecol 2003;**188**:1565–72

15. Vrouenraets FP, Roumen FJ, Dehing CJ, *et al.* Bishop score and risk of cesarean delivery after induction of labor in nulliparous women. Obstet Gynecol 2005;**105**:690–7

16. American College of Obstetricians and Gynecologists. Obstetric Care Consensus No 1: Safe prevention of the primary cesarean delivery. Obstet Gynecol 2014;**123**:693–711

17. Kozhimannil KB, Law MR, Virnig BA. Cesarean delivery rates vary tenfold among US hospitals; reducing variation may address quality and cost issues. Health Aff 2013;**32**:527–35

18. Cunningham FG, Leveno KJ, Bloom SL. Section IV. Labor and Delivery. In: *Williams Obstetrics*, 22nd edn. New York: McGraw-Hill; 2005:496

19. O'Driscoll K, Meagher D, Robson M. *Active Management of Labour*, 4th edn. London: Mosby; 2003

20. Pham JC, Aswani MS, Rosen M, *et al.* Reducing medical errors and adverse events. Ann Rev Med 2012;**63**:447–63

21. Chin GS, Warren N, Kornman L, Cameron P. Patients' perceptions of safety and quality of maternity

clinical handover. BMC Pregnancy Childbirth 2011;11:58

22. Chin GS, Warren N, Kornman L, Cameron P. Transferring responsibility and accountability in maternity care: clinicians defining their boundaries of practice in relation to clinical handover. Br Med J Open 2012;2(5):e000734

23. Martin JA, Hamilton BE, Ventura SJ, *et al. National Vital Statistics Reports.* Report No. 1. Hyattsville, MD: National Vital Statistics System; 2012

24. The Health and Social Care Information Centre. *NHS Maternity Statistics 2011–2012 Summary Report.* Geneva, Switzerland: National Health Service; 2012. Available at: http://www.hscic.gov.uk/hes

25. Australian Institute of Health and Welfare, Li Z, Zeki R, Hilder L, *et al. Australia's Mothers and Babies 2010.*

Canberra, ACT: Australian Institute of Health and Welfare; 2012. Available at: http://www.aihw.gov.au/publication-detail/?id=60129542376

26. EURO-PERISTAT Project. *European Perinatal Health Report.* Paris: EURO-PERISTAT; 2008. Available at: http://www.europeristat.com

27. Wing DA, Lockwood CJ, Barss VA. Induction of labor. UpToDate. Accessed November 2014

28. Agency for Healthcare Research and Quality. Maternal and neonatal outcomes of elective induction of labor. AHRQ Evidence Report/Technology Assessment No. 176. Rockville, MD: AHRQ; 2009 (Systematic review)

29. ACOG Committee on Practice Bulletins. Induction of labor. ACOG Practice Bulletin No. 107; 2009

Harmful birth care practices

There is an undeniable trend worldwide toward the acceptance and even the pursuit of medicalized childbirth. Giving birth is increasingly perceived as a risky experience for which only the hospital seems to be adequately equipped. Technological advances and possibilities are highlighted in the media, are framed as safety, and appear unlimited. Supply generates demand, and the client demands as much security as possible. To this end, many women and providers have the false assumption that the utmost in diagnostic and medical precautions guarantees the best chance of health. The extent to which the reverse is true is largely underestimated. Along with the benefits, resulting from the proper use of technology for women with real pregnancy and birth complications (the minority), have come the unnecessary medicalization and the high price of iatrogenic complications in healthy pregnancies (the majority). Undue medicalization causes anxiety and stress, thereby directly and indirectly creating problems in the dynamics of labor and delivery (Chapter 7). In this way, doctors create and maintain their own patient population.

The medical paradox

For women with a complicated pregnancy (the minority) there is no better place to give birth than a hospital. However, for women with a normal, healthy pregnancy (the majority), hospitals can be very dangerous.

4.1 Idle faith in technology

Obstetricians often claim that the use of high-tech maternity care equates with real progress, but the scientific evidence indicates otherwise. Over the past 40 years, no significant improvement has been demonstrated in highly industrialized countries in the reduction of cerebral palsy.[1] The decline in the perinatal mortality rates in the past four decades is attributable not to obstetrical improvements or to any decrease in fetal mortality but to a slight drop in neonatal mortality associated with neonatal intensive care. Indeed, all attempts to associate lower perinatal mortality rates with the higher obstetrical intervention rates in developed nations have failed.[2] Notzon comments in a US National Center for Health Statistics study that "the comparisons of perinatal mortality ratios with cesarean and operative vaginal rates find no consistent correlations across countries."[3] A review of the scientific literature on this issue by Lomas and Enkin states: "A number of studies have failed to detect any relation between crude perinatal mortality rates and the level of operative deliveries."[4] The US Centers for Disease Control and Prevention found a threefold risk of neonatal death for infants born by cesarean section to low-risk mothers and an alarming rise in US maternal mortality rates.[5-7] These findings suggest that we have now passed the point at which the benefits of development and technology outweigh the adverse effects.

High-tech childbirth is thought to be real progress, but the scientific evidence indicates otherwise.

4.1.1 The cesarean boomerang

In the past, cesarean section was used exclusively in perilous situations to save mother or baby from injury or death. Today, as indications broaden, and rates continue to go up, lives are saved in a smaller and smaller proportion of all cesarean deliveries. But the risks of this major abdominal surgery do not decrease with increasing rates, and, consequently, a rate has been reached at which cesarean section inevitably inflicts more harm on babies and mothers than it prevents. What once was a remedy has now become a major disease.

Uncritical use of cesarean delivery causes more harm to women and babies than it prevents.

4.1.2 Technical excess and harmful rituals

So far, mainstream obstetrics has not been able to exploit the advantages of medicalized pregnancy while avoiding the drift to medical excess. Technological advance has led to the almost automatic use of new, primarily diagnostic techniques without any therapeutic options except termination of pregnancy. Prenatal diagnosis, routine ultrasound, and electronic fetal monitoring have, aside from misinterpretations, also led to new questions and problems that may become unmanageable for pregnant women and providers. The latter must translate their findings into practice, and dubious information often creates more insecurity than confidence for both mothers and caregivers. This leads to the unnecessary medicalization of essentially healthy women.

Routine rituals in the labor ward – repeatedly taking blood pressure and temperature, restricting fluids and food, prohibiting a woman from wearing her own nightgown, restricting movement, routine insertion of fetal scalp electrodes and intrauterine lines, use of enemas, shaving the perineum, requiring personnel to wear scrubs, cap, and masks, and so forth – substantially increase the stressfulness of labor. Many labor disorders are indirectly caused by these routines with no recognition of the negative effects of this clinical excess on the dynamics of the parasympathetic birth process. Stress inhibits labor (Chapter 7).

Moreover, systematic reviews incontestably demonstrate that all the routines listed above lack any clinical benefit and should therefore be abandoned.[8] Even simple procedures during prenatal care as seemingly innocent as a routine vaginal examination in late pregnancy – to determine whether the cervix is "ready for labor" or "stripping" the membranes (digital separation of the fetal membranes from the lower uterine segment) – cause more problems than one realizes. False labor, from the anticipation created when a vaginal examination reveals "cervical ripeness" or from sweeping the membranes, is rarely recognized as iatrogenic (Chapter 23).

4.2 Negative psychology

The detrimental influence of negative psychology on the course and outcome of labor is greatly underestimated. Providing the woman with explanations and guidance is a must, but the manner in which they are presented is everything. Well-meaning information regarding possible risks, when presented with undue emphasis and without professional tact, casts a shadow of doubt on a woman's trust in a good outcome. Now the worm is in the apple and starts to grow. When a woman becomes alarmed, falsely or not, her anxiety progressively erodes her motivation and the self-confidence that are essential for creating the best condition for a safe and spontaneous birth (Chapter 7).

The psychological "black worm" metaphor
Like a tiny worm in a flawless apple, undue perception of risk progressively eats away a person's confidence and mental well-being. Both are difficult to restore.

4.2.1 Discouraging stories

As it is now, negative psychological impulses are freely spread on Internet blogs and by the woman's everyday surroundings. One out of two of her friends is likely to be an expert-by-experience in an operative delivery and is only too happy to share: "A whole day of suffering, and still a cesarean." What about sensational tabloid headlines such as "Actress's Baby Dead," or the pseudo-informative division of serious media, "The Truth about Uterine Rupture," or flatly distasteful reality-TV shows which spend two minutes on the dilatation stage and half an hour on misrepresentative and demeaning shrieks and growls in the second stage?

4.2.2 The culture of fear

Beyond this, it is the care providers themselves who unwittingly plant the blackest of psychological worms. Routine ultrasound often leads to dubious interpretations of "abnormal" findings. A leading expert in sonography described this as "the best way to terrify a pregnant woman."[9] Unnecessary uncertainty is aroused when the estimated fetal weight (mostly inaccurate) is printed on the sonography report that the parents take home – a prediction taken as an indication of likely birth outcome. A large baby diagnosed, and a worried look on the doctor's face during the pelvic examination are not motivating. The "trial of labor" is likely to fail, not because of fetopelvic disproportion but because of ineffective uterine action triggered by anxiety and the induction procedure.

> *The term "trial of labor" should be deleted from our vocabulary. All labors are trials, but calling them trials turns them into trial and error, with the error being the dominant part of the equation.*

Similarly, it does not build a woman's confidence when her providers schedule preparations for induction of labor when pregnancy is only one week overdue "because your baby is now at risk" (Chapter 23). Other findings such as a small belly, low-lying placenta, low amniotic fluid index, and so forth often lead to intensive observation by medical staff and readying of cross-matched blood and an IV line during labor as well as food restriction, "just in case." None of these actions has proven therapeutic benefits.[8,10] On the contrary, when performed thoughtlessly or with negative body language these precautionary actions generate undue stress and anxiety, which is the best way to provoke undesirable interventions and outcomes.

Likewise, well-meaning warnings in the woman's chart in red, such as "BEWARE" or "low-threshold for C section," are not conducive to the creation of a positive attitude among the on-duty staff who must convey to the woman in labor that she is perfectly capable of a safe, spontaneous delivery. It is much easier to make the prediction of a problematic birth come true than to prevent it. Women in labor do not benefit from the insecurities created by the overt anticipation of problems that have yet to occur. A risk factor is still not an illness – a distinction that is not immediately clear to most pregnant women and many "care" providers.

> *Unfavorable predictions are self-fulfilling prophecies.*

There is considerable evidence of the harmful effects of psychological "black worms" in clinical practice worldwide. For example, an American trial showed that false positive prediction by ultrasound of fetal macrosomia provoked a 50% increase in cesarean delivery of same-weight babies.[11] A Canadian trial revealed that labeling a woman as gestational diabetic conferred a doubled cesarean delivery rate, regardless of the fetal or maternal condition and with no relationship to birth weight.[12] In a German study, the label "growth retardation" biased interpretation of and action taken for fetal monitoring and led to twice as many cesarean sections as occurred in undetected cases of growth restriction.[13] An Israeli study observed that pregnancies of macrosomic fetuses, unrecognized upon admission, are more likely to end up with a normal vaginal delivery, in contrast to suspected macrosomia, which raises induction of labor and cesarean delivery rates without benefits for maternal and fetal outcomes.[14] A twin study from Iceland and Scotland revealed no difference in outcome for "naturally conceived" twins as compared with twins after "assisted conception," except that the cesarean rate was twice as high in the assisted-conception group.[15] In a Swedish study, older nulliparas had greatly increased odds of cesarean delivery regardless of maternal or fetal condition.[16] A Canadian study of the definition and management of dystocia found that among the strongest determinants of a decision for cesarean delivery were acquisition of a dystocia perception and label in the mind of the physician, although a significant proportion of such decisions were made during the "latent phase" of labor.[17]

> *Technical excess, clinical routines, discontinuous care, and psychological "black worms" create physical and emotional stress leading to a cascade of adverse effects that are hardly ever recognized for what they are: iatrogenic labor disorders.*

4.2.3 Professional daunting

Downright discouragement of vaginal birth may be part of pre-labor counseling to protect the hospital or obstetrician against liability suits. An expectant woman has to sign a document of consent after being informed that she is likely to have an episiotomy, that she might severely tear her vulva and pelvic floor, that she might bleed profusely, that she might need an emergency surgical delivery, and that she might lose her baby. Little wonder some people feel hospitals try to bully them into cesarean delivery.

> *Scare-care is a poor substitute for healthcare.*

4.3 Clinical ambience

For many women, pregnancy is the most amazing and wonderful time of their lives and its conclusion by giving birth should be an intimate experience leading to an ultimate sense of accomplishment and satisfaction. The vast majority of women, though, are not properly educated and thus not adequately prepared for this job; during labor, they are just told by staff to "get on with it." In many hospitals, routine procedures more often give rise to ambiguity and the feeling that one is neither being heard nor taken seriously. Added to this, the clinical outfit and attitude of providers and the "functional" and sterile furnishing of many delivery rooms may often act as potent tocolytic (labor-suppressant) methods.[18] Stress, as we have said, inhibits labor (Chapter 7). The result is iatrogenic dysfunctional labor.

4.3.1 Women's sense of isolation

The more efficiently the hospital seems to be organized, the more rapidly women feel reduced to a number. From time to time a nurse looks in, but most of the time women lie alone enduring the first stage of labor. Many caregivers do not realize how lonely women in labor may feel, especially in a busy labor unit, and how frightful loneliness can be. The women's partners, if in attendance, feel equally helpless.

The sense of isolation and the reality of being left alone, even momentarily, are often compounded by the appearance and disappearance of a rapidly changing cast of students, midwives, interns, residents, and occasionally consultants. Several survey studies report that a low-risk mother having her first child is attended by from 5 to 15 unfamiliar people (dubbed by one author as "masked intruders") but is still left alone most of the time.[19]

Medical equipment is used just because it is present or for reasons of efficiency only. Personal attention and supportive care are replaced by watching the fetal monitor screen in the coffee room. This method of "care" requires fewer personnel, convenient from a budget perspective but disastrous to the provision of real care. It seems that the main "advantage" of the introduction of routine electronic fetal monitoring has been that women in labor can be left unattended by nursing care.

It is not too fanciful to compare the state of laboring women nowadays with that of the absolutely terrified pregnant monkeys so often cited in relation to psychological stress, failed deliveries, and fetal distress.[18]

4.3.2 Frustratingly casual attitudes

In orthodox medical circles, recognition has come slowly that women may experience medicalized childbirth as genuinely traumatic. Failure to pay nearly enough attention to this important issue has been attributed to the fact that, until recently, obstetricians were mostly men. Ironically, however, the recent, rapid feminization of the profession has not resulted in more woman-friendly provisions, attitudes, and approaches.

Rarely is human consciousness more susceptible to impressions than during labor, and the all-too-common casual approach by professionals – both male and female – burdens women with frustrated feelings of dismissal.[20,21] Things as seemingly trivial as leaving the woman lying naked after an examination, thoughtless remarks, conversations about other patients in her presence, bloodstained clothing, unconsidered answers, inconsistent explanations by ever-changing staff, delays in giving her test results, concealing one's actual intentions, leaving her alone for long periods of time, not keeping appointments – to the woman, all these seem like personal insults. For obvious reasons, she interprets this behavior as indifference on the part of precisely the people in whom she has put her trust during the most vulnerable hours of her life.

In reality, however, indifference is not the problem. Most providers are devoted to the women in their care. Many seemingly thoughtless actions are rather the result of the lack of a central birth-plan and tolerance of long labors. An unclear perspective on how to proceed when black clouds are gathering and labor becomes increasingly difficult has a demoralizing effect not only on the parturient and her partner but also on the nursing staff. As a result, labor room staff consciously or unconsciously avoid the birthing room and frequent the coffee room.

Lack of personal attention and deficient care from all providers are the inevitable result of unnecessarily long labors and vice versa.

4.3.3 Divided attention

Many conventionally supervised first births take far longer than the length of one work shift. This means that it is increasingly rare for women to have continuous and personal attention from one and the same care provider throughout their labor. What is more, the nurse-midwife must equally divide her attention among several laboring women while frequently attending to responsibilities that have nothing to do with birth, but by which nearly every labor ward is plagued, such as (semi)-emergency consultations, small tasks, antenatal non-stress tests, external cephalic versions of breech, etc. And many a labor and delivery ward is abused as a gynecological first-aid facility.

The personal attention the nurse-midwife can provide to women in labor is further hampered by modern hospital rules regarding "quality assessments," which essentially require the keeping of extensive records of mostly irrelevant data at the expense of basic care. Defensive medicine dictates silly administration: "If you don't document it, preferably in triplicate, it wasn't done." In addition, understaffing in the interest of efficiency has taken over hospital policies. It is in this way that the backlash of budget cuts ("lean" or so-called "managed care") and supposed but irrelevant "quality demands" are felt most profoundly in labor rooms. Managers and policymakers seldom realize that indispensable personal attention throughout labor requires sufficient personnel at the bedside, whose focus should be on direct supportive care for each woman in labor.

Fundamental problem 9

Personal one-on-one support extended to all women in labor is critical to providing high-quality care, but it is a requirement that hardly any hospital meets.

It is increasingly difficult for midwives and nurses to provide really supportive care, and this affects their work satisfaction and increases burn-out rates. In times long gone, the mother–midwife relationship used to be an intimate one, with both parties emotionally involved. This emotional involvement – deeply appreciated by either party – has proven unsustainable in large organizations when operating in the absence of a clear strategy for supportive care in labor. Midwives and nurses react by detaching themselves emotionally, and mothers in the meantime have become socialized to expect little from hospital care and to submit to impersonal medicalized care.[22] Evidently, this vicious circle must be broken, and personal, supportive care in labor needs to be rediscovered and facilitated.

4.4 Care of fetus versus care of mother

Obstetrics has evolved from maternity care toward perinatology, and prevention of perinatal morbidity and mortality is at present its dominant benchmark. However, this also poses a significant risk to women. "Somehow the idea has gained ground that a conflict of interest exists between mother and child during labor and that mothers can be subjected to almost any form of indignity or discomfort provided it is well intentioned and undertaken on behalf of her baby."[23] Concerns about liability, whether real or remote, play an increasingly greater role in the defensive interpretation of indications used to justify aggressive interventions. As the saying goes: "When in doubt, get it out." Numerous inductions of labor or cesarean deliveries are performed on the basis of "fetal compromise," with the nature and validity of that generalization undefined. Most fetuses supposed to be compromised are most likely not, but are "rescued from normalcy" by induction and/or operative delivery for enhanced provider and patient anxiety.[24]

Modern birth care has surpassed the point at which the benefits of medical technology have reached their limits. By now, the negative effects of medical excess are prevailing.

4.4.1 Fetal trauma

Acceleration of slow labor is often postponed because of a supposedly negative effect on fetal oxygen supply, as though the interests of mother and child were opposed. This widespread misconception leads to therapeutic paralysis. On the one hand, caregivers are hesitant to accelerate labor, especially in the so-called latent phase, but, on the other hand, long labor does not benefit the fetus either. On the contrary, exhaustion after too long a labor is strongly associated with instrumental vaginal delivery. These interventions are the predominant cause of serious fetal injuries such as fetal skin lacerations, bone fractures, bleeding, paralyses, and lethal rupture of tentorium cerebelli (references in 2.2). Strangely, a paradoxical discrepancy continues to exist between the fear of fetal hypoxia and the failure to anticipate mechanical birth injuries. These birth traumas are rarely seen in children delivered spontaneously but nearly always result from instrumental delivery.[25]

The trauma paradox

The precautions against fetal hypoxic damage contrast sharply with the failure to foresee fetal birth traumas caused by forced traction with vacuum extractor or forceps.

4.4.2 Safety for mothers and babies

In essence, fetal trauma can be discussed under the same heading as severe birth injuries to the mother such as cervical laceration, vault rupture, and fourth-degree lacerations that need extensive surgical repair as well as damage to the pudendal nerve, levator ani, and fascial pelvic organ supports, which may result in life-long dyspareunia and urinary or fecal incontinence. These injuries occur in second-stage labor, and the circumstances that give rise to severe maternal trauma are essentially the same as those which give rise to severe fetal trauma – i.e. instrumental traction.[25] In reality, the interests of mother and child are parallel in that both profit from a strategy of care specifically focused on preventing an overly long labor that ends in a forced instrumental delivery (Section 3).

Excellent care in childbirth serves the best interests of both mothers and their babies.

References

1. Nelson KB. Can we prevent cerebral palsy? N Engl J Med 2003;**349**:1765–9

2. Matthews TG, Crowley P, Chong A, *et al.* Rising caesarean section rates: A cause for concern. Br J Obstet Gynaecol 2003;**110**:346–9

3. Notzon FC. International differences in the use of obstetric interventions. JAMA 1990;**263**: 3286–91

4. Lomas J, Enkin M. Variations in operative delivery rates. In Chalmers I, Enkin M, Keirse MJ, eds. *Effective Care in Pregnancy and Childbirth*, Vol. 1. Oxford: Oxford University Press; 1998

5. MacDorman MF, Declercq E, Menacker F, Malloy MH. Infant and neonatal mortality for primary cesarean and vaginal births to women with "no indicated risk," United States 1998–2001 birth cohorts. Birth 2006;**3**:175–82

6. Centers for Disease Control and Prevention. http://www:cdc.gov/nchs/data/series/

7. Harper MA, Byington RP, Espeland MA, *et al.* Pregnancy-related death and health care services. Obstet Gynecol 2003;**102**:273.

8. Chalmers I, Keirse MJNC, Enkin M, eds. *Effective Care in Pregnancy and Childbirth*, Vol. **2**: Childbirth. Oxford: Oxford University Press; 1998

9. Filly RA. Obstetrical ultrasonography: the best way to terrify a pregnant woman. J Ultrasound Med 2000;**19**:1–5

10. Wood L, Newton JM, Wamg L, Lesser K. Borderline amniotic fluid index and its relation to fetal intolerance of labor. J Ultrasound Med 2014;**33**:705–11

11. Levine AB, Lockwood CJ, Brown B, Lapinski R, Berkowitz RL. Sonographic diagnosis of the large for gestational age fetus at term: does it make a difference? Obstet Gynecol 1992;**79**:55–8

12. Naylor CD, Sermer M, Chen E, Sykora K. Cesarean delivery in relation to birth weight and gestational glucose tolerance: pathophysiology or practice style? JAMA 1996;**275**:1199–2000

13. Jahn A, Razum O, Berle P. Routine screening for intrauterine growth retardation in Germany: Low sensitivity and questionable benefit for diagnosed cases. Acta Obstet Gynecol Scand 1998;**77**:643–8

14. Sadeh-Mestechkin D, Walfisch A, Shachar R, *et al.* Suspected macrosomia? Better not tell. Arch Gynecol Obstet 2008;**278**:225–230

15. Agustsson T, Geirsson RT, Mires G. Obstetric outcome of natural and assisted conception twin pregnancies is similar. Acta Obstet Gynecol Scand 1997;**6**:45–9

16. Cnattingius R, Cnattingius S, Notzon FC. Obstacles to reducing cesarean rates in a low-cesarean setting: the effect of maternal age, height and weight. Obstet Gynecol 1998;**92**:501–6

17. Stewart PJ, Duhlberg C, Arnett AC, Elmslie T, Hall PF. Diagnosis of dystocia and management with cesarean section among primiparous women in Ottowa Carleton. CMAJ 1990;**142**:459–63

18. Foureur MJ, Leap N, Davis DL, Forbes IF, Homer C. Developing the Birth Unit Design Spatial Evaluation Tool (BUDSET) in Australia: a qualitative study. HERD 2009;**3**:43–57.

19. Enkin M, Keirse MJNC, Neilson J, *et al.* Hospital practices. In: *A Guide to Effective Care in Pregnancy and Childbirth*, 3rd edn. Oxford: Oxford University Press; 2000

20. Simkin P. Just another day in a woman's life? Women's long-term perceptions of their first birth experience. Part I. Birth 1991;**18**:203–10

21. Simkin P. Just another day in a woman's life? Women's long-term perceptions of their first birth experience. Part II. Birth 1991;**19**:64–81

22. Hunter B, Deery R. *Emotions in Midwifery and Reproduction*, 1st edn. Palgrave Macmillan; 2009

23. O'Driscoll K, Meagher D, Robson M. *Active Management of Labour*, 4th edn. London: Mosby; 2003

24 Menticoglou SM, Hall PF. Routine induction of labour at 41 weeks gestation: nonsensus consensus. Br J Obstet Gynaecol 2002;**109**:485–91

25. Keriakos R, Sugumar S, Hilal N. Instrumental vaginal delivery – back to basics. J Obstet Gynaecol 2013;**33**:781–86

Chapter 5

Destructive territorial disputes

Women's critique of the excessive medicalization of childbirth has led to reactionary calls for the return of independent midwifery and home births. The question is whether this post-modern trend will provide proper solutions. Answers can be found by examining western childbirth systems that formally include autonomous midwifery care. In this context, some fundamental differences between midwifery and the medical approach must be illuminated. Strong prejudices and emotions are involved here, and disputes are often characterized more by heat than by light: the debate is usually about choice of caregiver and place of birth, rather than about labor.[1]

5.1 Controversial birth philosophies

Unlike obstetricians and hospital managers, who generally see childbirth as a standard medical problem subject to the paradigm of "managed care", most midwives typically approach labor and delivery as a natural process and a highly personal experience, sometimes even compounded with a spiritual, near-mystical atmosphere. An exemplary quote: "[labor,] … it is predictable that it will occur, but unpredictable and idiosyncratic in its actual occurrence. Despite attempts to package labor into discrete phases and stages, it is better understood as a whole, with ebb and flow and rhythms of its own. It is intensely physical and emotional, consuming all of one's attention and energy; yet life-giving and empowering in that intensity. How then is it possible to 'manage' labor?"[2]

5.1.1 Adverse working relations

The typical role of the midwife is to provide strong supportive care and to preserve a woman's place in the group categorized as "normal" for as long as possible without intervention. In contrast, obstetricians focus on risks and pathological conditions, want to be in control, and put trust in technology. The differing starting points that typically characterize the two professions have often made for tense and even hostile working relations.

Obstetricians accuse midwives of backwardness, blocking progress, and trusting recklessly in biology. One obstetrician best summarizes the general sentiment of many: "Nature is a lousy obstetrician." On the other hand, midwives reproach obstetricians for providing interventional, impersonal, and technocratic care, for having a lack of faith in nature, for overriding biology, and disempowering women. The abundance of seditious manifestos and Internet blogs by "home birth activists" attests to a lot of furor, rancor, and frustration. Sadly, reactionary fantasists and zealots can be found on both sides of the debate. They resemble marine iguanas of the Galapagos Islands: all on the same beach but facing different directions and spitting at one another constantly. In some countries there is even, as it seems, a political "birth-war" going on, with the re-emergence of autonomous, "radical midwives" attracting more and more women who are fed up with the medicalized birth system.[3-6] Who is to blame?

> *Sadly, the debate is usually about choice of caregiver and place of birth, rather than about labor.*

Stuck between polarized positions, it is the mothers who draw the shortest straws. In reality, women's preferences and needs contain many elements of both midwifery and medical styles of care, and all laboring women should benefit from what are, in fact, the complementary skills of both professional groups. Clearly, both obstetricians and midwives – and foremost all laboring women – have much to gain from a childbirth system that combines the best of midwifery and medicine, and places pregnant women first (Section 3).

> *Women's preferences and needs include many elements of both midwifery and medical styles of care.*

5.2 Cross-cultural differences

Reforming childbirth services is not an easy task. No single component of healthcare is influenced more by culture, tradition, social pressures, politics, and litigation issues than pregnancy care. Consequently, there are three established forms of maternity services in the western world: the fully medicalized, doctor-centered childbirth system typically found, for example, in the USA, France, and Spain; the midwife-centered system almost exclusively found in New Zealand, the Scandinavian countries and the Netherlands; and a mixture of both systems, found, for example, in the UK, Canada, Australia, Germany, and Japan. Evidently, the defined role of midwives varies significantly throughout the western world. As a result, the disputes between midwives and obstetricians are at dissimilar levels in different countries. We will briefly discuss the extremes of the spectrum at the risk of caricaturing.

> For a detached woman having her first baby, it can be difficult to believe how culturally shaped the childbirth service can be.

5.2.1 Disputes in medicalized countries

Like in most western countries, home births are actively discouraged in the USA, and 99% of all births there take place in hospitals. Independent, community-based midwives have been marginalized or even pushed into illegality. Strikingly, the term "midwife" is not mentioned once in the 1376 pages of the leading US textbook *Williams Obstetrics* (2014). Pregnant women are patients, and birth is the responsibility of doctors. Auxiliary personnel are called "nurse-midwife." American midwives practice under the strict authority of the obstetricians, but for the convenience of the doctor they are given a high degree of their own responsibility. "Nurse-midwives" assess the "patient" and then contact the obstetrician, who is mostly not in the hospital, seeing patients in her or his office. The midwife, of course, knows the proclivity of each doctor, and so how she presents her findings is influenced by this knowledge. Despite the claim that they are "a team", they all know that the obstetrician is the boss. An insider explained it thus: "It is like a marriage where the husband and wife are a 'partnership', but the husband is ultimately in charge. The wife resorts to all kinds of trickery and manipulation to get the husband to do what she wants. That is what the relationship is like in the US between nurse-midwives and obstetricians." Midwives have to fight for every inch of bringing midwifery care back to American childbirth. In practice, many resort, as it seems, to everyday acts of resistance to put off unnecessary interventions. Clearly, there is an urgent need to redefine the professional relationships between obstetricians and midwives in the USA and many other countries (Chapter 25).

5.2.2 Disputes in midwife-centered systems

An example at the other end of the spectrum is the renowned childbirth system in the Netherlands. Midwifery has a long history there as an established and independent profession. Midwife-led home birth is still valued as part of a cultural heritage. Midwives stake their claim to an autonomous existence in isolation from the medical department on the premise that pregnancy and birth are natural processes, not illnesses. So, in those midwives' eyes, the pregnant woman is not a patient but a client. Although all Dutch midwives are well trained and legally certified, their education in the supervision of labor is based on the philosophy of expectancy. As a matter of principle, labor and delivery are approached conservatively. Since they attend only "normal labor" and are taught not to intervene, the bounds of "normal" are then widely overstretched. Labors lasting up to 24 hours are accepted as normal. In this way, the strict separation between midwifery and medical obstetrics creates illogical barriers against the small and timely corrections of slow labor that could forestall far more intrusive interventions at a later stage. Typically, a woman is transferred to the hospital only if she and the midwife no longer see the possibility of a natural end to labor. In this way, hospitals function as a safety net, and obstetricians obviously address problems only after the fact. Too many out-of-control labors – often dubbed "a total loss" or "a train wreck" – are transferred. What essentially was a dynamic problem is then solved mechanically: by an operative delivery.

> Autonomous midwifery creates a barrier to minor and timely corrections of slow labor that can prevent the need for far more invasive interventions at a later stage.

Unlike the situation in the USA – where midwives have not reached the point of practicing independent midwifery, and quality of childbirth might surely benefit from a reappraisal of various aspects of midwifery care – the discussion in the Netherlands is at a different level. Dutch obstetricians feel the need to have more input in the decision making about when a woman has crossed the line from normal to abnormal labor. Clearly, in both doctor- and midwife-centered systems much better cooperation is needed. Provider-centered care must be replaced by mothers-centered care.

5.3 Myths and facts of autonomous midwifery

While most readers will be familiar with medicalized childbirth systems and recognize the need for structural reforms, most are unaware of the ins and outs of a formal midwifery-centered system. Since the childbirth organization in the Netherlands is often extolled as a "midwives' Mecca" that deserves to be copied elsewhere, the facts and myths of the Dutch childbirth system need to be put into proper perspective.

5.3.1 Gatekeepers

The Dutch system seems to embody what many midwives worldwide are struggling for, and that is acknowledgment of the appropriateness and self-proclaimed superiority of midwifery care for normal pregnancy and birth. In the Netherlands, primary (midwifery) care has a gatekeeper role: healthy women with an uncomplicated pregnancy are directed into primary care, whereas women facing some kind of risk are referred to secondary (medical) care. A formal list of indications defines the conditions that require a referral from primary to secondary care.[7]

Primary care is practiced independently in a primary birth center or at the birthing woman's home. Only a minority of Dutch midwives work in hospitals as "clinical midwives" and report to an obstetrician as is typical in most countries. The majority still work independently in that they are self-employed, work outside of the hospital, carry independent insurance, and are paid directly through their clients' insurance. The Dutch government assures the midwives' job security; under health insurance law, healthy pregnant women are reimbursed only if they see a midwife for their care. In other words, midwifery is the system for normal childbirth in Holland.[8,9] Obstetricians supposedly are not involved in the care of normal pregnancy and childbirth, unless the midwife requests their help. That is the story, now the facts.

5.3.2 Transfer rates

Serious doubts must be raised about the gatekeeper role of independent primary care, in particular with regard to first pregnancies. In reality, the primacy of Dutch midwifery does not prevent the medicalization of birth. No less than 80% of all Dutch nulliparas eventually end up in the secondary care division.[10] Thirteen percent begin their antenatal care with an obstetrician because of a pre-existing condition or risk factor, and another 33% are referred during pregnancy. Of the remaining 54% who planned a midwife-led delivery at home or in a birth center, more than half are transferred during labor to the hospital where an obstetrician (or rather the youngest resident) takes over their care. The main indications for intrapartum referral include requests for epidural pain relief, failure to progress in the first stage (but often quite late), meconium passage, abnormal fetal heartbeat counts, second-stage arrest, and afterbirth disorders. In summary, only 20% of all nulliparas (and 35% of all multiparas) in the Netherlands remain exclusively in primary care at home or in an independent midwifery birth center. Under 10% of all nulliparas and about 20% of all multiparas now deliver at home in the Netherlands.[10]

> There are many misguided ideas abroad about the effectiveness, cost-benefits, safety, and woman-friendliness of independent midwifery care in the Netherlands.

These exorbitant transfer rates seriously question the efficiency and cost-to-benefit ratio of independent primary care, in particular for first-time mothers. The main risk factor for birth problems proves to be first labor, but the majority of nulliparous "clients" in Dutch midwifery care are unaware of the high likelihood of becoming a "patient." The result is a disappointing mismatch between prior expectations of an intimate delivery at home and the actual course of events. This explains why women who are transferred to the hospital during labor (>50%) report significantly less satisfaction with the childbirth experience than those who planned a hospital birth in advance.[9,11]

Most labor disorders arise in healthy, first-time mothers after a completely uneventful pregnancy. A strict division between midwifery care and secondary obstetrical care cannot cope with this phenomenon.

5.3.3 Discontinuous and unsafe care

Unlike the midwives of earlier times – who worked around the clock and stayed with laboring women from beginning to end – modern midwives have their own family life, often disallowing continuous labor attendance at their clients' home. As a result, periodic visits at intervals of three hours or more during the first stage of labor are now standard practice. Support and care – and thus responsibility for maternal and fetal well being – are left to the woman's partner, a relative, or a friend. Clearly, this situation is far from ideal and proves, indeed, irresponsible: the perinatal mortality rate for term babies in Holland, albeit low, exceeds that of most other European countries, and this reflects, at least in part, its divided childbirth system.[1,12] Fifty percent of all term babies admitted to Dutch neonatal intensive care units – in most cases for meconium aspiration, post-asphyxia syndrome, or neonatal sepsis – are born to women whose "low-risk labor" at home or in alternative birth centers was, initially or until the end, attended by independent midwives.[13] Even more striking, the perinatal mortality rate in the selected "low-risk" population under independent midwifery care is twice as high as that of the at-term "medium- and high-risk" pregnancies under hospital care.[13] Clearly, adequate pre-labor risk selection remains illusory. When labor attendance at home or in a birth center is intermittent, a serious perinatal complication in so-called "low-risk pregnancies" is not assessed in time for safe and timely transfer to the hospital. Simply put: if you are not there, you don't give care.

Advocates of home births should be cautioned not to replace obstetric excess by non-attendance and undertreatment.

However, those who advocate the spread of the Dutch midwife-centered system in other countries never mention these practices and key figures. The superiority of autonomous midwifery care often resembles the story of the emperor's new clothes. The Dutch example disproves the premise that midwifery care during a first labor at home is personal, superior, and safe. A 50% transfer rate during labor – sometimes compounded with a nerve-racking ambulance drive – whereby care is taken over by strangers, no longer supports the proposition that a trial of labor at home is an empowering experience, enhancing women's self-esteem and self-confidence. The unique Dutch system is actually on the verge of a breakdown unless the working relationships between midwives and obstetricians change radically. Recently, the Dutch government has taken initiatives to promote integration of midwifery and medical services that should place women first instead of caregiver interests. Paradoxically, in other countries with doctor-centered childbirth systems, reactionary calls for independent midwifery and home births refer to the Dutch system and increasingly resonate with politicians and healthcare policymakers.

Independent midwifery does not prevent the medicalization of birth, whereas safety issues are insufficiently appreciated.

An autonomous midwifery service for normal pregnancy and childbirth is often claimed to have psychological advantages, but the Dutch reality has developed into the opposite in recent decades. More than 80% of all nulliparas end up in the secondary care division and are implicitly told they have to deliver in the hospital because their pregnancy or labor is now "at risk" or "abnormal." The mismatch between prior expectations and actual place of birth surely contributes to disappointments and dissatisfaction with the labor experience.[11]

5.4 Universality of childbirth

Although normal childbirth is the same physiological process worldwide, there are important cross-cultural differences in childbirth systems. Territorial disputes – prevalent all over the western world, albeit on different levels – are destructive of the quality of birth care and block improvements. The universality of childbirth and solid evidence should eliminate territorial struggles and refocus attention on the real issue: the interests of pregnant women whose needs and preferences include many elements of both midwifery and medical styles of care. Both the exclusively medical interventional approach and the hands-off midwifery approach unsupported by congenial medical back-up lack a scientific basis. Conclusions from clinical studies in high-risk pregnancies have been inappropriately extrapolated to low-risk care, mostly resulting in medicalization of normal childbirth without improving outcomes. Fully medicalized obstetrics easily results in *mismanagement* of labor with spiraling cesarean rates. On the other hand, independent midwifery care that avoids intervention may easily result in *non-management* of labor with equally unintended effects.[1] Clearly, radical reforms at both ends of the spectrum are needed. Cultural prejudices and entrenched positions must be overcome. The interests of birthing women are universally the same. Maternity care should be woman-centered instead of provider-centered in its approach (Chapter 25).

> Both the medicalized and the non-interventional midwifery care must be seen as two opposite but equally uninformed approaches. A compromise is urgently needed.

5.4.1 In search of the evidence

Debates are being dominated by emotions clouding facts.[1] Until now, most midwives have not been educated in the creation and critical review of scientific studies, resulting in a paucity of scientific work originating at the level of primary care. This has hindered the achievement of scientifically founded professional midwifery standards. In fact, well-founded, truly evidence-based guidelines on labor supervision of initially low-risk pregnancies are non-existent. In the Netherlands, independent midwives' claims of providing superior care are not supported by higher spontaneous delivery rates and/or better fetal outcomes of women who begin their labor under their supervision.

Quality assessments reliably exploring women's satisfaction with autonomous midwife-led childbirth are not available either. Home delivery is advocated on the basis of biased sentiments rather than solid arguments. In conclusion, there are no valid reasons to support initiatives for introduction of the Dutch system in other western countries. The Dutch system with a strict division between primary and secondary care is a vestige rather than a vanguard. That is not an argument, however, to defend the medicalized systems elsewhere. In countries with a fully medicalized birth system, the evidence seems to support midwifery-led care for low-risk women,[14] and

obstetricians should accept this evidence. However, indiscriminate antipathy of "radical midwives" against all obstetricians will not help to find a compromise between "medicalized" and "all natural" birth. The advantage of a reappraisal of midwifery, often disparaged by obstetricians, is the pregnant and birthing woman's satisfaction with her care, at least when all goes well. Their "holistic" approach prioritizes women's feelings and the midwifery literature seems to be overwhelming: midwife-led continuity models of birth care is claimed to be more satisfying to the woman and her family than doctor-centered care.[15] This claim is most likely valid in birth settings in which there is close cooperation between midwives and obstetricians. The literature concerning independent midwifery, however, is troublingly confused by disregard of parity, client selection-bias, and the focus on choice of provider or place of birth, rather than on the method of labor supervision. Gross but inaccurate generalizations and extrapolations are then easily made.[1]

> **Fundamental problem 10**
>
> In current debate, where and by whom the cord is cut seems to be more important than the circumstances preceding and surrounding it, let alone adequate assessment of safe selection criteria.

5.4.2 Bridging the controversies

Ironically, the majority of protraction disorders of labor, as well as cases of intrapartum fetal distress, occur in completely healthy women giving birth to their first child, and most of these complications arise gradually in the first stage of labor. This makes a clear-cut distinction between the need for primary or secondary care virtually impossible, especially in nulliparous labor.

> The most important risk factor for labor complications is nulliparity.

Evidently, high-quality care requires much closer cooperation and mutual respect among all birth care providers and a redefinition of professional working relationships (Chapter 25). In fact, a new balance must be found so that all women in labor will benefit from the complementary skills of both professions. To develop the team spirit that is vital to high-quality care, the professional relations between nurses, mid-wives, and obstetricians must be redefined in a mutually satisfactory manner. This emphasizes the need for a collective plan for the supervision of normal childbirth that stimulates a synthesis of the managerial and medical approach of obstetricians and the individual attention so typical of midwifery care (Section 3). This is an issue of great practical importance in all childbirth services all over the world. Section 3 of this book will demonstrate how organizational reforms and well-defined mutual responsibilities can improve maternity care immensely. This collective purpose is one of the greatest challenges for obstetricians, midwives, nurses, hospital managers, and health officials.

Maternity care should be woman-centered instead of provider-centered. All pregnant women should benefit from the complementary skills of midwives and obstetricians.

References

1. Keirse MJNC. Home births: gone away, gone astray, and here to stay. Birth 2010;**37**:341–6

2. Kaufman KJ. Effective control or effective care. Birth 1993;**20**:150–61

3. Block J. Pushed: The Painful Truth about Childbirth and Modern Maternity Care. Cambridge, MA: Da Capo Press; 2007

4. Wagner M. Born in the USA: How a Broken Maternity System Must Be Fixed to Put Women and Children First. Berkeley, CA: University of California Press; 2007

5. Lake R, Epstein E. The Business of Being Born (documentary film) (2007) www.thebusinessofbeingborn.com/about.htm.

6. Tritten J. The miracle of homebirth. Midwifery Today Int Midwife 2010;**93**:5

7. Verloskundig vademecum 2003 – Eindrapport van de Commissie Verloskunde van het College voor zorgverzekeringen. [Obstetric vademecum 2003 – Final report of the Committee Obstetrics of the College of health insurances]. De verloskundige-indicatielijst 2003. [List of obstetric indications 2003] Accessed October 2014. Available at: http://www.knov.nl/vakkennisenweteschap/richtlijnen/verloskundigeindicatielijst

8. Stubbs V. Working relations: midwives and obstetricians in the Netherlands. Midwifery Today Int Midwife 2003;**67**:52–5

9. De Vries R. Midwifery in the Netherlands: vestige or vanguard? Med Anthropol 2001;**20**:277–311

10. Perinatal care in the Netherlands 2012 (in Dutch). Stichting Perinatale Registratie Nederland. www.perinatreg.nl

11. Rijnders M, Baston H, Schönbeck Y, et al. Perinatal factors related to negative or positive recall of birth experience in women 3 years postpartum in the Netherlands. Birth 2008;**35**:107–16

12. Zeitlin J, Mohangoo AD, Delnord M, Cuttini M. EURO-PERISTAT Scientific Committee. The second European Perinatal Health Report: documenting changes over 6 years in the health of mothers and babies in Europe. J Epidemiol Community Health 2013;**67**:983–5

13. Evers AC, Brouwers HA, Hukkelhoven CWPM, et al. Perinatal mortality and severe morbidity in low and high risk term pregnancies in the Netherlands: prospective cohort study. Br Med J 2010;**341**: c5639

14. Olsen O, Clausen JA. Planned hospital birth versus planned home birth. Cochrane Database Syst Rev 2012; Cochrane Library DOI: 10.1002/14651858. CD000352.pub2

15. Sandall J, Soltani H, Gates S, Shennan A, Devane D. Midwife-led continuity models versus other models of care for childbearing women. Cochrane Database Syst Rev 2013

Self-sustaining mechanisms

Birth professionals – be they doctors, midwives, or nurses – often fail to see the adverse effects their care may have on women's childbirth experiences and the outcomes of labor. "Fish can't see water", as the saying goes. Providers are caught up in complex systems hiding several intrinsic mechanisms that sustain the current methods of childbirth. If the much-needed changes are to be made, these hindering values need to be identified, explored, and overcome.

6.1 The applause phenomenon

Modern intervention possibilities allow those professionals who lack elementary labor and delivery skills to achieve what appears to be the best result: the birth of a living child. Indeed, there are few problems of labor that cannot be simply resolved by cesarean section. In this way, blasé practitioners may quickly come to think they are good care providers and will not recognize the need for proper evaluation of their care. The truth is that labor disorders are much easier to create than to prevent, and although each traumatic birth experience is unintentional, nonetheless it is often the result of factual mistreatment and violation of a woman in an exceedingly vulnerable position. No matter how empathetic, friendly and kind the birth professional remains through all this, the end-result is utterly unfriendly to a woman. And yet, there is nearly always applause…

In the delivery room, even after a mediocre performance, a round of applause typically follows.

After the cesarean or instrument-assisted delivery of a healthy baby, the professional is almost always regarded as having done a good job, or at least the "policy" of care is sold as that. "With the midwife's patience, has the woman not had the best prospect of a natural birth?" Because it is she who "could not do it herself," was the vacuum or cesarean delivery not "truly

inevitable?" Did not the despairing woman herself literally plead for the mercy of surgery? Ironically, after a long and failed induction, the obstetrician is not recognized as the originator of the woman's ordeal but is thanked as her savior for performing the relieving cesarean. When the fetus that was supposedly "in distress" was operatively delivered, and the child was born in good condition, "the intervention was performed in good time"; and for the newborn with a poor start, "the intervention was well-indicated." What can we professionals possibly do wrong?

Professional satisfaction resulting from a deftly performed operative delivery and the self-image of the heroic, right-on-time obstetrician push the willingness to reflect on the real cause of the problems to the back burner. And performing a surgical intervention is ultimately sexier than waiting around for a spontaneous birth. The negative result of all this is positive reinforcement of the non-management or mismanagement of labor. Furthermore, "black worm psychology" (see 4.2) is bolstered by the unmerited applause: the more forcefully an obstetrician stresses the possibility of an unfavorable outcome, the more thankful the parents will be for the operative birth of a healthy baby. One cowboy-colleague once whispered in our ear: "Just scare the hell out of those 'clients,' do a cesarean, and you'll have happy 'patients' for sure."

Undeserved compliments and daily affirmation do not inspire self-evaluation but fuel the continuation of this sort of "care". Childbirth services desperately need new quality-control criteria that will make providers accountable not only for perinatal morbidity and mortality, but also for superfluous interventions, iatrogenic complications, avoidable operative deliveries, physical and psycho-emotional trauma, and the (dis)satisfaction of the women subjected to their care (Chapters 26 and 27).

Obstetrics needs new quality-control criteria.

6.1.1 Remuneration practices

In many countries, surgery is far more lucrative for doctors. They get a higher fee for a quick operation than for the much more time-consuming attendance of a spontaneous labor and delivery. And many hospitals are more than happy to comply since they get paid more than twice as much by insurance companies for a cesarean as for an uncomplicated vaginal birth. What is more, in some countries mothers can get a few additional weeks of paid maternity leave from their employers after a cesarean. Clearly, these provisions do not stimulate changes in the right direction. Policymakers in governmental health departments, insurance companies, labor unions, and employer organizations should wake up and realize that they are promoting improper medical care.

Current financing and insurance systems promote improper incentives for cesarean delivery.

6.2 Consumerism

Undue medicalization of birth is also the result of changing attitudes of pregnant women themselves. The body is increasingly regarded as something we can control to the extent that discomforts inherent to late pregnancy and birth are no longer acceptable. Today's parents have busy jobs and have children along the way. They regard the free choice of a medical intervention as their God-given right. More and more women request an induction of labor or even a cesarean delivery at the time that best suits both their schedule and that of the physician. This is the patient or client as the modern consumer. Some women go from one doctor to another until they get what they want. And doctor shopping surely biases the responsiveness to the desires of a woman: "If I don't do it, my colleague/rival in another hospital most certainly will."

Sadly, some leading feminists who fight for women's rights have been drawn into believing biased information. As a result, they have unwittingly promoted the right of women to demand elective obstetric procedures that are potentially dangerous to themselves and their babies. Ironically, their rightful appeal to self-determination is completely nullified by making themselves totally dependent on the operative skills of doctors. In reality, their claim to self-determination and autonomy rather stands for the right to harm themselves and their babies. Obstetricians are now increasingly confronted with impassioned requests from women who have been overwhelmed by biased and ill-founded information from the media and the Internet, the sheer volume of which renders the information completely incoherent. Compelling demands for an induction of labor or a cesarean delivery without any identifiable medical indication create a strange excuse for the complications resulting from these interventions. In the final analysis, however, it is not the clients who are responsible for this, but the specialist who allows it to happen.

Women's ill-informed preferences and wishes are no excuse for the excessive medicalization of birth. The key problem is that professionals do not have the right answers and create most insecurities, anxieties, and demands themselves.

6.2.1 Biased information

The issue of possible damage to the pelvic floor in childbirth is attracting more and more attention among laypersons and caregivers alike.[1] Cesarean delivery is often assumed to protect against pelvic floor and sexual dysfunction after childbirth, but this assumption is not supported by evidence.[2,3] Real risk factors for relevant pelvic morbidity have repeatedly been defined and include long second-stage labor and operative vaginal delivery.[4,5] Identified prevention strategies include pre-labor and postpartum pelvic floor exercises, restricted use of episiotomy, and avoiding instrumental vaginal deliveries. The preventive role of elective cesarean delivery, however, seems very tenuous.[4,6,7]

There is no evidence to support the widespread assumption that cesarean delivery effectively protects women from long-term sexual and pelvic floor dysfunction.

Advertisements in women's magazines, offering cesarean delivery ("spare your love channel") serve the bank accounts of private doctors much more than the health of their potential clients. For now, the stereotypical profile of the primigravida who opts for the knife without any medical indication seems to be a professional woman, accustomed to having control over her life and those of others. These suited executive women have even spawned a label seen in the medical literature and the lay press: "too posh to push." But also pop idols (often more celebrated than cerebrated) and movie stars – role models for many young women – frequently set insidious examples. Each report of a cesarean on celebrity-request in tabloids and magazines encourages thousands more 'unnecesareans.' Popular magazines never write about disfiguring scars, persisting abdominal pain owing to adhesions and scar tissue, decreased fertility, or life-threatening complications in following pregnancies.

> *Reduction of surgical consumerism requires the provision of honest and factual information to the general public.*

All doctors once solemnly swore the Hippocratic oath not to harm their patients ("primum non nocere"), so they should ensure that any intervention does more good than harm. However, cesarean on request has become widely disseminated without any proof of benefit and before the potential risks to women have been carefully determined. And once introduced and accepted in routine practice, interventions tend to persist. With more doctors willing to do a cesarean on request, and increasing numbers of women seeing it as a personal choice, the incidence of associated complications rises proportionally.

6.3 Overdiagnosis and overtreatment

There is a fundamental difference between the practice of science and the practice of medicine: to generate and test hypotheses scientists must believe they do not know, whereas practicing doctors, to have the confidence to make life and death decisions, pretend they know. In reality, however, practitioners often do not know the exact risks in individual cases. Intensified by the culture of blaming and litigation, adversity odds are then readily overestimated, and normalcy odds even more significantly underestimated, eliciting overdiagnosis and overtreatment. Numerous pregnant women are subjected to a potentially hazardous form of treatment in the hope that a few might benefit (Chapter 23).

> *Doctors readily overestimate adversity odds and underestimate normalcy odds. Clinical decision-making may be seriously warped as a result.*

6.3.1 Invalid excuses

Despite the movement toward evidence-based medicine, still many doctors simply reject the evidence in their practice. Common excuses are: "The evidence is out of date; collecting evidence is too slow and prevents progress; evidence erodes physician autonomy; I am an experienced specialist, so trust me and stop doctor-bashing." Some practitioners use anecdotal horror stories trying to prove the need for an intervention that the evidence has shown to be unnecessary. Others quote evidence of poor or inadequate quality, for example the false "evidence" from disputable meta-analyses claiming a tempering effect of induction of labor on cesarean delivery rates, more of which will be discussed in a moment.

The first response of most obstetricians whose intervention rates are compared unfavorably with those of their peers is: "My patients are more complicated than average" (is that so?) or "Our women have smaller pelvises" (nonsense), or "Our babies are getting bigger" (not true), and "Our population is not as homogeneous" (no evidence). Such uncritical attitudes, paired with omitting to audit their own practices in a reliable way (Chapter 27), explain the tenacity of current methods of "care" and the persistent gap between obstetric practice and the overall evidence.

> *The explosion of cesarean delivery rates is the greatest uncontrolled experiment in modern medicine.*

6.4 Liability concerns and control

Clearly, high-quality maternity care is a skilled art, but doctors increasingly circumvent this challenge and take refuge in surgery when labor gets tough. Many obstetricians feel they regain control with a cesarean, a move that might cut down on malpractice litigation.

6.4.1 Defeatism

Within the spiral of medical excess and intervention, the treacherous waltz of obstetrics with litigation goes on. The more that obstetricians intervene in pregnancy and childbirth, the more complications occur, the more obstetricians get sued, and the more they intervene. Cesarean birth seems to be safer legally while it is not so medically. There are even obstetricians who say, "The only cesarean I have ever been sued for is the one I didn't do." Such a striking remark not only echoes frustration within medical circles but also reflects the widespread defeatism with respect to the spiraling cesarean rates. Such attitudes, however, seriously call into question whether these physicians operate on the basis of a consistent policy of care for short and safe labor. Structural improvement of labor care is indeed possible (Section 3) if there is the professional will to do so, and this will no doubt coincide with diminishing litigation threats.

6.4.2 Convenience

A surgical intervention in labor not only decreases the chance of being sued but is also far more convenient to the doctor and much more efficient from a time-management perspective than waiting around for natural birth. But the trend goes even further with the avoidance of labor altogether. Birth is rapidly becoming a 9-to-5 business, circumventing the burden of working at night. What once used to be an emergency intervention is now often a scheduled procedure, and parents' biased wishes are a welcome excuse.

It is much easier and less time-consuming to fulfill misinformed and biased requests than to guard the medical necessity of inductions and cesarean deliveries.

Women are more educated and assertive about their healthcare decisions, and read Internet blogs and magazines that provide unbalanced information from biased patients and doctors. So, more and more women are demanding a cesarean without any medical reason rather than undergoing a vaginal birth. They, too, feel in control, knowing in advance the date of their delivery, which can be helpful in planning the multitude of activities, from career issues to child care, that surround a birth. Since everyone seems to be content, why bother?

6.4.3 False information

The crucial questions, however, are whether such practical advantages outweigh the risks and whether women are honestly informed. The key moral issue is not the right to choose or demand a major intervention for which there is no medical indication, but the right to receive and discuss full, unbiased information prior to any medical or surgical procedure. The rise in inductions and cesarean deliveries on-demand in

low-risk pregnancies is actually a reflection of being told by the medical community, "This is a quick fix without risk, why wouldn't you?" But it is highly unlikely that such women would ever consider choosing that intervention if they were given the honest information on the direct and indirect risks for themselves and their (future) babies (Chapter 2). The obstetrician who readily accepts the risk of a failed induction or conveniently decides for an elective cesarean delivery actually remains co-responsible for all uterine scar-related complications in the woman's future pregnancies and childbirths. But by the time women (and lawyers) figure that out, these doctors are going to be long gone.

Women considering elective cesarean delivery should be counseled on the basis of the evidence: no extra safety for their baby and significantly more short- and long-term problems for themselves, not only now but in particular in their next pregnancies.

Since serious maternal and neonatal morbidity and even death may occur in association with repeat cesareans or VBACs in next pregnancies (Chapter 2), all studies on the short-term effects of primary cesarean delivery underestimate the total morbidity and mortality. Despite this, ACOG has released a formal opinion supporting obstetricians who honor a woman's request for cesarean delivery in the absence of any medical indication, citing the ethical premise of patient/client autonomy and informed consent.[8] Strangely, the question of free choice asks only whether a woman should have the right to choose a cesarean, whereas a woman's right to choose vaginal delivery is not addressed.[9] Paradoxically, the choice of women for VBAC or vaginal breech-delivery is bluntly overruled in many hospitals, although these options can be safe in selected cases.[10,11]

The key ethical issue is not the right to choose a cesarean delivery, but the right to receive and discuss full, unbiased information prior to any medical procedure.

6.4.4 Inflation

The more readily an obstetrician honors requests for a cesarean delivery without any identifiable medical indication, the lower becomes his/her threshold for surgical solutions for minor problems in labor. Such inflation is especially worrying in teaching hospitals, where residents no longer master prevention and appropriate handling of labor disorders, and grow permanently malconditioned by the liberal operative practices of their teachers. The vicious circle is closed, and it is increasingly difficult to break it.

Clearly, reduction of medical excess is as much about education of the general public as about re-education of knife-loving doctors. This is a painful but necessary undertaking for the obstetrical community. Change has a chance of success only if birth professionals can offer an acceptable alternative promoting a safe, vaginal delivery (Section 3).

> Promoting normal labor and delivery is as much about re-education of the general public as about re-education of childbirth professionals.

6.5 EBM: merits, pitfalls, and misunderstandings

Evidence-based medicine (EBM) – which claims to define the value of interventions in terms of empirical evidence from clinical trials – was particularly designed to reduce practice variation and overtreatment. Since its introduction in the mid-1980s, EBM has gradually evolved into a powerful tool indeed, with a profound effect on both medical education and clinical practice. Its potential benefits are obvious and well described. The intrinsic limitations, however, as well as the counterproductive effects of uncritical use are now surfacing.[12–14] Abuse even gives rise to new and dangerous vicious circles.

> Like any powerful instrument, EBM can be used for good or bad. As it is now, widespread misapplication leads to self-sustaining untoward effects.

Despite its promises, EBM still fails to provide an adequate account of optimal medical education and practice, and has even made some problems worse. This is apparent from the overall "meta-meta-analysis" showing an ever-increasing intervention rate in healthy, term pregnancies since the advent of EBM without any tangible improvements in maternal and perinatal outcomes (Chapter 2). Manifestly, something is going terribly wrong here.

> The practice of EBM turns out not to be evidence-based: there remains a lack of high-quality evidence that EBM has resulted in substantial population-level health gains.[14]

6.5.1 Warped medical education

Medical expertise begins with a thorough academic education, which is now increasingly under threat. Owing to educational reforms ("competences") and the gradual change from science-based into "evidence-based" medicine, there is now less curriculum time available for the basic biological sciences than ever before. Medical schools have shifted the focus from transfer of thorough scientific knowledge towards empirical clinical data ("evidence") and how to find it (on the smart-phone). Also clinical training tends to overappreciate immediately usable information and "practical" protocols and undervalues the importance of developing intelligent clinical reasoning skills built on a solid theoretical foundation of in-depth bio-scientific knowledge, reflection, and comprehension.

> "Science is a way of thinking much more than it is a body of knowledge" (Carl Sagan). In this respect, academic education and medical training are worryingly in decline.

As a compounding factor, tried-and-true educational methods such as apprenticeship under a master have fallen into disrepute. It is, therefore, increasingly difficult for medical students and residents to gain a proper academic understanding of relevant medical knowledge and proven clinical concepts. Certainly, modern doctors are very adept in instantly finding mountains of data on any topic on the Internet, but it remains fragmented information, lacking structure, cohesion, and interpretation. Scientific understanding and concept-based medicine are out; browsing disconnected data on the Internet is in. Personal mentorship is out; impersonal education behind the computer is in. Studying textbooks and thematic academic treatises that make sense of medicine is out; scanning summaries and key points of "evidence-based" guidelines is in. Scientific illiteracy is increasingly common among students and medical professionals, and, alas, scientific illiterates do not know what they don't know. Young doctors may now enter the clinic more or less devoid of elementary knowledge of the physiology of the human body, let alone of pregnancy and parturition. As a result, childbirth professionals increasingly lack the theoretical basis for sound clinical reasoning from basic science. By default, they seek an anchor in "evidence-based" guidelines and simplified protocols.

Increasingly, doctors are uncritical consumers of guidelines and protocols. Today's doctors need to regain a broader understanding of medical knowledge and reasoning.

6.5.2 Guideline culture

Many professionals draw security from "evidence-based" guidelines. Some even put blind trust in the "evidence" and feel comfortable under the self-degrading assumption that "the thinking has been done by the intellectual elite; we just have to follow the protocols." These doctors are like an airplane pilot who knows the manuals but does not understand why and how a plane flies. This ignorance might even be excusable if all guidelines were entirely trustworthy, but this is a far cry from reality. A recent study evaluating the evidence underlying the Royal College of Obstetricians and Gynaecologists (RCOG) guidelines found that only 9–12% of the recommendations are based on the best-quality evidence.[15] Strict followers of guidelines apparently prefer adherence to poor "evidence" to tolerance of uncertainty, which is an inevitable fact of real life that has to be met with acumen, wisdom, and experience.

While official guidelines are touted as "evidence-based" they often lack a sound evidence base.

To complicate matters further, the volume of "evidence" being produced is by now unfathomable, and the number of guidelines and their size is becoming unmanageable.[16] NICE (the UK National Institute for Health and Care Excellence) for instance, published a guideline on intrapartum care exceeding 300 pages with countless stand-alone recommendations, but lacking a structured biological base and a central strategy for care aimed at a rewarding, safe, and spontaneous delivery.[17] What is more, the very production of guidelines is the *raison d'être* of "quality" institutions and professional task forces, and the flood

of publications helps to promote funding and individual careers ("publish or perish"), regardless of clinical relevance. Meanwhile, the search for evidence increasingly proves an activity with marginal gains, since the low-hanging fruit (interventions that promise substantial improvements) were picked long ago.[14] The literature now teems with studies addressing questions as irrelevant and unanswerable as whether one should drive a BMW or a Mercedes to get from A to B. Not surprisingly, busy clinicians get turned off.

The volume of alleged "evidence" is now unmanageable and makes daily birth care needlessly complex. Frontline caregivers cannot see the forest for the trees anymore.

6.5.3 Opposition

EBM is now imperative, but more and more practitioners and scientists revolt, identifying the guideline culture itself as the real new problem that fuels harmful overdiagnosis and overtreatment. EBM, in its present form, is dubbed a "poisoned chalice" rather than "the Holy Grail" and perceived as "a loaded gun at clinician's heads" leaving no room for discretion or clinical judgment.[18] Indeed, harmful effects of official guidelines in a medico-legal context have been repeatedly exemplified in various situations.[19–21]

EBM is further criticized for misappropriation of the evidence-based quality mark by vested interests.[14] These interests may be territorial (Chapter 5) and commercial, but also include managers and insurers who increasingly use guidelines to control practitioners.

There is a disconcerting misappropriation of the EBM brand by vested interests that backfires on professionals and patients.

6.5.4 Dodgy evidence

Concerns and resistance are growing, and critical minds, who support EBM in principle, challenge the validity of a large proportion of "clinical evidence" altogether. For instance, meticulous meta-research by the well-respected Ioannidis group at Harvard, examining numerous studies in different fields of medicine, suggests that a large part of the reported "evidence" is based on poorly designed studies flawed by poor case selection, sham diagnoses, inadequately defined controls, surrogate or ill-defined outcomes, a short follow-up, flukes, data manipulation, other unintended or unconscious irregularities, and occasionally even fraud. Under forensic scrutiny, over 75% of observational studies and 25% of supposedly gold-standard randomized trials turn out to be wrong.[22] There is no reason to assume that this is any different in obstetrics.

> It is high time to acknowledge the limited validity of much of the reported "evidence".

That does not mean, of course, that we may simply throw the literature overboard. It rather emphasizes the grave responsibility for guideline-makers to exercise extreme caution. Not surprisingly, they go awry at times, with dire consequences for uncritical users and their patients/clients.

The irony in this context is that the once-derogatory notion "armchair scholarship" has been rehabilitated, it appears, since it is increasingly epidemiologists and other desktop scientists, far removed from clinical practice, who select the studies for meta-analyses and distill the evidence that is subsequently used in guidelines. As a result, statistically significant but clinically irrelevant benefits are being exaggerated, while disrupting repercussions of "evidence-based" recommendations on the individual and the healthcare service as a whole are systematically overlooked (as will be shown). In the same vein, direct and indirect harms are being underestimated because adverse events tend to be underreported in the studies reviewed, and long-term adverse effects remain undetected altogether.[14,23–25] Most worryingly, the central mission of frontline obstetricians and midwives – namely how to promote safe and rewarding childbirth – gets buried under a mass of heterogeneous and nebulous "evidence" of isolated issues.

> Official guidelines are often dictated by epidemiologists with impressive skills in inferential statistics, but far removed from clinical practice.

One of the most influential biases in the acquisition of "evidence" is the choice of the question, and the best evidence in answer to the wrong question is pointless. The place of birth and choice of caregiver are two of the many examples that will follow in the next sections of this book. Moreover, the methods of EBM itself are subject to several limitations, biases, and shortcomings that are insufficiently acknowledged.

6.5.5 EBM: ideological bias

EBM has gradually shifted the focus away from the care of individuals towards the care of populations, neglecting the complex nature of sound clinical judgment and devaluing the individuality of both patients and doctors.[26] There is a fundamental mismatch between the evidence produced and the complex demands of clinical practice, where pregnant women present with a complex mix of psychological, physiological, and social problems, as well as various co-morbidities.

It is often overlooked that clinical trials are dichotomous by design whereas patients/clients in the real world represent numerous shades of grey. The tendency in practice is now that patients must comply with the "evidence" of isolated issues rather than the evidence fitting the individual case. Both logic and clinical behavior may be seriously warped as a result. A pregnant woman is not a number, and a good care provider is not a robot, and neither should be expected to behave accordingly.

> With the evolution of EBM, the focus of medical education and clinical practice is subtly shifted away from the care of individuals towards the care of populations.

Admittedly, bodies issuing guidelines routinely remind users (in small print) that the recommendations should not replace clinical judgment. But, by now, the cart is before the horse, as the scientific knowledge and academic skills required for sound clinical reasoning and expert judgment are rapidly declining, not least because of the EBM primacy in current medical education. As a result, clinical "evidence" is uncritically accepted even when it is fundamentally inimical to universally valid bio-scientific knowledge and understanding. The false evidence that induction of labor protects against cesarean delivery is a disastrous example that will be discussed below in more detail.

What is more, EBM has drifted from investigating and managing established disease towards detecting risk and intervening in non-disease. Risk assessment using "evidence-based" scores and algorithms now occurs on an industrial scale, with scant attention to the opportunity costs or unintended human and financial consequences.[27]

> *The focus is gradually shifted away from the detection and treatment of disease towards "risk factors" leading to adverse interference in healthy pregnancies.*

6.5.6 EBM: cultural bias

Under the narrow understanding of EBM, "evidence" purely rests on clinical research and, therefore, on clinical practice, which in turn is rooted in structural arrangements and cultural ideas. Obviously, cultural, social, and judicial backgrounds vary significantly across the globe, and this diversity puts big question marks behind the potential for generalization of "clinical evidence" from diverse cultural contexts. Yet uncritical extrapolations are readily made.[28]

> *While confirmed evidence from bio-scientific laboratory research is universally valid, clinical "evidence" is strongly dependent on cultural, social, and judicial contexts.*

What is more, the relative emphasis placed on particular "evidence" strongly depends on what individuals or communities think is most important. This may range from enjoyment of the experience of childbirth to the pretension of shaving another fraction of a percentage point off the perinatal mortality rate, no matter what the costs in terms of disturbance of intimacy, intervention-associated maternal morbidity, and rocketing financial expenses. As a result, conflicting views will persist.[28] People and professional groups with opposite convictions may even use the same "evidence" to support their ideas, only differently interpreted and differently ranked. Analysis of "the best available evidence" from the debate over home delivery versus hospital birth, for instance, shows that the "evidence" is mainly the product of the researcher's assumptions about the practice in question.[28,29] In this way, "evidence" rather becomes a rhetorical justification for whatever particular groups are going to do anyway.

> *Differences in culture and tradition give rise to irresolvable disagreements about what constitutes evidence and how that evidence is to be interpreted and ranked.*

6.5.7 EBM: philosophical bias

Clearly, clinical "evidence" cannot settle scientific disputes in any simple way. Clinical research only describes what happens, not why. Science, however, is not about mere fact-finding but implies careful interpretation and explanation. Real medical science combines biological, epidemiological, psychological, and clinical knowledge, and constructs sensible clinical concepts explaining isolated findings and facts. Scientific concepts are the framework for organizing relevant knowledge that should guide medical practice.

In this respect, it might even be doubted whether EBM is a science in the strict sense. Clinical research, when performed in isolation, neither develops nor challenges scientific constructs. EBM is rather a quality assessment technique, and potentially very useful indeed, if used correctly for the evaluation of carefully defined interventions in specific situations. EBM is designed to establish the relative effectiveness of different forms of clinical interventions. It can and should be used for vindication or rejection of specific clinical actions in particular circumstances. It explains little to nothing, though.

> *Clinical research only describes what happens, but not why.*

Genuine medical science is aimed at exploration, explanation, and innovation. It should be noted that all major breakthroughs in medicine (e.g. antisepsis, antibiotics, blood-typing, anesthesia), and the related reduction in perinatal and maternal mortality, are science-based and stem from the era before EBM. However important it is as a quality control instrument, EBM cannot be expected to contribute substantially to the advancement of medical knowledge and practice. To the contrary, to overrate the precepts of EBM and underrating the relevance of biological science may even lead to counterproductive effects (as will be seen). Ironically, leading medical journals now prefer to publish randomized controlled trials (RCTs), whereas basic scientific research and intelligent comments that enhance scientific and clinical understanding are virtually banished to journals with lower impact factor.

> *EBM is aimed at justification and exoneration, rather than exploration, interpretation, and explanation.*

6.5.8 Limitations of RCTs

EBM may be further criticized for the methodological shortcomings of the technique. Under the dominant understanding of EBM, RCTs are at the top of the evidence pyramid, superior to all non-randomized evidence, so it is claimed. This assumption, however, is not always justified. "Evidence" is not necessarily reliable just because it is borne out by randomized trials. In order to provide reliable results, RCTs need to meet a number of preconditions that many of them fail to satisfy. It is important to note that the method is copied from laboratory research where all conditions are identical and under strict control, and only a single variable is examined, a situation very different from clinical settings. Humans are no laboratory guinea pigs.

An RCT is indeed the gold standard for clinical evidence, provided that the trial is used for the evaluation of a singular intervention in a standardized population. The ideal RCT is, of course, double-blinded and placebo-controlled, examining a singular, uniform, well-described intervention in adequately sized, accurately diagnosed and homogeneous study groups, using unequivocal and relevant primary outcomes. Whether prophylaxis with antibiotics during cesarean section is a useful precaution or not is a feasible example.

However, the validity of RCTs is subject to severe limitations when used for the evaluation of complex procedures in heterogeneous populations with varying and often unquantifiable medical conditions. Yet, examples abound of RCTs addressing complex clinical issues that are wholly unsuitable for this method of research.[23–25,30–32] Many obstetric policies, of which induction of labor is a good example, depend on intricate interactions between medical, psychological, and organizational factors. Using RCTs to examine the effectiveness and safety of such a complex procedure overestimates the possibilities of this research method and oversimplifies the complicated clinical problems. Conclusions drawn from such inappropriate trials are at best confusing and at worst dangerous.

> As RCTs continue to ascend in the evolution of EBM, we must recognize and respect their limitations when examining complex phenomena in heterogeneous populations.

6.5.9 Perverted use of EBM: induction of labor

Some authors manage to step into all pitfalls at once and falsely claim to have found revolutionary evidence against commonly accepted clinical ideas. Misleading meta-analyses denying the existence of failed induction of labor is a good example. This topic needs to be discussed in some detail as it focuses the general criticism – relating to medicine as a whole – on the management of labor, the subject of this book.

Induction of labor has profoundly adverse effects on women's childbirth experience and the supervision of labor. Induction causes long labors, disturbs the individual, and disrupts the entire delivery service (Chapter 23). There is also a wealth of consistent evidence, albeit from non-randomized studies, that an induction of labor is associated with cesarean delivery, in particular with nulliparas (abundance of references in Chapter 23). Every physician with some basic background knowledge of the physiology of parturition also understands why (Chapter 8). And surely, every observant practitioner with experience at the labor ward is familiar with the embarrassing problem of failed inductions. Every knowledgeable obstetrician realizes that elements such as indication, gestational age, parity, and cervical status play a crucial role in the decision-making on whether induction of labor is a feasible proposition or not. And every clinician is aware of the relative nature of "indications" ranging from maternal requests for any but a medical reason to severely pathological conditions, and all permutations in between.

Yet clinicians are told they have been entirely wrong all along in "believing" that induction of labor increases cesarean delivery odds. "It is the other way around: induction prevents cesarean deliveries," epidemiologists preach to us now.[33] And they reach pregnant women, of course, who read the headlines in magazines and retweet the 140-character messages from customer organizations, medical agencies, and even prestigious journals on Twitter: "Cesarean deliveries drop 12% with induction of labor" and "induction protects against cesarean delivery, the 'evidence' says".[34,35]

The recent "evidence" comes from a new meta-analysis,[33] the method generally regarded as the platinum standard for clinical evidence. Safe behind their computer, statistical magicians fished in the same pond with ill-designed and poorly executed RCTs as four previous meta-analyses[36–39] that have been deeply questioned.[30] For the latest review, the epidemiologists searched six electronic databases, identifying 2894 potentially relevant studies. Subsequently, they "winnowed" that assortment down to 157 RCTs that compared labor induction with placebo or expectant management – whatever that may be – and simply dismissed all non-randomized studies as irrelevant. Their findings are truly extraordinary: "in uncomplicated, term pregnancies with no medical reason for induction, the risk of cesarean delivery plummeted by 19% on average after induction"[33] (sic!).

Meta-analyses of poor RCTs on complex clinical issues provide at best confusing and at worst dangerously misleading information.

Interestingly, the number of studies included in the five reported meta-analyses varied significantly, owing to different selection criteria. Be that as it may, a significant part of the evidence in all five is derived from a single, Canadian, multi-center RCT, comparing induction at 41 weeks with expectant management.[40] This RCT has been profoundly questioned with respect to the evidence for a lower cesarean rate associated with induction.[24,30,41] For a starter, nulliparas and multiparas were lumped together and cervical status was not taken into account. What is more, only about one-half of the eligible women were randomized. The other half "elected" not to participate, or the caregiver decided for non-clarified reasons to refrain from recruitment. Has this, perhaps, something to do with cervical status? The analysis according to the intention-to-treat denominator was correct for assessing *what* happened, not for evaluation of the effectiveness and safety of the induction procedure in its own right. One-third of the women randomized to induction were not induced, and one-third of those randomized to expectant management were induced. The randomization itself might have instigated concerns and anxiety in the controls because their pregnancy was apparently "at risk" (because "overdue"!?) but not scheduled for induction. And anxiety is a powerful trigger for interventions, indeed, poised to follow what is more "management" than "expectancy."[30] The result is a (reversed) Hawthorn effect.

Analysis according to the intention-to-treat denominator is correct for assessing what happens in practice, not for the evaluation of the physical effects of induction per se.

These inevitable flaws illustrate why an RCT cannot reliably examine complex issues such as indication and execution of induction. To add to the confusion, the women who were induced in the control group of this RCT did not have the choice of induction methods that were available to women in the induction group, for reasons that have remained poorly justified other than that the trial was sponsored by the manufacturer of one of the induction agents.[24,30,41] To confound matters even further, the labor management in the control group, if any, was completely undefined. In the end, only half of the women in the trial achieved a spontaneous vaginal birth with only a marginal difference between those assigned to induction (51.0%) and those assigned to "expectant management" (49.2%).[24,30,41] Clearly, the results do not justify the authors' conclusion that inducing labor at 41 weeks results in a decreased cesarean section rate. The trial provided more evidence on the high overall intervention rates in the participating hospitals than on whether induction increases or reduces cesarean rates.[24]

No meta-analysis can be stronger than the (poor) studies that contribute to it.

No single other RCT included in the five meta-analyses was of any better quality. All trials had different entry criteria and different induction methods, but shared the omission of clarifying the "expectant management" and the labor strategies in the controls. So it remains a complete mystery what was compared with what. The controls in some of the trials even included an unknown number of women with a uterine scar, a powerful trigger on a scalpel. The background cesarean rate in the diverse hospitals was unknown, and the absolute cesarean rates in the study arms of each separate RCT were not mentioned in the meta-analyses, only the relative risks between study arms. Almost all trials neglected cervical status and parity, the two major predictors of success of any induction. Yet all women and all induction methods were jumbled up in the RCTs, and subsequently in the meta-analyses, disallowing any sensible conclusions.

Lumping inappropriate RCTs together in a meta-analysis is a dangerous misapplication of EBM: "garbage in, garbage out."

43

The latest meta-analysis[33] reported a subgroup analysis pretending to make pudding out of these muddy data. At first sight, the statistics may look impressive, but no statistical method can improve the quality of the individual studies, of course. Tellingly, women in the subgroup "alternative induction methods" – acupuncture, homeopathic preparations, nipple stimulation, castor oil, bath, enema, or sexual intercourse – had a 34% lower cesarean rate when "induced" with one of these methods than the controls (RR 0.66, 95% CI 0.50–0.86). Studies of this nature strain credibility to the max. Nevertheless, these trials were used and contributed significantly to the overall result of the meta-analysis (pooled RR 0.88, 95% CI 0.84–0.93). Even more bizarre is the finding that in women with an "unfavorable cervical status" significantly fewer cesarean deliveries were observed after induction than after expectant management (RR 0.87, 95% CI 0.81–0.94) whereas women randomized with a "favorable cervix" did not show significantly different cesarean rates (RR 0.83, 95% CI 0.60–1.14).[33] So, the covert or overt message of the meta-analysis is: "one is better to induce labor with an unfavorable cervix than with a favorable cervix if one wants to prevent a cesarean delivery." Credibility is now strained beyond all limits. Meta-analyses like these have engendered new meanings to the acronym EBM, such as Evidence-Biased Misguidance or Evidence-Based Madness.

The RCTs on induction of labor compare mismanagement with undefined non-management in heterogeneous populations, disallowing any conclusions about the safety and effectiveness of the intervention per se.

No meta-analysis can be stronger than the studies that contribute to it, and lumping inappropriate studies together is what has given meta-analyses their undeserved reputation of "garbage in, garbage out." This is surely not what icons like Sacket, Chalmers, Enkin, and Keirse had in mind when they introduced the utterly useful precepts of EBM. Keirse rightly commented: "It is not the garbage bin that is at fault, but the people who fill it or those who empty it, as well as what is being put into it."[30]

Yet the epidemiologists claim they provided "a robust answer to the disputed question of risk of cesarean delivery associated with induction of labor."[33] They even waived the usual plea for more

evidence with which the other meta-analyses concluded. Discussion closed, is the message. Even ACOG, as it appears, tacitly accepts this fallacy. In the 2014 consensus statement on the prevention of primary cesarean delivery[42] the task force cites the Cochrane meta-analysis[37] and fails to advise restricted use of induction as a relevant method to reduce overall cesarean rates, a deplorably missed opportunity.

Misapplication of the laudable techniques of EBM – and going public with unfounded messages that induction protects against cesarean delivery – augments exactly the problems that EBM aims to combat: unnecessary interventions with harmful effects.

What is more, the meta-analyses selectively focused on cesarean delivery but entirely neglected the detrimental effects of induction on women's labor experience and the childbirth service as a whole (Chapter 23).[43–48] Despite this gross omission, authors claim their findings "are important when selecting candidates for labor induction" (all women beyond 37 weeks we presume?), and "when advising women on the risks of induction."[33]

None of this could be further from the truth, of course. The only honest way of counseling women is providing them with the data of the institution where they will give birth (Chapter 27). Ironically, many obstetricians do not know the outcomes of inductions in their own unit. Instead, they buy this stuff at face value, and use this misinformation. If they only looked into their own data, they would be flabbergasted by the number of cesarean deliveries for failed induction in their practice, especially in nulliparas (Chapter 27). Moreover, to overlook all other adverse effects of induction (Chapter 23) divulges a worryingly narrow-minded view of childbirth.

The debate about induction should include much more than associated cesarean rates, such as prolonged labors, instrumental deliveries, traumatic birth experiences, and the disruption of the labor and delivery service as a whole.

The most upsetting downstream effect of this kind of pseudo-research, published in prestigious journals, is that it catches the public eye. Papers like these undoubtedly enhance the CVs of authors but are not helpful to clinicians. Obstetricians who know better are now confronted with misguided women who demand an induction of labor to prevent a cesarean section, meanwhile handing over a copy print from PubMed. Critical doctors have a lot to explain, and who wants to listen to tiresome naysayers anyway? The self-sustaining mechanism discussed previously in this chapter will further increase the induction rates, adding more momentum to the march of folly.

RCTs cannot settle scientific disputes on complex clinical issues in any simple way.

6.5.10 The "E" of EBM

The dominant narrow view of EBM is dangerous indeed. The fundamental issue is that – given the poor selection and management criteria – none of the above-discussed studies and meta-analyses would have seen the light of day in a prestigious journal, for sure, if the trials had not been randomized. Marc Keirse, one of the very founders of EBM, captured the misunderstanding in a few lines: "Anything randomized controlled became the gospel and anything else has become either poor evidence or lack of evidence. Of course, nothing is wrong with advocating or promoting randomized trials. There is a great deal wrong, though, with the perception that evidence, to be evidence, needs to be randomized evidence." The EBM expert further comments: "There is also a great deal wrong with the belief that only evidence is an e-word that deserves to be written with a capital E, whereas other e-words, such as education, experience, expertise, and even excellence, are merely ignominious."[25] At the end of the day, the most relevant e-word for any professional unit should be "evaluation" of processes and outcomes at the hospital level on a continuous basis (Chapters 26 and 27).

In its current misapplication, EBM is a dead-end street. There is an urgent need for a renaissance of Real-EBM.

6.6 Turning the tide

The world of childbirth faces huge challenges. Many vicious circles need to be broken, and core values – safety, simplicity, and high quality in childbirth – need to be reinstated. Much of the reported "evidence" needs to be re-evaluated, separating the wheat from the chaff,

and expert labor and delivery care needs to be rediscovered.

To this end, medical and midwifery education and practice need to re-orientate and revalue basic knowledge of the physiology of pregnancy and birth. To help in finding feet in the mass of complex scientific data, Section 2 will analyze and organize the biology of human parturition in a structured manner, identifying the essential biological principles that should direct expert care in childbirth. Section 2 will also debunk several tenacious misconceptions and unfounded dogmas that needlessly thwart current care in labor and delivery.

Secondly, the narrow understanding of EBM – which promotes prescriptive protocols encouraging "cookbook" practice – needs to be broadened, refocusing on proven physiological and psychological concepts, and embracing usable and reliable clinical evidence that can be combined with context so that individual women get optimal guidance and care. Real EBM accommodates basic scientific knowledge, clinical evidence, common sense, and the clinical and personal idiosyncrasies of the patient/client.[14] Clinical "mind-lines" or "patterns of thought" – based on proven scientific concepts and supported by real clinical evidence – should govern birth care, rather than protocols.

Real EBM in childbirth promotes logic and consistency in care and clarity for all women in labor and for all caregivers as well. The overall plan of *proactive support of labor* will undoubtedly help to apply real evidence-based care in childbirth and to hone labor and delivery skills (Section 3).

The mind-lines of proactive support of labor provide a framework for organizing relevant bioscientific knowledge and reliable clinical evidence, promoting safe, simple, and high-quality care in everyday childbirth.

References

1. Murphy M, McDonagh Hull P. Choosing Cesarean Delivery: A Natural Birth Plan. Prometheus Books; 2012

2. McKinnie V, Swift SE, Wang W, *et al.* The effect of pregnancy and mode of delivery on the prevalence of urinary and fecal incontinence. Am J Obstet Gynecol 2005;**193**:512–7

3. Barret G, Peacock J, Victor CR, Manyonda I. Cesarean section and postnatal sexual health. Birth 2005;**32**:306–11

4. Handa VL, Brubaker L, Falf SJ. Urinary incontinence and pelvic organ prolapse associated with pregnancy and childbirth. UpToDate. Accessed October 2014

5. Bahl R, Strachan B, Murphy DJ. Pelvic floor morbidity at 3 years after instrumental delivery and cesarean delivery in the second stage of labor and the impact of a subsequent delivery. Am J Obstet Gynecol 2005;192:789–94

6. Durnea CM, Khashan AS, Kenny LC, et al. The role of prepregnancy pelvic floor dysfunction in postnatal pelvic morbidity in primiparous women. Int Urogynecol J 2014;25:1363–74

7. Stafne SN, Salvesen KÅ, Romundstad PR, et al. Does regular exercise including pelvic floor muscle training prevent urinary and anal incontinence during pregnancy? A randomised controlled trial. Br J Obstet Gynaec 2012;119:1270–80

8. ACOG Committee Opinion. Surgery and patient choice: the ethics of decision making. Obstet Gynecol 2003;102:1101–6

9. Leeman L, Plante LA. Patient-choice vaginal delivery? Ann Fam Med 2006;4:265–8

10. Metz TD, Scott JR. Contemporary management of VBAC. Clin Obstet Gynecol 2012;55:1026–32

11. Kotaska A, Menticoglou S, Gagnon R, et al. Maternal Fetal Medicine Committee; Society of Obstetricians and Gynaecologists of Canada. Vaginal delivery of breech presentation. J Obstet Gynaecol Can 2009;31:557–66, 567–78.

12. Cohen D. FDA official: "clinical trial system is broken". Br Med J 2013;347:f16980

13. Spence D. Evidence based medicine is broken. Br Med J 2014;348:g22

14. Greenhalgh T, Howick J, Maskrey N; Evidence Based Medicine Renaissance Group. Evidence based medicine: a movement in crisis? Br Med J 2014;348:g3725

15. Prusava K, Churcher L, Tyler A, Lokugamage AU. Royal College of Obstetricians and Gynaecology guidelines: How evidence-based are they? J Obstet Gynaecol 2014;12:1–6 (Epub ahead of print)

16. Allen D, Harkins K. Too much evidence? Lancet 2005;365:1768

17. NICE-guidelines. Intrapartum care: care of healthy women and their babies during childbirth. 2007. RCOG press. Updated 2010 www.nice.org.uk/guidance/cg55

18. Howick J. The evidence based renaissance: Holy Grail or poisoned chalice BioMed Central Blog 2014. http://biomedcentral.com/bmcblog

19. McIntyre KM. Medicolegal implications of consensus statements. Chest 1995;108:502–5

20. Hyams AL, Brandenburg JA, Lipsitz SR, et al. Practice guidelines and malpractice litigation: a two-way street. Ann Intern Med 1995;122:440–5

21. Hirshfeld EB. Should practice parameters be the standard of care in malpractice litigation? JAMA 1991;266:2886–91

22. Ioannidis JP. Why most published research findings are false. PLoS Med 2005;2:e124

23. Kotaska A. Inappropriate use of randomised trials to evaluate complex phenomena: case study of vaginal breech delivery. Br Med J 2004;329:039–42

24. Menticoglou SM, Hall PF. Routine induction of labour at 41 weeks gestation: Nonsensus consensus. Br J Obstet Gynaec 2002;109:485–91

25. Keirse MJ. Commentary: the freezing aftermath of a hot randomized controlled trial. Birth 2011;38:165–7

26. Tonelli MR. The philosophical limits of evidence based medicine. Acad Med 1998;73:1234–40

27. Moynihan R, Doust JC, Henry D. Preventing overdiagnosis: how to stop harming the healthy. Br Med J 2012;344:e3502

28. Keirse MJNC. Home births: gone away, gone astray, and here to stay. Birth 2010;37:341–6

29. Devries RG. The warp of evidence-based medicine: lessons from Dutch maternity care. Int J Health Serv 2004;34:595–623

30. Keirse MJ. Elective induction, selective deduction, and cesarean section. Birth 2010;37:252–56

31. Bewley S, Shennan A. HYPITAT and the fallacy of pregnancy interruption. Lancet 2010;375:119

32. Greene MF. Delivering twins. N Engl J Med 2013;369:1365–6

33. Mishanina E, Rogozinska E, Thatthi T, et al. Use of labour induction and risk of cesarean delivery: a systematic review and meta-analysis. CMAJ 2014;168:665–73

34. Inducing labour reduces risk of caesarean delivery by 12%, finds analysis. Br Med J 6 May 2014; www.bmj.com/content/348/bmj.g2960/rr/696718

35. Cesarean deliveries drop 12% with induction. Medscape 2014; www.medscape.com/viewarticle/824211

36. Caughey AB, Sundaram V, Kaimal AJ, et al. Systematic review: elective induction of labor versus expectant management of pregnancy. Ann Intern Med 2009;151:252–63

37. Gülmezoglu AM, Crowther CA, Middleton P, et al. Induction of labour for improving birth outcomes for women at or beyond term. Cochrane Database Syst Rev 2012; CD004945

38. Wennerholm UB, Hagberg H, Brorsson B, *et al.* Induction of labor versus expectant management for post-date pregnancy: Is there sufficient evidence for a change in clinical practice? Acta Obstet Gynecol Scand 2009;**88**:6–17

39. Wood S, Cooper S, Ross S. Does induction of labour increase the risk of caesarean section? A systematic review and meta-analysis of trials in women with intact membranes. Br J Obstet Gynaec 2014;**121**:674–85 discussion 685

40. Hannah ME, Hannah WJ, Hellmann J, *et al.* The Canadian Multicenter Post-term Pregnancy Trial Group. Induction of labor as compared with serial antenatal monitoring in post-term pregnancy. A randomized controlled trial. N Engl J Med 1992;**326**:1587–92

41. Keirse MJ. Postterm pregnancy: New lessons from an unresolved debate. Birth 1993;**20**:102–105

42. American College of Obstetricians and Gynecologists. Obstetric Care Consensus No. 1: Safe prevention of the primary cesarean delivery. Obstet Gynecol 2014;**123**:693–711

43. Henderson J1, Redshaw M. Women's experience of induction of labor: a mixed methods study. Acta Obstet Gynecol Scand 2013;**92**:1159–67

44. Hildingsson I, Karlström A, Nystedt A. Women's experiences of induction of labour–findings from a Swedish regional study. Aust N Z J Obstet Gynaecol 2011;**51**:151–7

45. Enabor OO, Olayemi OO, Bello FA, Adedokun BO. Cervical ripening and induction of labour awareness, knowledge and perception of antenatal attendees in Ibadan, Nigeria. J Obstet Gynaecol 2012;**3**:652–56

46. Shetty A, Burt R, Rice P, Templeton A. Women's perceptions, expectations and satisfaction with induced labour—a questionnaire-based study. Eur J Obstet Gynecol Reprod Biol 2005;**123**:56–61

47. Nuutila M, Halmesmäki E, Hillesmaa V, Ylikorkala O. Women's anticipations of and experiences with induction of labor. Acta Obstet Gynecol Scand. 1999;**78**:704–9

48. Bramadat IJ. Induction of labor: an integrated review. Health Care Women Int. 1994;**15**:135–48

Forgotten lessons from nature

"The real act of discovery is not in finding new lands, but in seeing with new eyes."
–Marcel Proust

Our cultures, ways of life, judicial systems, and religions are parts of the ecological niche in which we human beings live. In biological terms, however, every human being is a product of millions of years of evolution. Accordingly, the basic biological processes of parturition are essentially the same in different higher mammalian species.[1]

7.1 Comparative biology

Comparative studies have shown that most mammals, including *Homo sapiens*, exhibit increased activity prior to the onset of labor; they are busy gathering nesting materials.[1] Apparently, the hormonal changes in late pregnancy that prepare the uterus for the forthcoming birth (Chapter 8) also set the behavioral nesting impulse in motion. The preparation of the female body for labor is normally not unduly taxing. Despite pre-labor bodily changes and latent uterine contractility, the expectant mother takes and gets sufficient rest to be fit enough to begin the real exertion of birthing.

7.1.1 Duration of natural birth

A laboring animal is extremely vulnerable to predators. That is why the process of birth in nature is short. Most observers of domesticated mammals estimate a duration of total parturition of a couple of hours, even for the first offspring.[1–6] Although observations of primates giving birth in the wild are rare, we know that diurnal monkeys give birth within the confines of one night, whereas nocturnal species such as prosimians usually give birth during the restricted hours of daylight – so within the timeframe of half a day at the most.[7] There is no precedent in the animal world to indicate that the fetus benefits from an overlong endeavor to escape from the womb. And there is no evidence that the time required for human childbirth must

necessarily be different from that required for the birth process in other higher mammals: less than half a day. Procreation in the wild is, above all, a selection process, and nature is a bad obstetrician indeed. As a renowned scientist in comparative biology pointed out: "The only obstetric help in nature is that offered by predators who will shorten the period of pain by killing the laboring female and eating her."[1] Nature is cruel.

> Advocates of "natural childbirth" should know the true nature of biological labor and delivery: in the animal world, the whole process takes no more than a few hours.

7.2 The biological functions of labor pain

In the western world, human procreation has long ceased to present a serious threat to the lives of healthy women, but the emotional impact of labor remains a matter of common concern. As a human physiological process, natural childbirth is intensely physical, immensely emotional, and painful. No good purpose is served by pretending otherwise. Labor pain is a phenomenon embedded in the very nature of human female existence. Unlike other acute and chronic pain experiences, labor pain is not associated with pathology but with the most basic and fundamental of life's experiences: the bringing forth of new life.[8]

> Giving birth is the only physiological process in nature that causes pain. As with everything in biology, pain in childbirth has specific functions.

Pain in childbirth is a ubiquitous biological phenomenon: all mammals deliver their young with great effort, and most species show signs of discomfort and even severe pain.[1] Why the physiological process of birth should cause pain has been the subject of philosophic and religious debate. The biological explanation, however, is simple: labor 'hurts' so that the pregnant woman has adequate warning to get to a place of safety in which to birth her infant. In addition, the pain-related production of endorphins strongly promotes maternal behavior. Both effects are critical for survival of the helpless newborn in nature and the preservation of the species.

7.2.1 Warning sign

The pain of contractions warns laboring animals to go and find a place where predators are least likely to be around. They instinctively seek the isolation and security of their den and stay there, whereas humans call for professional help. Women will also instinctively seek surroundings in which they feel safe. For some this is the sanctity of their home and for others it is a hospital. Nearly all mammals that live in groups are protected during labor and delivery by their group members. Unrest, a change in the environment, or simply being left alone can so disturb the autonomic vegetative balance that labor stalls. This effect is no different in humans.

7.2.2 The role of endorphins

Females of all mammalian species show maternal behavior immediately after birth, which is vital to the survival chances of the offspring and thus for the preservation of the species. Maternal nursing performance is a critical biological effect promoted through the natural pain of labor.

Labor pain induces the production of large amounts of endorphins in the mother's brain, and these endorphins play a crucial role in the instant establishment and maintenance of maternal nursing response. Moreover, maternal endorphins cross the placenta and promote sucking behavior in the newborn.[1]

In wildlife, endorphins are critical for effective mother–child bonding. Again, there is no reason to assume that this should be any different in the human species. In fact, human studies show that after analgesic medication during labor, the neonates exhibit decreased alertness,[9] inhibition of sucking,[10] lower neurobehavioral scores,[11] and a delay in effective feeding.[12–15]

The natural pain of labor has important biological functions, especially for mother–child bonding. Endorphins encourage the natural establishment of a bilateral sucking–suckling relationship.

7.3 Psycho-vegetative regulation

Whenever an animal in labor is disturbed, uterine contractions are inhibited so that she can run and find a safe place before she gives birth. This adaptive mechanism shows the importance of the perception of security and avoidance of disturbance during birth.[16]

7.3.1 The parasympathetic system

From the biological point of view, labor is a parasympathetic process, a physiological condition that requires quietude, ease, comfort, confidence, and a feeling of security.[16] Our species is not an exception, and for this reason home birth is in greater accord with people's basic instincts than is going out in the dark to a hospital, unless faith in medicine so exceeds trust in nature that the expectant mother perceives the hospital to be safer. For many women, however, leaving home is the greatest stress of the whole process of parturition.[17]

The change of the environment is the reason why ineffective labor occurs more frequently since hospitals have replaced the home as the place for birth, though this is not always recognized by clinicians.[18] Birth attendants should make more allowances for the basic conditions of natural birth and instinctive behavior.[19] Doing so would create an intimate, safe, and private atmosphere. The serious lack of this in many birth settings was documented in Chapter 4.

Giving birth is a parasympathetic process: labor is easiest during parasympathetic dominance, whereas sympathetic stimuli inhibit labor.

7.3.2 Biological effects of stress

Environmental disturbances strongly affect the course and outcome of labor and delivery in all mammalian species. Anxiety and fear invariably lead to prolongation of labor.[1] A laboring wild mare, for instance, is capable of stopping labor and running for her life when she observes wolves. As soon as the cause of anxiety has disappeared, she resumes her discontinued activity. If the disturbance is too long, she loses her unborn foal and sometimes even her own life.

Anxiety and stress invariably lead to prolongation of labor.

An epinephrine (adrenalin) surge from fear or anxiety has the biological effect of weakening and even stopping contractions. Stress hormones suppress the oxytocin receptor's activity and lower the concentration of free calcium ions in the myometrial cells. As a result, the frequency and force of contractions decrease and may completely stop.[16,20,21]

Suppression of uterine activity is a life-saving adaptation for the laboring animal, developed through evolution – *fright: fight or flight*. In this way, mammals halt birth when they feel threatened.[16] The sympathetic control system is primarily activated by fear.[22] What was originally a protective mechanism has in the human situation – where it is not necessary to flee to protect one's life – turned against the parturient. Human studies in low-risk pregnancies showed that the pre-labor level of anxiety is an independent predictor of long dilatation time during labor.[23]

> Stimulation of the stress response is one of the most important causes of (iatrogenic) dynamic birth disorders.

After many millions of years of evolution, human biology cannot change as quickly as can civilization and patterns of culture, and the biological stress response is, without a doubt, a factor of major importance in the currently high incidence of iatrogenic birth disorders. A strange environment, discontinuity of care, negative psychological conditioning, crippling uncertainty, and indecisive conduct and care not infrequently play a pivotal role in dysfunctional, protracted labor (Chapter 4). All standards of *proactive support of labor* – as will be explained in Section 3 – aim to prevent, overcome, and end this vicious circle of undue stress.

References

1. Naaktgeboren C. The biology of childbirth. In Chalmers I, Keirse MJNC, Enkin M, eds. Effective Care in Pregnancy and Childbirth, Vol. **2**: *Childbirth*. Oxford: Oxford University Press; 1998

2. Parkes AS. Marshall's Physiology of Reproduction 4th edn, Vol. **2**. London: Longmans, Green; 1958:504–5

3. Young IR. The comparative physiology of parturition in mammals. Front Horm Res 2001;**27**:10–30

4. Fortman JD, Hewett TA, Bennet BT. The Laboratory Non-Human Primates. Boca Raton, FL: CRC Press; 2000

5. Jensen P. The Ethology of Domestic Animals: An Introductory Text. New York: CABI Publishing; 2002

6. Nagel C, Erber R, Bergmaier C, *et al.* Cortisol and progestin release, heart rate and heart rate variability in the pregnant and postpartum mare, fetus and newborn foal. Theriogenology 2012;**78**:759–67

7. Jolly A. Primate birth hour. Int Zoo Yearb 1973;**13**:391–7

8. Lowe NK. The nature of labor pain. Am J Obstet Gynecol 2002;**186**:16–24

9. Belsey EM, Rosenblatt DB, Lieberman BA, *et al.* The influence of maternal analgesia on neonatal behaviour: I. Pethidine. Br J Obstet Gynaecol 1981;**88**:398–406

10. Kron RE, Stein M, Goddard KE. Newborn sucking behavior affected by obstetric sedation. Pediatrics 1966;**37**:1012–16

11. Hodgkinson R, Bhatt M, Wang CN. Double-blind comparison of the neurobehaviour of neonates following the administration of different doses of meperidine to the mother. Can Anaesth Soc J 1978;**25**:405–11

12. Righard L, Alade MO. Effect of delivery room routines on success of first breast-feed. Lancet 1990;**336**:1105–7

13. Nissen E, Lilja G, Matthiesen AS, *et al.* Effects of maternal pethidine on infants' developing breastfeeding behaviour. Acta Paediatr 1995;**84**:140–5

14. Matthews MK. The relationship between maternal labour analgesia and delay in the initiation of breastfeeding in healthy neonates in the early neonatal period. Midwifery 1989;**5**:3–10

15. Crowell MK, Hill PD, Humenick SS. Relationship between obstetric analgesia and time of effective breastfeeding. J Nurse Midwifery 1994;**39**:150–6

16. Nagel C, Erber R, Ille N, *et al.* Parturition in horses is dominated by parasympathetic activity of the autonomic nervous system. Theriogenology 2014;**82**:160–8

17. Friedman DD. Conflict behavior in the parturient. In Hirsh H, ed. The Family. Proceedings of the 4th International Congress of Psychosomatic Obstetrics and Gynecology. Basel: Karger; 1975:373–6

18. Newton N, Foshee D, Newton M. Experimental inhibition of labor through environmental disturbance. Obstet Gynecol 1966;**27**:371–7

19. Rosenberg K, Trevathan W. Birth, obstetrics and human evolution. Br J Obstet Gynaec 2002;**109**:1199–206

20. Lopez Bernal A. Overview of current research in parturition (Uterine Contractility Symposium of the Physiological Society). Exp Physiol 2001;**86**:213–22

21. Nathanielsz PW. Comparative studies on the initiation of labor. Eur J Obstet Gynecol Reprod Biol 1998;**78**:127–32

22. Lawrence AB, Petherick JC, McLean K, *et al.* Naloxone prevents interruption of parturition and increases plasma oxytocin following environmental disturbance in parturient sows. Physiol Behav 1992;**52**:917–23

23. Wijnen HA, Denollet J, Essed GG, *et al.* High maternal anxiety during late gestation predicts protraction of labor. In Wijnen HA, ed. The Kempen Study. Academic Thesis 2005, University of Tilburg, The Netherlands

8

Elementary biophysics of birth

Although the basic physiology of parturition is a permanent design of nature, the conduct and care of normal childbirth vary significantly (Chapter 5). This diversity reflects differences in appreciation or knowledge of the elementary processes that control birth. By and large, interventionist obstetricians tend to override biology, whereas conservative caregivers who eschew interventions often allow labor to derail from the physiological track for too long. If scrutinized, both dogmatic approaches allow professionals to attend birth with neglect or even ignorance of the basic natural science of parturition.

Rational care must be based on a solid understanding of the biology of birth, and this is precisely the hallmark of *proactive support of labor* (Section 3). For the comprehension of the physiological basis of this method of care, this chapter is of critical importance to all professionals involved in childbirth. Laypersons without a medical background, however, might be discouraged from further reading by the biotechnical aspects of birth and may wish to scan only the boxed key points and proceed directly to Chapter 9.

> Basic knowledge of the biophysics of birth is a prerequisite for understanding labor.

8.1 The pre-labor preparation of the uterus

The function of the uterus changes radically at the end of pregnancy. For nine months, the uterus maintains a state of functional quiescence. The natural contractility of the myometrium is effectively suppressed and the resistance of the cervix is kept high enough to ensure that the fetus remains safely inside the womb. At the end of pregnancy, however, the uterus must suddenly recover its contractile competence and effectively expel the fetus.

> **The biological transformation**
>
> *At term, the uterus changes radically from being a safe, inert cocoon to a powerful expulsive organ.*

Slow growth in our understanding of pre-labor uterine transformation and the onset of labor reflects the difficulty in extrapolating from the control mechanisms in animal models to human parturition, a process that in humans precludes direct investigation.[1] Although the exact starting signal of parturition seems to vary, the final common pathway from the functional progesterone withdrawal and estrogen activation is probably common in all mammalian species, including humans. The science of the complex interactions between the paracrine, autocrine, and inflammatory pathways involved has been reviewed by several distinguished researchers in this field.[1–15] This chapter summarizes and structures – in a simple and comprehensible way – those essentials needed for an appropriate clinical understanding of the physiological process of human birth.

8.1.1 The fetal trigger

Considerable evidence suggests that, under physiological conditions, the fetus is in control of the uterine preparation for labor and the timing of birth. The signals that initiate the functional transformation of the uterus represent the expression of the fetal genome acting through endocrine pathways involving the maturing fetal brain, adrenal glands, and placenta, as well as mechanical signals acting directly on the myometrium (distension and stretch) as a result of the growth of the fetus. Together, these fetal signals contribute to the timely, safe, and effective birth at term.

> *In the weeks preceding birth, it is the fetus itself that triggers the preparation of the uterus for labor.*

8.1.2 Biochemistry

With advancing pregnancy, the placenta and fetal membranes increasingly produce corticotropin-releasing hormone (CRH). Weeks before there is any indication of labor onset, maturation of the fetal neuro-endocrine system activates the fetal pituitary gland to respond to CRH with the production of ACTH. This hormone, in turn, activates the fetal adrenal glands to produce and release corticosteroids and DHEAS.

Fetal cortisol and cortisone trigger the production of phospholipids and surfactant proteins in the fetal lungs. Surfactant not only prepares the fetal lungs for extra-uterine life but also enters the amniotic fluid and reaches the fetal membranes. Surfactant elicits membrane activation with the attraction of leukocytes and production of prostaglandins and cytokines that are transmitted into the myometrium and cervix. The pro-inflammatory cytokines cause tissue remodeling, building up contractibility of the myometrium and simultaneously degrading the dense collagen network of the cervix. In addition, cytokines attract more leukocytes, creating a positive feedback loop.

Added to that, the placenta and amniotic membranes convert fetal DHEAS into estrogens. The conversion of DHEAS to estrogen at the level of the fetoplacental unit is critical for the preparation of the uterus for labor; the progesterone to estrogen ratio begins to decline at the level of the uterine tissues. Functional withdrawal of progesterone may also be effected through blockade of progesterone receptor action at the level of the genome. The decrease in functional progesterone and the relative rise in estrogens induce intricate biochemical changes in both the cervix and the myometrium.

The activation of the fetal endocrine system initiates both fetal lung surfactant production and uterine transformation, synchronizing fetal lung maturation and the preparation of the uterus for labor.

8.1.3 Transformation of the uterus at two distinct levels

To achieve a proper understanding of the physics of birth, we must first of all distinguish between the pre-labor transformation of the cervix and that of the myometrium, because labor relies on the balance between myometrial force and the resistance of the cervix. This balance is orchestrated physiologically, but the two events are not necessarily synchronous (Chapter 14).

Pre-labor biophysical transformation

The cervical transformation determines how much resistance must be overcome to open the womb. The myometrial transformation determines how much force can be exerted to achieve this.

8.2 Pre-labor transformation of the cervix

The process of pre-labor cervical maturation is a complex enzymatically controlled process with substantial remodeling of the cervical extracellular matrix. In brief, the decrease in inhibitory progesterone activity and the rise in amniotic surfactant trigger leukocyte invasion and production of inflammatory cytokines, particularly in the area of the internal os of the cervix. These cytokines (especially IL-8) attract granulocytes that release collagenases and elastases acting to break down the mucopolysaccharide bonds both in the cervix and the fetal membranes. As a result the cervical collagen fibers begin to shift in relation to one another, with a resultant softening (ripening) and shortening (effacement) of the cervix. In the same way, the fetal membranes develop a weakened area that is to become the site of rupture.

8.2.1 Cervical ripening

The term effacement refers to the incorporation of the cervix into the lower segment of the uterus. This process begins at the internal os of the cervix and gradually proceeds downward to the external os, at which point the cervical body has disappeared and effacement is complete (Fig. 9.1 in Chapter 9).

Effacement begins several days to weeks before the end of pregnancy and progresses slowly to the time of labor.[16] Effacement is mostly, but not always, complete before the clinical onset of labor.[16]

In this context, it should be noted that complete effacement and beginning of dilatation of the cervix are not requirements for the clinical diagnosis of labor (Chapter 14). However, the birth process is likely to be prolonged if effacement has not taken place to a substantial degree beforehand. These are usually the troublesome labors. When the cervix is fully effaced at the start, labor can be expected to proceed smoothly and without any intervention. In this situation, progress is usually rapid, and the woman is likely to deliver spontaneously within a matter of hours (Chapter 10).

Adequate pre-labor cervical transformation is essential for effective labor.

8.3 Pre-labor transformation of the myometrium

Labor should be regarded as an event initiated by the removal of the inhibitory effects of pregnancy on the myometrium rather than as an active process governed by uterine stimulants. The maintenance of the state of uterine quiescence during pregnancy involves active blockade of the expression of genes that govern myometrial contractility. In particular, progesterone inhibits contractibility, cell–cell coupling and responsiveness to endogenous stimulants such as oxytocin and prostaglandins.

The preparation for labor involves a remarkable change in the phenotype of the myometrium, restoring uterine contractile competence. Functional progesterone withdrawal and the relative increase of estrogens stimulate hypertrophy of the myometrial cells. In addition, pro-inflammatory cytokines enhance calcium entry in the myometrial cells, increasing the myotropic effect. Cytokines also trigger the production of prostaglandin E_2 (PGE_2) in the myometrium. PGE_2 in turn activates the formation of mRNA that codes for specific intercellular proteins (*connexons*).[17] The widespread deposit of connexons between the myometrial cells is the final and crucial step in the preparation of the myometrium for effective labor.

The uterine preparation for labor involves a remarkable change in the phenotype of the myometrium (uterine muscle) near term.

8.3.1 Braxton Hicks contractions

The beginning of myometrial transformation often becomes clinically apparent when the pregnant woman experiences intermittent periods of discomfort from contractions at irregular intervals, often 10–30 minutes apart. Such periods of Braxton Hicks contractions that come and go may be noticed for

several weeks before true labor begins. Every myometrial cell can act as a pacemaker and stimulate nearby muscle cells to contract, but there is still no coordination; therefore, Braxton Hicks contractions have no substantial effect on the cervix.

8.3.2 The activation of the myometrium

During labor, the uterus must produce forceful contractions to overpower the resistance of the cervix. To this end, radical changes take place in the myometrium during the last days of pregnancy. The rise of estrogen levels in the myometrium and the relative decrease of progesterone activate the expression of a cassette of genes encoding contraction-associated proteins (CAPs), including oxytocin receptors, prostaglandin receptors, and connexons. Oxytocin levels do not rise significantly prior to or during labor, but the effect of endogenous (and exogenous) oxytocin on uterine contractility becomes stronger as the number of oxytocin receptors increases.[18,19] The binding of oxytocin to its receptors enhances the production of PGE_2 at the precise location where it must act: in the myometrium. PGE_2 reinforces the production of connexons deposited between the myometrial cells.

After passing a threshold of the hormonal and inflammatory processes, these connexons are capable of quickly creating stimulus-conducting connections between the myometrial cells, known as *myometrial gap junctions*. These are small, intercellular channels that have a low resistance to ions and a high electrical conductivity for action potentials. This cell–cell conduction system develops suddenly (within a few hours) and is essential for the coordination of myometrial cell contractions and thus for the achievement of forceful contractions and effective labor.

Pre-labor deposition of connexons – the precursors of gap junctions electrically connecting myometrial cells – is essential for an effective start and adequate progression of early labor.

8.4 The onset of labor

The final step of myometrial activation – the sudden formation of the myometrial gap junctions – takes only a few hours. Prior to labor, gap junctions are scarcely present, if at all. In fact, it is precisely the sudden and widespread formation of gap junctions that triggers the onset of clinical labor. The orchestration of myometrial cell contractions occurs in a very short time, resulting in propagated contraction waves, and the newly coordinated contractions begin to have an impact on the softened cervix. In this way, the physical connection between the fetal membranes and the lower decidua is disrupted, stimulating PGE_2 production on the spot. The weakened membranes may rupture, and the production of PGE_2 further increases. The formation of gap junctions accelerates rapidly, and the process reinforces itself through positive feedback: labor has begun.

> *The sudden formation of the myometrial gap junctions triggers the onset of labor.*

8.4.1 Electromechanical coupling

As with other types of muscle contractions, uterine action potentials must be generated and propagated to yield effective contractions in a process known as electromechanical coupling. Uterine action potentials during labor occur in bursts originating in one of the fundal corners. Here, cells have a higher resting potential than other myometrial cells, and act as "pacemakers." Contraction waves propagate through the myometrial gap junction-conduction system, and the electrical activity supplies the uterine force exerted on the contents of the uterus. The electrical orchestration determines the number of myometrial cells recruited for action, which in turn determines the strength of each contraction. A refractory period of the myometrial cells for at least one minute after each excitation wave secures uterine relaxation between the contractions needed for adequate fetal oxygenation (8.7).

> *The efficiency of labor contractions relies on the degree and quality of the pre-labor myometrial transformation.*

8.5 Physics of effective labor

For labor to be effective, uterine force must overpower the resistance of the cervix. In terms of physics, force is a vector, meaning it has a particular direction. This elementary principle is all too often forgotten in obstetrics. From a physics point of view, the vector uterine force is a fundamentally different parameter from uterine tone assessed by manual palpation and from intrauterine pressure measured with intrauterine catheters. Pressure is not the measure, force is the course.

8.5.1 Uterine coordination

To gather effective, directional force, contractions must propagate in a coordinated fashion. Coordination, in turn, requires a functional electrical conduction system and thus a fully and adequately transformed myometrium. Pacemaker cells in the right cornu usually predominate over those in the left and start the vast majority of contractions. The excitation wave first propagates laterally and subsequently downward toward the cervix at 2 cm/s, depolarizing the whole organ within 15 seconds. In this way, the uterine tube first stiffens and then shortens, producing effective traction on the dilatation ring and thrusting force on the cervix via the fetal head or the bulging amniotic sac (wedging action). Only electrically orchestrated contractions are efficient, and efficient contractions are needed for effective labor. The overall effectiveness of labor depends on the frequency and the efficiency of the contractions versus the cervical resistance.

> **Efficient and effective contractions**
>
> *Only coordinated contractions are efficient contractions, and only efficient contractions can be effective.*

8.5.2 Cervical resistance in labor

The resistance of the cervix determines how much cumulative force the uterus must generate to accomplish full dilatation. Direct measurement of the cervical resistance is not possible. Clinical assessment of cervical softness provides only an indirect and subjective impression. This is true both prior to and during labor. One way to overcome slow progress in labor is to enhance uterine force by rupturing the membranes and by the use of oxytocin. Another approach would be to reduce cervical resistance. Several methods for influencing cervical resistance to accelerate slow labor have been tested.[20] These techniques include parenteral administration of porcine relaxin, local cervical injections of hyaluronidase, electrical vibration of the cervix, and local application of prostaglandins. To date, however, controlled trials have not demonstrated any significant advantage in the use of these methods, whereas the safety of these measures needs further assessment.[20]

> There are no effective and safe measures to reduce cervical resistance in labor. The only safe and effective way of accelerating slow labor is enhancing uterine force.

8.5.3 Uterine force

Uterine force comprises two components: pulling and pushing forces.[21] In a physical sense, the combination of pulling and pushing is comparable to what happens when one pulls on a sock: there is traction on the cervix and, subsequently, a pushing force is applied to the cervix by the presenting part. In other words, cervical dilatation is achieved by traction combined with hydrostatic action of the intact membranes or, after their rupture, by direct pushing of the descending fetal head against the cervix. The presenting fetal part functions as a blunt wedge.

As in pulling on socks, the initial force in the dilatation process is predominantly traction in order to allow entrance of the blunt end of the wedge into the partially dilated cervix. The contribution of the pushing (descending) component gradually increases in importance later in time; descent is required for adequate wedging action needed to complete the last centimeters to full dilatation (Chapter 10).

> Uterine force comprises two components: pulling and pushing forces.

In an in-vivo experimental setting, the "head-to-cervix force" (HCF) has been measured with a sensor between the caput and the cervix.[22–25] HCF estimates uterine force and is shown to be lower in long labors. During normal contractions, HCF increases before intrauterine pressure does. Oxytocin treatment in slow labor increases both the frequency of contractions and HCF. Most importantly, HCF is a better predictor of the achievement of vaginal birth than is intrauterine pressure or even dilatation rate.

These findings support the assertion that uterine force and not intrauterine pressure is the most important factor for a successful birth, and, by extension, that efficient coordination of contractions is the deciding factor in the effectiveness of labor.

> Force is a vector with a particular direction. Uterine force is a fundamentally different parameter from the clinical measures of uterine tone or intrauterine pressure.

8.5.4 Exhaustion of the myometrium

Prolonged labor leads to accumulation of lactic acid in the myometrium and a progressive loss of oxytocin receptors.[26] In addition, belated and prolonged oxytocin treatment results in myometrial desensitization through a significant reduction in both oxytocin-binding sites and receptor mRNA.[27,28]

Consequently, the uterus gradually loses its ability to respond to oxytocin stimulation – this effect is sometimes described as oxytocin-resistant dystocia. Alternatively, the uterus may react like any overburdened muscle with disorganized hypertonia (tetanic spasms), leading to fetal distress. This is the exhausted, refractory uterus; a common though often unrecognized complication when acceleration of slow labor is postponed too long (Chapters 15, 17, 21).

> **The refractory uterus**
>
> In slow labor, the uterus gradually loses its ability to respond to oxytocin stimulation.

8.5.5 Disorganized uterine action

In other non-physiological conditions, uterine relaxation may be compromised through random excitation of myometrial cells by meconium, intrauterine infection, or free blood, leading to dysfunctional labor and fetal distress. The fetal bowels contain bile acids and salts that render meconium very corrosive.[29] As in cases with intrauterine infection, fresh meconium may induce the production of excessive amounts of inflammatory cytokines in the fetal membranes and the decidua.[29–35] These cytokines may randomly stimulate myometrium cells, thereby disturbing electrical coordination in a similar way as in cases of intrauterine infection. Disorganized myometrial activity, in turn, results in inefficient contractions in conjunction with hypertonia in the inter-contraction intervals. A vicious circle of fetal distress and dysfunctional labor may ensue (Chapters 21 and 24). Free blood *in utero* due to (partial) placental abruption may have a similar effect.

Hypertonic dystocia

Fresh meconium, intrauterine bacteria, or free blood may lead to a vicious circle of fetal compromise and dysfunctional labor through inflammatory cytokines instigating disorganized uterine hypertonia.

8.6 First labor compared with subsequent labors

The most significant difference between nulliparous and parous labor is the relatively long duration of first births.[36] Effacement and dilatation evolve slower in first labors, because of the relatively higher resistance-to-force ratio. There are two sides to this equation:

1. The average resistance of the nulliparous cervix is higher because it has never before been stretched and opened.
2. The absolute force the nulliparous uterus is initially able to generate is usually less because the contractions often are less efficiently coordinated.[21,37,38]

Both factors explain why early dynamic dystocia frequently occurs in first labors. The key factor seems to be the less-efficient contractions because, even after correcting for cervical ripeness at the onset of labor, the nulliparous uterus has to produce twice as much work (in terms of physics and as inferred by intra-uterine pressure readings) as its multiparous counterpart to effect vaginal delivery.[38] It appears that the myometrial activation – like so many other complex biological processes – is not always executed as swiftly and as well on the first attempt as it is on subsequent occasions. One could say that the nulliparous myometrium still has to learn how to birth. While for some scientists it may still be open for debate whether the relatively longer duration of nulliparous labor is predominantly a result of higher cervical resistance or mainly the result of less force per contraction, the clinical point remains that ineffective early labor is a problem specific to first labors. Parous women do not suffer from dynamic dystocia to any significant extent, unless their labor is induced (Chapter 10, 21, 27).

The fundamental parity difference

Ineffective labor (dynamic dystocia) is a problem specific to first labors.

8.7 Fetal oxygenation during labor

The importance of the myometrial gap junction system is electrical orchestration, establishing forceful contractions and regulating interval uterine relaxation. Adequate inter-contraction relaxation of the uterus is a prerequisite for adequate fetal oxygenation during labor and delivery.

8.7.1 The placental reserve capacity

A healthy fetus is exceptionally well equipped to endure the stress and pressures of normal labor. Fetal blood flow through the placenta remains unimpeded during contractions, unless the umbilical cord is compressed by accident. In contrast, the maternal blood supply to the placenta is blocked during each normal contraction owing to external compression of the spiral arteries in the myometrium. The normal, healthy fetus is perfectly able to tolerate this potentially stressful situation because the placental circulatory system has a functional reserve capacity. The maternal blood pool within the placenta is sufficiently large and saturated to maintain a positive maternal-fetal oxygen gradient throughout a normal contraction, thereby ensuring normal fetal oxygenation. During the intervals between contractions, the spiral arteries open again and maternal–placental blood is refreshed. In other words: both placental reserve capacity and adequate uterine relaxation in the intervals between contractions are essential for the fetus to survive labor. These obligatory intervals are secured by a physiological refractory period of the myometrium for at least one minute after each excitation wave.

Reserve capacity of the placental circulation

The healthy fetus is well equipped to tolerate the arrest of maternal blood flow to the placenta during contractions. Interval uterine relaxation is vital to fetal oxygenation.

8.7.2 Interval uterine relaxation

The force of contractions poses no threat to a healthy fetus, but insufficient uterine relaxation in the intervals between contractions certainly does. Good uterine relaxation depends on adequate electrical orchestration, which means a completely transformed myometrium. Even in a healthy fetus with adequate placental circulatory reserve, insufficient interval uterine relaxation (uterine hypertonia) invariably leads to fetal hypoxia. Uterine hypertonia is a frequent complication particular to induction and is attributable to an attempt to force a non-transformed or incompletely transformed myometrium into contractions. The clinical implication is clear: a safe labor involves waiting for the spontaneous onset of labor and refraining from induction.

The vicious circle of fetal distress (meconium) and hypertonic dystocia was mentioned above (8.5.5). Inter-contraction uterine hypertonia may also result from the accumulation of lactic acid. In order to avoid this fetal predicament, dysfunctional labor is best corrected in time (Chapters 15, 17, 21).

> *Exogenous oxytocin may cause inter-contraction hypertonia and related fetal distress when used for induction or if used too late in cases of protracted spontaneous labor.*

8.8 Acceleration versus induction

The foregoing analyses reach the core of most problems encountered in daily birth care with both overuse and underuse of oxytocin. Doctors with liberal induction policies override biology and ignore the physiological preconditions for a smooth and safe birth. On the other hand, conservative caregivers, who tolerate slow progress in spontaneous labor much too long, overlook the problem of gradual exhaustion of the myometrium.

Care providers go awry because of a misunderstanding about the true nature of induction of labor and acceleration of slow labor after spontaneous onset often referred to as labor "augmentation". As both procedures use amniotomy and subsequently oxytocin, caregivers and mothers may assume that induction and acceleration (augmentation) are somehow extensions of the same procedure, merging imperceptibly into each other. Nothing could be further from the truth. The logic behind this assumption is comparable to the conclusion that fighting a fire and watering the flower garden is the same thing because both actions use water and hose.

> *There should be no confusion between induction of labor and acceleration as they concern two fundamentally different procedures with overall opposite effects.*

8.8.1 Acceleration of slow spontaneous labor

Once labor has begun spontaneously, oxytocin receptors are abundant, and the cervix and myometrium have transformed at least to the point that the physiological circle has started: contractions → *myometrial gap junctions* → electrical orchestration → effect on the cervix → prostaglandin release → contractions, and so forth. The already laboring but ineffective uterus reacts in a predictably favorable fashion to amniotomy and oxytocin (Chapter 15). Acceleration of slow labor greatly improves a physiological process that has already begun spontaneously.

> **Fundamental distinction**
>
> *Timely acceleration normalizes slow labor whereas induction usually causes a slow and difficult labor.*

8.8.2 Induction of labor

In contrast, induction interrupts the natural course of pregnancy. The transformation of the uterus is by definition not complete, and gap junctions are not yet formed. The amount of precursors required (connexons) may be low or even absent. The same holds for oxytocin receptors. This explains why the uterus reacts unpredictably to oxytocin when used for induction. The myometrium may completely fail to respond, or the induced contractions may have little effect because of poor electrical coordination. At the same time, the cervix is not yet optimally transformed. This means that the cumulative force the uterus has to exert to effect dilatation is always more than would be necessary if one had waited for the spontaneous onset of labor. The intended effect – progress in dilatation – is extremely varied with inductions: mostly progress is much too slow and occasionally even entirely absent, especially in nulliparas. Induction sets in motion effects that are the exact opposite of those of acceleration of spontaneous labor in nearly every respect.

While it is true that locally applied exogenous prostaglandins may sometimes soften an unripe cervix, this so-called "cervical priming" is often ineffective in achieving the activation of the myometrium. Quite often the proteins (connexons) needed for the formation of gap junctions are simply not yet present.

Oxytocin is not nearly so predictably effective and safe in initiating the process of labor as it is in accelerating progress after labor has already started spontaneously.

Asynchronous cervical and myometrial transformation also explains why induction may lead to ineffective labor despite "cervical ripeness." In nulliparous women with a "ripe" cervical score, too, induction significantly increases cesarean delivery odds as compared with controls with spontaneous labor onset (Chapter 23).

8.9 Expert care in childbirth

Thorough knowledge and understanding of the biology of parturition is a prerequisite to a rational approach to the conduct and care of labor and delivery. The complex basic biology discussed in this chapter will be translated into simple clinical mind-lines guiding expert care (Section 3). The main theme, constantly emphasized throughout this book, is a sharp distinction between nulliparous and parous labor and between acceleration and induction of labor. Before the overall plan for expert care can be explained, though, we first need to re-examine several (false) ideas and dogmas dominating current care.

References

1. Norwitz ER, Robinson JN, Repke JT. The Initiation of Parturition: A Comparative Analysis Across the Species. New York: Mosby; 1999

2. Smith R. Parturition. N Engl J Med 2007;**356**:271–83

3. Liao JB, Buhimschi CS, Norwitz ER. Normal labor: Mechanism and duration. Obstet Gynecol Clin N Am 2005;**32**:145–64

4. Lye SJ, Challis JRG. Parturition. In: Harding R, Bocking AD, eds. Fetal Growth and Development. Cambridge University Press; 2001:241–66

5. Challis JGR, Matthews SG, Gibb W, *et al*. Endocrine and paracrine regulation of birth at term and preterm. Endocr Rev 2000;**21**:514–20

6. Norwitz ER, Robinson JN, Challis JRG. The control of labor (review articles). N Engl J Med 1999;**341**:660–6

7. Makieva S, Saunders PT, Norman JE. Androgens in pregnancy: roles in parturition. Hum Reprod Update 2014;**20**:542–59

8. Kamel RM. The onset of human parturition. Arch Gynecol Obstet 2010;**281**:975–82

9. Gomez-Lopez N, Tanaka S, Zaeem Z, *et al*. Maternal circulating leukocytes display early chemotactic responsiveness during late gestation. BMC Pregnancy Childbirth 2013;**13** Suppl 1:S1–S8 Epub 2013 Jan 31

10. Mesiano S, Wang Y, Norwitz ER. Progesterone receptors in the human pregnancy uterus: do they hold the key to birth timing? Reprod Sci 2011;**18**:6–19

11. Golightly E, Jabbour HN, Norman JE. Endocrine immune interactions in human parturition. Mol Cell Endocrinol 2011;**335**:52–9

12. You X, Liu J, Xu C, *et al*. Corticotropin-releasing hormone (CRH) promotes inflammation in human pregnant myometrium: The evidence of CRH initiating parturition? J Clin Endocrinol Metab 2014;**99**:199–208

13. Smith R, Van Helden D, Hirst J, *et al*. Pathological interactions with the timing of birth and uterine activation. Aust N Z J Obstet Gynaecol 2007;**47**:430–7

14. Shynlova O, Tsui P, Jaffer S, Lye SJ. Integration of endocrine and mechanical signals in the regulation of myometrial functions during pregnancy and labour. Eur J Obstet Gynecol Reprod Biol 2009;**144** Suppl 1: S2–10

15. Lopez Bernal A. Overview of current research in parturition (Uterine Contractility Symposium of the Physiological Society). Exp Physiol 2001;**86**:213–22

16. Hendricks CH, Brenner WE, Kraus G. Normal cervical dilatation pattern in late pregnancy and labor. Am J Obstet Gynecol 1970;**106**:1065–82

17. Chow L, Lye SJ. Expression of the gap junction protein connexin-43 is increased in the human myometrium toward term and with the onset of labor. Am J Obstet Gynecol 1994;**170**:788–95

18. Shojo H, Kaneko Y. Characterization and expression of oxytocin and the oxytocin receptor. Mol Genet Metab 2000;**71**:552–8

19. Blanks AM, Thornton S. The role of oxytocin in parturition. Br J Obstet Gynaecol 2003;**110** (Suppl 20):46–51

20. Enkin M, Keirse MJNC, Neilson J, *et al*. A Guide to Effective Care in Pregnancy and Childbirth, 3rd edn. Oxford: Oxford University Press; 2000:332–40

21. Buhimschi C, Buhimschi IA. The forces of labour. Fetal and Maternal Medicine Review 2003;**14**:273–307

22. Gough GW, Randall NJ, Genevier ES, Sutherland IA, Steer PJ. Head-to-cervix forces and their relationship to the outcome of labor. Obstet Gynecol 1990;**75**:613–18

23. Antonucci MC, Pitman MC, Eid T, Steer PJ, Genevier ES. Simultaneous monitoring of head-to-cervix forces, intrauterine pressure and cervical dilatation during labour. Med Eng Phys. 1997;**19**:317–26

24. Allman AC, Genevier ES, Johnson MR, *et al.* Head-to-cervix force: an important physiological variable in labour. 1. The temporal relation between head-to-cervix force and uterine pressure during labour. Br J Obstet Gynaecol 1996;**103**:763–8

25. Allman AC, Genevier ES, Johnson MR, Steer PJ. Head-to-cervix force: an important physiological variable in labour. 2. Peak active force, peak active pressure and mode of delivery. Br J Obstet Gynaecol 1996;**103**:769–75

26. Quenby S, Pierce SJ, Brigham S, Wray S. Dysfunctional labor and myometrial lactic acidosis. Obstet Gynecol 2004;**103**:718–23

27. Phaneuf S, Asboth G, Carrasco MP, *et al.* Desensitization of oxytocin receptors in human myometrium. Hum Reprod Update 1998;**4**:625–33

28. Phaneuf S, Rodriguez Linares B, TamByraja RL, *et al.* Loss of oxytocin receptors during oxytocin-induced and oxytocin-augmented labour. J Reprod Fertil 2000;**120**:91–7

29. Pariente G, Peles C, Perri ZH, *et al.* Meconium-stained amniotic fluid – risk factors and immediate perinatal outcomes among SGA infants. J Matern Fetal Neonatal Med 2014;**30**:1–4

30. Matsubara S, Yamada T, Minakama H, *et al.* Meconium-stained fluid activates polymorphonuclear leucocytes; ultrastructural and enzyme cytochemical evidence. Eur J Histochem 1999;**43**:205–10

31. Anahya SN, Kakshmanan J, Morgan BL, Ross MG. Meconium passage in utero: mechanisms, consequences, and management. Obstet Gynecol Surv 2005;**60**:45–56

32. Mark SP, Croughan-Minihane MS, Kilpatrick SJ. Chorioamnionitis and uterine function. Obstet Gynecol 2000;**95**:909–12

33. Edwards RK. Chorioamnionitis and labor. Obstet Gynecol Clin N Am 2005;**32**:287–96

34. Rauk PN, Chiao JP. Oxytocin signaling in human myometrium is impaired by prolonged exposure to interleukin-1. Biol Reprod 2000;**63**:846–50

35. Rauk PN, Friebe-Hoffman U. Interleukin 1-beta down regulates the oxytocin receptor in cultured uterine smooth muscle cells. Am J Reprod Immunol 2000;**43**:83–9

36. NICE guidelines. Intrapartum care: care of healthy women and their babies during childbirth. RCOG Press; 2007. Updated 2010; www.nice.org.uk/gui dance/cg55

37. Fairlie FM, Phillips GF, Andrews BJ, Calder AA. An analysis of uterine activity in spontaneous labour using a microcomputer. Br J Obstet Gynaecol 1988;**95**:57–64

38. Arulkumaran S, Gibb DM, Lun KC, *et al.* The effect of parity on uterine activity in labour. Br J Obstet Gynaecol 1984;**91**:843–8

Definitions and verbal precision

9

One of the major impediments to improvements in labor care is the lack of definitions (3.1.2). This is true not only of common clinical conditions, of which "normal labor" is a good example, but also of the elementary parameters that describe the basic processes marking the onset and progression of labor. In daily practice, the terms effacement and dilatation are constantly used, but they are seldom accurately defined. As a result, many poorly defined concepts such as the "latent phase" of labor serve as a cloak for clinical indecision. Even worse, ambiguous locutions such as "failure to progress despite good contractions" convey a blatant ignorance of the situation.

Most problems in labor have their origin in inaccurate diagnosis; unwittingly, various labor disorders are seen as one and the same problem and classified as "dystocia," the most frequently reported indication for operative delivery. Although its common definition – abnormal progress in labor – seems simple, there is an endless variation in the interpretation of what abnormal progress means. This explains the wide variation in the reported incidence and related operative delivery rates in hospitals that appear similar in all other aspects. Dystocia is, in fact, a syndrome, heterogeneous in its manifestation and causation, and should, therefore, be examined in detail. Detailed analysis, in turn, first requires strict definitions of the basic parameters of birth.

> *Most of the problems encountered in the supervision of labor originate in inaccurate diagnosis, primarily because the elementary parameters marking the onset and progression of labor are poorly defined.*

9.1 Elementary parameters of parturition

To avoid semantic debates and confusion about various stages and components of labor, we will formulate unequivocal definitions of basic phenomena as "good" contractions, cervical effacement, and cervical dilatation. These definitions and their relationship to the definitions of separate clinical events – such as the onset of labor, normal progression, false labor, effective labor, and dystocia – are critical for expert birth care. Genuinely science-based and real evidence-based obstetrics begins with strict definitions.

9.1.1 Labor pains = contractions of labor

Although labor pains are painful contractions, painful contractions are not necessarily labor pains. In Germanic languages, e.g., German and Dutch, different words exist for labor pains (*Wehen*), meaning labor contractions, and uterine contractions in general but not specific for labor (*Kontraktionen*). A similar distinction between "contractions" (of labor) and uterine "contractures" (unrelated to labor) has been suggested in the English literature. In practice, however, these words with explicitly distinctive meanings are hopelessly mixed up. It is alarming how ambiguously the term "pains" (*Wehen*) is misused, confusing the question of whether or not a state of labor exists. Many professionals use extremely unprofessional terminology such as *"Vorwehen"* (pre-labor pains), *"Übungswehen"* (practice pains), etc. This confusing use of language can only lead to uncertainty and lack of clarity at the bedside because the only thing that matters to the woman in question is whether she does or does not have labor pains, because she either is in labor or she is not. For her, there is no in-between.

Absolute clarity regarding the onset of labor is a primary requirement for professional care. Labor pains, i.e. contractions of labor, are by definition uterine contractions that have a progressive effect on the cervix. Pains (*Wehen*) are inherent to labor. There is no labor without labor pains, and a woman does not have labor pains (*Wehen*) without being in labor.

Braxton Hicks contractions may indeed be painful, but by definition they are not labor pains (*Wehen*) because they do not have any short-term effect on the cervix. Labor is characterized by pains plus progression.

> **Definition**
>
> *Contractions of labor (labor pains) are regular uterine contractions with a progressive effect on the cervix, leading to complete effacement of the cervix followed by dilatation.*

The status of having labor pains can be objectively verified with cervical effacement and dilatation. These are two more everyday terms that are usually used in a careless and often fundamentally incorrect manner. O'Driscoll keenly observed: "In view of the paramount importance of the diagnosis of labor and the central role of the cervix in this decision-making, surprisingly little attention is generally directed to the understood meaning of the terms used to describe cervical behavior in early labor. Instead, the terms effacement and dilatation tend to be taken for granted and are quickly passed over as if everyone understood precisely what they meant."[1]

> **Cervix in labor**
>
> *Effacement and dilatation are consecutive and not simultaneous features of one and the same process: the incorporation of the cervix into the lower segment of the uterus.*

9.1.2 Effacement

Effacement refers to the inclusion of the cervical body into the lower uterine segment. This process begins at the internal os and proceeds gradually downward to the external os, at which juncture the cervical canal disappears, and effacement is complete (Fig. 9.1).

> **Definition**
>
> *Effacement is the shortening of the cervix through its incorporation into the lower uterine segment. With full effacement, there is no longer an internal os or a cervical body.*

9.1.3 Cervical accessibility versus dilatation

The antepartum cervical body is closed, but at term it often becomes weak enough to allow the easy passage of a probing fingertip. It is an endless source of confusion that this finding is considered the equivalent of 1 or 2 cm dilatation in an intact or halfway-effaced cervix. Since dilatation refers only to the external os of the fully effaced cervix, such a conclusion is by definition impossible and counter-informative. One should not call this dilatation but rather cervical accessibility.

The term "accessibility" is intended to convey an inert and temporary static situation, which provides information regarding the extent of pre-labor cervical weakening. In contrast, the term "dilatation" connotes an evolving, dynamic situation resulting from active uterine force. This distinction may seem to be semantic quibbling, but it is essential for avoiding the rampant verbal confusion and mistakes that occur in the diagnosis of labor. Of course, no problem in the diagnosis of labor exists when a well-dilated cervix accompanies regular and painful contractions. As always, the need for verbal precision is greatest in doubtful cases where diagnosis presents a genuine problem (Chapter 14).[1]

> *Cervical "accessibility" gives information about cervical ripening, "dilatation" about uterine force.*

9.1.4 Dilatation

The term cervical dilatation relates only to the active opening of the external os by uterine force. The external os can be actively pulled open only if the cervical body has completely disappeared into the lower uterine segment, i.e. if full effacement has occurred. It is essential to recognize that effacement is, by definition, completed before dilatation begins. To speak about dilatation before effacement is complete involves a direct contradiction in terms.

> **Definition**
>
> *Dilatation is the diameter of the external os of the fully effaced cervix.*

This definition holds true for both nulliparas and multiparas. The term dilatation is commonly used

Cervix in Labor
sequence of effacement and dilatation

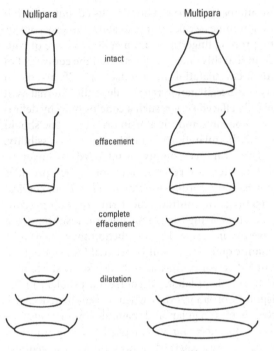

Figure 9.1 Cervix in labor: effacement and dilatation are consecutive effects.

incorrectly, especially in relation to multiparas because most standard textbooks mistakenly teach that the patulous parous cervix simultaneously effaces and dilatates. This is a persistent mistake, based on and leading to careless use of words: cervical accessibility is confused with dilatation.

In contrast to the situation with nulliparas, the parous cervical canal is cone-shaped, and the external os may freely admit one or two examining fingertips in late pregnancy while the internal os may still be closed (Fig. 9.1). Thus, by definition, there is still no dilatation, only accessibility. Contractions do not yet stretch the external os because the body of the cervix must first vanish completely (full effacement) before the external os can be pulled open. Accessibility only then becomes dilatation. In practice, full effacement is the equivalent of 1 cm of dilatation in a nullipara because the external os is always open to this extent. In multiparas dilatation begins only at 2 or 3 cm (Fig. 9.1) and in grand multiparas the dilatation scale could begin at an even larger value.

> *Imprecision in describing the cervical changes in early labor has led to fundamental and pervasive misapprehensions such as the false concept of the latent phase of labor.*

9.1.5 The transition at full effacement

The point at which effacement ends and dilatation begins requires special attention. At this juncture, the presence or absence of painful contractions is decisive, and the practical consequence is straightforward: without regular contractions, there is no question of labor, whereas a woman with regular, painful contractions and a fully effaced cervix can be firmly declared to be in labor (Chapter 14).

> *The point at which effacement ends and dilatation begins is the practical demarcation line of whether a woman with contractions is in labor or not.*

9.2 The onset of labor

One of the most important decisions in labor involves recognizing whether or not labor has started. Many care providers avoid this dilemma by leaving this decision to the woman as a self-diagnosis on the basis of regular, painful contractions, at which point the so-called "latent phase" of labor begins (Chapter 10).[2]

However, this practice avoids a professional distinction between true and false labor. Even leading textbooks and official guidelines claim "the confirmation of labor is presumed to be reasonably reliable only once painful contractions have established at least 3 to 4 cm dilatation."[3] According to that proposition, the diagnosis of labor is confirmed only after the event. Even worse, primary dysfunctional labor is not recognized at all. O'Driscoll noticed: "an essential difference between theory and practice is that the doctor – or more likely the midwife – cannot enjoy the luxury of hindsight when an agitated woman presents late at night because she thinks she is in labor."[1] A firm and prospective decision is required in these circumstances, and full effacement plays a decisive role.

> *The greatest impediment to understanding labor is recognizing its start.*

Given the fundamental importance of accurate diagnosis in early labor, separate chapters will address the distinction between true and false labor and the timely recognition of primary ineffective labor (Chapters 14, 15, 21).

9.2.1 Crucial clarity

Poor definitions and resultant conceptual blurring hinder the transfer of knowledge and stand in the way of significant discussion on any aspect of labor. Most studies on labor-related issues in the obstetric and midwifery literature are more or less invalidated by imprecise definitions of elementary parameters of labor, such as its onset and thus the duration of normal labor (Chapter 10). By inference, guidelines based on systematic reviews of studies on the length of "normal" labor, dystocia, amniotomy, augmentation of labor, etc., are much less evidence-based than they pretend to be.

Even more worrying from the perspective of everyday practice is the use by professionals of ill-defined and equivocal terminology for basic parameters of birth, which hampers transfer of relevant patient information. Imprecision inevitably leads to inconsistent conduct and care by ever-changing staff, and hence to confusion at the bedside.

No one can deny that consistent policies and clarity at the bedside require cooperating providers to use the same definitions and unequivocal language.

Clear and consistent labor management benefits from the proper use of professional language; a woman either is in labor or she is not. Unprofessional phrases, such as "practice run", "labor not established", "rumbling", "niggling", "latent labor", "slow start", "beginning in labor", "passive labor", or "moderate labor", serve as a cloak for indecision or ignorance and are as empty as saying "a little bit pregnant", "somewhat sterile", or "moderately dead."

Nonetheless, one is regularly faced with a woman who considers herself to have been in labor for more than 24 hours while her primary birth attendant classifies her first 10–20 hours as "niggling", or "latent" labor. Such meaningless jargon only serves as a cover for hesitant and muddling demeanor, which in turn can only lead to chaos, misery, and despair. Thus, for clarity's sake:

- Strict definitions of the terms effacement and dilatation are the first requirement for the correct diagnosis of the onset of labor (Chapter 14).
- A careful diagnosis of labor is a *conditio sine qua non* to define the duration of labor.
- Only a strict definition of labor duration allows for objectively distinguishing between an acceptable and an unacceptable labor duration, which further supports objective criteria for adequate progress (Chapter 10).
- A clear definition of adequate progress is needed for determining departures from the norm and for evaluating treatment (Section 3).

Clinical science, too, begins with accurate definitions.

9.3 "Good" or "adequate" contractions

The sole purpose of uterine contractions in the first stage of labor is to dilate the cervix and, ultimately, to provoke descent and activate the pushing reflex. The sole objective of contractions in second-stage labor is to prompt the cardinal movements of the fetal head and to expel the fetus. Therefore, the quality of contractions should be evaluated exclusively as it relates to these effects. Unfortunately, too many care providers lose sight of these effect-criteria, using meaningless jargon such as "slow, prolonged, or protracted labor, despite 'good' contractions." This is a contradiction in terms. Careless use of words stems from – and leads to – failure to recognize dynamic birth disorders in time. The regrettable result is therapeutic paralysis by dithering and insecure providers in cases of ineffective labor, leading to a detrimental waste of time and an unnecessary exhaustion of both the woman and her uterus.

The effect-criterion

The quality of contractions must be evaluated exclusively in terms of their effect.

9.3.1 Futile external assessment

Conservative doctors and midwives traditionally evaluate the quality of labor with hand on abdomen, judging the intensity, tone, and frequency of the contractions and how the woman winces as her uterus contracts. When the contractions appear to be vigorous ("super strong contractions"), the common policy is to refrain from vaginal examinations – regarded as a burdensome interference – and to wait four hours or more. This is a common mistake. Both the subjective element of pain, as felt by the mother, and the intensity or tone of the contractions as assessed by ritual palpation correlate very poorly with dilatational progress.[4] Moreover, a period of four hours is much too long to discover that labor has hardly progressed (Chapters 10, 15, 21).

The clinical characteristics of uterine contractions – frequency, intensity, tone, duration, and painfulness – cannot be relied on as measures of effective labor or indices of normality. Only progress counts.

9.3.2 Intrauterine pressure readings

A similar misunderstanding flourishes in relation to Montevideo units (MU), which many clinicians assume can be used to evaluate the quality of uterine action. By this definition, uterine activity is the product of intrauterine pressure – peak pressure above baseline tone – of a contraction in mmHg multiplied by contraction frequency per 10 minutes. ACOG equates a score of 200 MU with "adequate" contractions and UpToDate falls into the same trap.[5,6] This is but one of the many examples of confusing verbal imprecision even used and endorsed by official bodies. It is not intrauterine pressure that determines whether contractions are adequate, but progression of labor. Moreover, in physical terms, pressure is not the measure; force is the course (8.5).

Pressure and force are two entirely different physical entities, and uncoordinated contractions can certainly build up pressure without exerting effective, directional force. Therefore, insufficient progress of labor is the only criterion on which to base a decision to start oxytocin or to refrain from treatment,

regardless of the amount of MUs. The same applies to the evaluation of treatment. Intrauterine pressure readings are redundant, not without complications, and sometimes misleading, as "adequate MUs" may unjustly lead providers to withhold treatment while it is clearly indicated (Chapter 15).[7]

Montevideo units are not as useful in the evaluation of uterine performance as they are typically believed to be. The only "adequate" contractions are those that lead to adequate progression of the birth process, irrespective of Montevideo units.

In order to define criteria for "normal" or "adequate" progress, we will have to discuss some more stubborn misconceptions and unfounded dogmas about the "normal" course of dilatation. That is the subject of the next chapter.

References

1. O'Driscoll K, Meagher D, Robson M. Active Management of Labour, 4th edn. London: Mosby; 2003

2. Friedman EA. Labor: Clinical Evaluation and Management, 2nd edn. New York: Appleton-Century-Crofts; 1978

3. Cunningham FG, Leveno KJ, Bloom SL, *et al.* Normal labor and delivery. In: Williams Obstetrics, 22nd edn. New York: McGraw-Hill; 2005:407–42

4. Arrabal PP, Nagey DA. Is manual palpation of uterine contractions accurate? Am J Obstet Gynecol 1996;**174**: 217–19

5. American College of Obstetricians and Gynecologists. Obstetric Care Consensus No 1: Safe prevention of the primary cesarean delivery. Obstet Gynecol 2014;**123**:693–711

6. Ehsanipoor RM, Satin AJ. Overview of normal labor and protraction and arrest disorders. UpToDate. Accessed November 2014

7. Pauli JM, Repke JT. Insertion of intrauterine pressure catheters. UpToDate. Accessed November 2014

Chapter 10

First-stage labor revisited

Although natural birth is a continuous process, labor traditionally has been divided into the first or dilatational stage and the second or expulsion stage with the transition at full dilatation. First-stage labor is conventionally subdivided into the slow "latent" phase up to 3 to 4 cm, followed by the relatively faster "active" phase of labor, and a final "deceleration phase" from 8 to 10 cm dilatation.[1]

These artificial divisions were originally designed to facilitate study and to assist in clinical management. Ironically, however, most problems encountered in the conduct and care of labor arise exactly from these classic subdivisions.

The physiological pattern of dilatation is much simpler than described in most textbooks and guidelines. In effective labor, dilatation progresses in a straight line.

10.1 The fallacy of the latent phase

The persistent idea of "latent labor" or "passive labor" followed by "active labor" is based on the work of Friedman,[2,3] who deserves credit for being pioneer in this field of research more than 60 years ago, but whose conclusions were factually incorrect.

10.1.1 Flawed source studies

Friedman's study included patients with twins, breech presentation, oxytocin, heavy sedation, and a high rate of forceps delivery, and thus did not represent a "normal" population. What is more, the study methodology was severely flawed: prior to the analysis, Friedman had arbitrarily divided the data into three artificial sections – from 0 to 3 cm, from 3 to 8 cm, and from 8 cm to full dilatation, and extrapolated zero dilatation back to time zero. Subsequently, means and standard deviations were calculated, a novelty in those days. Predictably, the separate analysis of three prefixed sections yielded three phases in first-stage labor,

a clear example of a self-fulfilling prophecy. Friedman claimed that the latent phase lasts 8.6 hours on average in nulliparas (+2 SD 20.6 hours), and that the range varies from 1 to 44 hours with a maximum of 20 hours still accepted as statistically normal (sic!).

However, labor and delivery times do not follow a symmetrical distribution, indicating that the use of parametric mathematics (means) is not correct; it falsely lengthens the estimated "normal" duration of labor. Another crucial shortcoming was the lack of a clear diagnosis of labor. Friedman had vaguely defined labor onset as the reported moment "regular" contractions had begun. The decisive significance of full effacement was entirely overlooked. As a result, no distinction was or could be made between "latent" labor and primary dysfunctional labor. This omission, added to the retrospective extrapolation of zero dilatation to time zero, inevitably resulted in an overestimation of the duration of "normal" labor.

The concept of the "latent phase" lacks a scientific basis and should be discarded.

Since the introduction of the "latent" phase, similar mistakes flawed virtually all studies describing early labor or constructing reference labor curves. Moreover, in all studies, the term dilatation was ill-defined, so that cervical accessibility was likely misinterpreted as dilatation (9.1.3). And when the fundamental parameters are poorly defined, the conclusions can be wide of the mark.

Despite the lack of a reliable scientific basis, the concept of the latent phase has been widely accepted and proves to be long-lived. Even authoritative guidelines still fail to question the Friedman doctrine and take the latent phase for granted.[4–6] Guideline-makers quote "evidence" from retrospective survey studies of mainstream practices wherein providers had not defined the diagnosis of labor and had acknowledged a "latent phase."[7] Akin to the original source study, such "evidence" is based on circular reasoning, of course, and thus delusive, however large the studies.

> Dividing first-stage labor into a latent and an active phase constitutes a persistent misconception, invalidating most studies on labor-related issues and blocking competent management of early labor. There is no recognizable latent phase of labor.

10.1.2 The latent phase defeated

Unfortunately, the vague concept of the latent phase has taken on a life of its own and blocked the understanding and management of early labor for a long time. Apart from the misinterpretations and methodological flaws in the reference studies, there are several more arguments for radically erasing the concept of the "latent phase" from our vocabulary and our practice:

- Hendricks *et al.* were the first to dispute the very existence of a latent phase because they carefully observed that contractions in late pregnancy may come and go, and cervical effacement and incipient dilatation – presumed to be typical of the "latent phase" of labor – occur during the final four weeks before women go into labor.[8]
- Most women go into effective labor without any significant warning and with an already completely effaced cervix. In Hendricks' study, the average dilatation of nulliparas at the clinical onset of labor was 2.5 cm while that of multiparas was 3.5 cm.[8]
- The beginning and the end of the presumed latent phase of labor is utterly vague and "defined" as one pleases.
- The notion of a latent phase allows care providers to circumvent the diagnosis of labor. As a result, primary dysfunctional labor is misconstrued as "latent labor." It is the false idea of the latent phase in particular that provides a cover-up excuse for indecision and ambiguity, delaying treatment when it is clearly indicated.
- These omissions are the most common and persistent shortcomings in conventional birth care, leading to unnecessarily long labors with all the related complications.
- Little wonder that acceptance of a (long) "latent phase" (viz. neglect of a clear diagnosis of labor) is strongly associated with poor outcomes: more

fetal distress, more maternal exhaustion and dissatisfaction, more interventions, and more operative deliveries.[9–18]

For these reasons, we had better dismiss the concept of the latent phase entirely, and use, instead, strict criteria – based on accurately defined parameters – to assess the clinical onset of labor, as well as adequate progression (Section 3).

> The latent phase of labor is a persistent echo from the past, and it is prudent to discontinue the clinical use of this misguided and misleading concept altogether.

10.2 The S-shaped reference curve refuted

Separate analysis of three artificial sections (Friedman's research and nearly all studies thereafter) predictably created the illusion of a sigmoid dilatation curve. Friedman stated: "a characteristic pattern for the first stage of labor [becomes manifest] when cervical dilatation is graphed against time. [The average dilatation curve] takes on the shape of a sigmoid curve: a relatively flat latent phase, followed by the acceleration phase, a steep phase of maximum slope, and ending in a deceleration phase."[3] As so often in a new field of research, first ideas, once introduced, tend to persist, despite later emergence of convincing counter-arguments. Indeed, the classic Friedman curve is still reproduced today in most textbooks, manuals, and official guidelines as the reference curve of "normal labor", despite the abundance of evidence of its invalidity.

10.2.1 No deceleration phase

The sigmoid curve is incorrect at both ends. Friedman had included patients with dysfunctional labor in the computation of his reference curve and, therefore, the graph inevitably flattened out in its final proportion. The curve thus computed is clearly not representative of the mean *normal* cervical dilatation curve. A recent retrospective US study by the 'Consortium on Safe Labor' analyzed labor progression in 62,415 singleton term first labors with spontaneous onset, cephalic presentation, vaginal delivery, and a normal perinatal outcome, and used more correct statistics: repeated-measures analysis with interval-censored regression, stratified by cervical dilatation centimeter by centimeter.[7] Apart from the omission of a strict diagnosis of labor and unjust recognition of a latent phase that flawed this study too, the researchers found a linear or continuously accelerating dilatation rate beyond 6 cm, disproving the S-shaped curve. In conclusion, there is no deceleration phase in normal first-stage labor, only in abnormal labor.

> When dilatation is graphed against time, normal progress is linear or accelerative.

Several reference labor graphs have been published since the work of Friedman, and the principal difference between these graphs is contingent on when labor is determined to begin.[19] When a latent phase is excluded, a remarkable similarity of individual labor curves becomes apparent, with dilatation proceeding in a straight or even accelerative line to full dilatation. ACOG Task Force on Cesarean Delivery Rates respectfully concluded a systematic review with the understatement: "the [S-shaped] Friedman curve may not be as applicable today as it once was thought to be."[20]

> The characteristics of first-stage labor are far less complex than suggested by the sigmoid dilatation reference curve; there is no latent phase, and there is no deceleration phase in normal labor. Furthermore, normal labor is short.

10.3 Duration of labor

Our perception of the duration of labor may be clouded not only by the alleged latent phase but also by the many clinical variables and routine measures that disturb the natural course of labor in modern maternity units (Chapters 3 and 4). As a result, conflicting views on the "normal" duration of labor dominate fruitless debates (Chapter 5).

10.3.1 Deluding studies

Several studies[4,7,21,22] have attempted to define the boundaries distinguishing between a normal and an abnormal duration of labor, but have proved to be pointless exercises. The upper limit for "normality" varied significantly because of divergences in the definition of labor onset and the inclusion or exclusion of an ill-defined "latent phase". Moreover, no single study allowed all labors to continue endlessly without any intervention. There was a wide variance in the time criteria used for starting oxytocin treatment or other measures such as operative delivery. These interventions influence the subject under investigation. Added to that, most studies used incorrect mathematics with means and standard deviations in skewed distributions.

10.3.2 Confirmation bias

As ever, when the science is complicated, the confirmation bias tends to kick in to suit ideological convictions and to claim vocational domains. This form of bias directs the mind to seek and find confirming facts and ignore disconfirming evidence. Even official agencies issuing "evidence-based" guidelines neglect the methodological errors in the studies meta-analyzed, in order to reach a politically correct compromise in otherwise incompatible points of view. NICE, for instance, shows no compunction in pooling the above-mentioned sloppy studies and concludes – against its better judgment – "first ['established'] labors last on average 8 hours and are unlikely to last over 18 hours. Subsequent labors last on average 5 hours and are unlikely to last over 12 hours."[4]

As a meta-analysis cannot be stronger than the studies that contribute to it, these statements clearly do not hold water. Unfortunately, when given an official status in authoritative guidelines, such false contentions look convincing to uncritical readers and are readily accepted, effectively blocking progress in the understanding and professional management of labor.

> Statements in official guidelines on the "normal" duration of labor are based on a non-sensus consensus, rather than on solid science.

Computing percentiles – the best approach when analyzing asymmetrical distributions – offers no solution, as virtually no births in the upper quartile of labor duration are completed without extraneous measures. An alternative method is in analogy with the approach in a marathon or long cycle race, where a "broom-wagon" sweeps up the stragglers who are unable to make it to the finish in time. The maximum time permitted is then usually defined as twice the time span in which half of all contenders have reached the finish. In the context of labor, it should be noted that half of all nulliparas who deliver their baby spontaneously under (Dutch) midwifery care give birth within six hours without any form of medical intervention.[23] This means that a labor lasting $2 \times 6 = 12$ hours could or should be accepted as being "normal".

10.3.3 Acceptable labor duration

Evidently, the definition of "normal" duration of labor remains an argument that cannot be resolved satisfactorily. Therefore, we had better define a clinical norm for the length of labor that is acceptable, rather than searching in vain for an arbitrary reference to a "normal" duration. What is clear is that the longer the labor lasts, the more complications gradually arise. Long labor is associated with more fetal distress, more infections, more postpartum hemorrhages, and poorer neonatal outcomes.[9–18] Most importantly, the longer the labors, the more frequent the need for surgical intervention simply because, with the passage of time, women increasingly fail to cope and to deliver by themselves. The high operative delivery rates today attest to this problem.

> Any attempt to define the range of "normal" labor duration is a mission impossible. Therefore, we had better define what duration is acceptable in terms of safety for mother and child, and women's gratification: a limit of 12 hours is a reasonable choice.

The impact of labor duration must be evaluated as much in emotional as in physical terms. The current intrapartum cesarean rates mainly reflect how long modern women (or providers) are willing to let labor continue. Although some women are already unduly perturbed at the point of admission, and others remain apparently unmoved after many hours have passed, most fall somewhere between these extremes. Nowadays, the majority of women typically endure the strain and pain of labor well for between five and seven hours. If a woman is well prepared and well supported and cared for, it is unlikely she will panic. As time passes, however, physical and emotional strength begins to weaken perceptibly. After 10 hours in pain, morale typically deteriorates exponentially. When the end is not yet in sight, a stage may be reached "in which the adult woman is reduced to pleading with anyone standing by for deliverance unless she is lulled into a would-be sense of security by epidural analgesia or rendered semiconscious by powerful sedatives into a degrading state of indifference."[24] Desperation, dehydration, salt depletion, ketoacidosis, and a humiliating loss of decorum complete her total disablement. The effects of such a trauma are likely to remain with her for the rest of her life (2.4.1).

> All relevant outcomes incrementally deteriorate with the length of labor. In emotional terms, a labor lasting 12 hours is close to or well beyond acceptability to most women.

Clearly, it is high time to replace "natural" and "normal" as our criteria for good practice in midwifery and obstetrics with an open concept of the good.[25] The physical and emotional impact provides the rationale for a prospective, safe, and woman-friendly standard for the duration of first-stage labor: 10 hours at the most. A policy aimed at this target ensures that women preserve their physical and emotional strength needed for a successful second stage. The whole process of labor and delivery is completed this way within the timeframe of 12 hours. As adequate dilatation proceeds at least in a straight line, progress in first-stage labor should be at least 1 cm/h from the very onset of labor. Slower progress should be accelerated without delay (Section 3).

> **Key point**
>
> An upper boundary of 10 hours for first-stage labor is a sensible, safe, and women-friendly policy objective. By implication, adequate progress is best defined as a minimum dilatation rate of 1 cm/h from the very start.

10.4 Fundamental biophysical reassessment

The S-shaped curve, found in most textbooks as the reference for "normal labor", lacks a scientific base and is confusing. Slow progress in early labor should not be considered to be "a normal latent phase", and secondary protraction should not be regarded as a "normal deceleration phase." Both signs are birth disorders ("dystocia") albeit different in causation. To really understand first-stage labor and to distinguish a physiological from a pathological course, the defining physics of good labor needs to be explored.

10.4.1 Dynamics and mechanics of labor

For labor to be effective, uterine force has to prevail over cervical resistance. This is initially accomplished by pure traction and, secondarily, by additional thrusting force of the descending fetal head functioning as a wedge (8.5.3). As the shape of the caput is blunt, it can only start to function as a wedge once the occiput enters and passes the dilatation ring, that is to say, once 6–7 cm has been attained.[26] For effective wedging action, progressive descent is needed, which in turn requires adequate driving force.

Initially, descent of the fetal head is not a factor for the progress of dilatation at all. However, completion of the last centimeters to full dilatation requires descent of the presenting fetal part, functioning as a blunt wedge.

Lessons can be learned from observations in the nineteenth century, when pelvic deformations were common (rickets) and hydrocephaly remained undetected until birth. When the fetal head could not possibly descend because of an absolute anatomical obstruction, dilatation progressed smoothly to about 6–7 cm (traction), but after that point progress slowed down and labor arrested (no wedging action).[27,28]

In conclusion, descent into the pelvis is needed for proper wedging action in order to reach full dilatation. And not until 6–7 cm has been reached do the fetopelvic proportions begin to play a role in the progress of labor.

10.4.2 Retraction phase and wedging phase

On these physical grounds, first-stage labor is better subdivided into two phases with its transition at about 6–7 cm (Fig. 10.1). The defining nomenclature is open to debate. We prefer the terms retraction phase and wedging phase because those are concisely factual. Other options could be the initial "dynamic phase" followed by the "mechanical phase" or "descent phase" or "pelvic phase". What label one prefers is not important. The crucial point is that – in the context of the dynamics and mechanics of first-stage labor – two distinct phases can and must be distinguished, with the transition at about 6–7 cm.

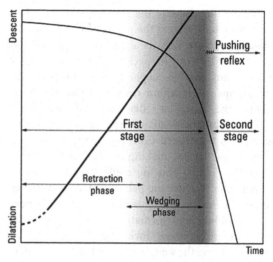

Figure 10.1 Relationship between dilatation and descent. Dilatation proceeds in a straight line. The anatomical fetopelvic proportions play a role in the (shaded) wedging phase only, when the fetal head needs to descend to accomplish full dilatation and, ultimately, to provoke the pushing reflex that marks the onset of the second stage of labor. These re-interpretations differ fundamentally from the classic contentions that wrongly recognize a latent phase and a deceleration phase, mistakenly define the second stage of labor to begin with full dilatation, and regard, in error, the second stage of labor as part of the mechanical (pelvic) phase of birth.

The first stage of labor is subdivided into the "retraction phase" and the "wedging phase", with the transition at 6–7 cm. This distinction, based on the dynamics and mechanics of labor, has significant clinical relevance in difficult labor only.

With effective labor, the transition from retraction phase to wedging phase typically goes unnoticed. In effective labor, dilatation proceeds in a straight line or is even accelerative for the final centimeters (Fig. 10.1). The wedging phase becomes clinically manifest only in *abnormal* labor. In that case, contractions have been strong enough to retract the cervix for 6 to 7 cm, but fail to provoke descent. As a result, progress slows down and may even stop completely. This is called secondary protraction or secondary arrest.

10.4.3 Fetal adaptations to negotiate the birth canal

Wedging action requires force, but the ability of the fetal head to descend also depends upon the cephalopelvic proportions. While the pelvic dimensions are essentially static, those of the fetal head are not. The largest diameter entering the pelvis is determined by the head's absolute size, its ability to mold, and the fetus's ability to bend its neck (flexion). In cases of relatively unfavorable cephalopelvic proportions, even extreme hyperflexion occurs so that the fetus presents the smallest diameter of its head (suboccipito-bregmatic diameter). The posterior fontanel is then positioned centrally in the pelvic axis (*extreme hyperflexion*) making the end of the wedge sharper (less blunt) and more effective. The largest head diameter to enter the pelvis is made as small as necessary by flexion or as possible by extreme hyperflexion. Molding and formation of caput succedaneum further enhances lock and impact on the cervix, enhancing the wedging action needed for dilating the last centimeters.

Compliance of the fetal head requires uterine force. This is a reciprocal phenomenon: substantial caput succedaneum formation, molding, and extreme hyperflexion offer clinical proof that uterine contractions are (or have been) forceful during the wedging phase. The reverse is also true: failure to descend and achieve full dilatation in the absence of these clinical signs indicates that the uterine force is insufficient (Chapter 15).

> Substantial caput succedaneum, molding, and extreme hyperflexion of the fetal head are clinical proof of strong uterine force.

10.4.4 Relationship between dilatation and descent

In the retraction phase, it is exclusively uterine force and cervical resistance that are the key factors for progress. There is no relationship between the degree of descent and the dilatation velocity of the first 6–7 cm. Force is the course (8.5).

Consequently, slow progress in the retraction phase is a purely dynamic labor disorder that must be treated accordingly: by enhancement of uterine force using amniotomy and oxytocin. Several factors may be involved, and prevention, early detection, and expert treatment will be elaborated in detail in Chapters 15 and 21. Crucial for now is the notion that mechanics does not play any role yet. Slow dilatation of the first 6 centimeters has nothing to do whatsoever with birth obstruction.

> Slow progress of the first 6 centimeters (retraction phase) is a purely dynamic labor disorder that must be treated accordingly. Mechanics does not play any role yet.

However, completing the last centimeters requires adequate wedging action, which in turn requires compatible cephalopelvic proportions as well as adequate thrusting force. In other words, anatomical proportions between the fetal head and the bony pelvis only play a role in the progression of birth in the wedging phase of first-stage labor (Fig. 10.1): from about 6 cm to the natural start of expulsion, never earlier and rarely later.

So, secondary slowing down beyond 6 cm indicates inadequate wedging action that may be caused either by dynamic or by mechanical problems or a combination of both. The station, presence or absence of substantial molding, caput succedaneum formation, and hyperflexion will provide the clinical information needed to distinguish between suboptimal dynamics (force) and anatomical obstruction (mechanics).

> Mechanical birth obstruction will manifest itself only in the wedging phase beyond 6 centimeters in the form of a secondary protraction and arrest, never earlier.

As anatomical deformities of the pelvis are extremely rare nowadays, birth obstruction is uncommon, occurring in fewer than 1% of all labors (Chapter 27). Obstructed labor may be caused by either malposition (asynclitism, deflexion attitude) or cephalopelvic disproportion (CPD). Expert diagnosis and treatment will be discussed in Chapter 22.

10.5 Transition from the first to the second stage

At the beginning of the wedging phase (6–7 cm), the fetal head is still relatively high in the pelvis (Fig. 10.1) with the caput in the transverse or diagonal position (Fig. 11.1 in the next chapter).[26] The fetal head only then begins to descend, wedging the cervix further open to full dilatation. Neither the parturient nor her attendant is aware of any significant change at that point. Indeed, the fact that the cervix has attained full dilatation passes entirely unnoticed, unless a chance vaginal examination is performed at this juncture.

10.5.1 Obsolete definition

Unfortunately, leading textbooks and official guidelines still mark full dilatation as the onset of the second stage of labor. This definition goes back to the Victorian era when nothing could be done to improve uterine force, and cesarean section was life-threatening to the mother. Hence, the approach to slow labor was expectant by default, and full dilatation – finally! – marked the point from which difficult labor could be resolved by high rotational forceps delivery.

10.5.2 Natural demarcation point

The obsolete definition of second-stage onset may lead modern care providers to instruct the woman to begin active pushing at full dilatation, even if she does not feel any inclination to do so. Here, obstetrics and midwifery stray far from biology. Full dilatation is not an end in itself nor is it a natural demarcation line between the first and the second stage of labor. In nature, no laboring mammal knows when she is fully dilated and neither do women who deliver their babies without professional help – in historical perspective all our female ancestors until recently.

> *Any interval between the chance assessment of full dilatation and the activation of the irresistible pushing reflex still belongs to the wedging phase of the first stage of labor.*

Every woman does, however, invariably notice the cataclysmic sensation provoked by the descending fetal head the moment it impacts on her pelvic floor. This arouses an uncontrollable reflex that compels her to bear down. Naturally, the second stage of labor begins at the moment the irresistible pushing reflex is activated, not earlier. This occurs initially at the top of the contractions when the fetal head reaches the level of the ischial spines to which parts of the levator ani muscle are attached (0-station).[26] Once the fetal head reaches the pelvic floor (and is visible when the labia are spread), the expulsion reflex usually becomes irrepressible during the whole length of the contractions, owing to enormous pressure on the rectum. It is not until the wedging action effects full dilatation and propels the head deep enough to activate the irresistible pushing reflex that the wedging phase ends and second-stage labor begins (Fig. 10.1).

> *It is not full dilatation that marks the transition from first- to second-stage labor, but the occurrence of the reflexive, irresistible urge to push after full dilatation has been reached.*

At the start of the true second stage of labor, the fetal head is by definition deep and fully engaged, meaning that its largest diameter has well-passed the pelvic inlet (Fig. 11.1 in the next chapter). Since a compatible pelvic inlet almost invariably implies an adequate mid-pelvis and pelvic outlet, functional pelvic capacity is now virtually proven, and a safe vaginal delivery is a near-certainty. From this point, the anatomical proportions do not play a decisive role anymore. Women who are carrying an exceptionally large baby or who have an exceptionally small pelvis (contracted pelvis) cease progressing at 6–7 cm and never reach the true expulsion stage (Chapter 22). The only resistance that remains to be conquered in true second-stage labor is that of the pelvic soft tissues (Chapter 11). In conclusion, the "mechanical" or "pelvic" phase represents the last phase of the first stage of labor and does not transgress into the second stage of labor (Fig. 10.1 and Table 10.1).

> *Once the true second stage of labor has been attained, the only remaining resistance lies in the pelvic soft tissues.*

10.5.3 Redefining passive and active labor

The persistent use of obsolete definitions and confusing terminology has greatly impeded improvements in the understanding and supervision of labor for many years. As demonstrated above, the classic distinction between "passive labor" (the "latent phase") and "active labor" (beyond 3–4 cm) lacks any scientific foundation and should be rigorously abandoned.

From a biological point of view, it is far more logical to distinguish between a *passive* first stage (dilatation and descent) and an *active* second stage of labor (expulsion). This re-definition is much more in accordance with biology and the mother's perception and instinctive behavior. At the transition, her hitherto passive role in labor – in terms of working to birth her child – suddenly changes by the natural expulsion reflex to active hard work in which she delivers her baby (Chapter 11).

Table 10.1 Physical factors that determine the progression of labor

FIRST (PASSIVE) STAGE	**Dynamics**: in both retraction and wedging phases	– Uterine force – Cervical resistance – Transmission of force onto the cervix
	Mechanics: in wedging phase only	– Pelvic size and structure – Dimensions and attitude of the fetal head – Compliance of the fetal head
SECOND (ACTIVE) STAGE	**Dynamics**:	– Force from the abdominal muscles – Uterine force – Resistance of the pelvic soft tissues

Fundamental redefinition

Labor is best divided into the passive first stage and the active second stage with the occurrence of the expulsion reflex beyond full dilatation as the transition point.

10.6 Parity and resistance-to-force ratios

In terms of physics, it is the ratio of resistance to force that determines whether or not labor will progress smoothly. This holds for both stages of the birthing process (Table 10.1).

Importantly, this ratio differs significantly between first and subsequent labors. A first labor is longer, because inefficient uterine contractions are common and the soft tissue resistance is significantly higher than that of its parous counterpart (8.6). This applies equally to the resistance of the cervix in the first stage and to the resistance of the vagina, pelvic floor, and vulva in the second stage.

The relatively high resistance-to-force ratio explains why dynamic dystocia is common in all stages and phases of nulliparous labor. In contrast, parous women do not suffer from ineffective labor to a significant extent, unless their labor was induced (8.8.2).

In first labors, secondary protraction and arrest may be indicative of fetal obstruction, but insufficient force is still the most likely explanation (Chapter 21). In contrast, the parous uterus is a highly efficient organ in exerting force, and cervical resistance is relatively low. Hence, the cause of secondary protraction of parous labor should be sought primarily with anatomical obstruction (Chapter 22).

Clearly, a strict distinction between nulliparous and parous labors is crucial for intelligent and safe

labor care. Thorough understanding of the dynamics and mechanics of labor will further guide expert diagnosis and management in cases of secondary protraction and arrest disorders (Section 3).

References

1. Cunningham FG, Leveno KJ, Bloom SL. Section IV. Labor and delivery. In: Williams Obstetrics, 22nd edn. New York: McGraw-Hill; 2005:423

2. Friedman EA. The graphic analysis of labor. Am J Obstet Gynecol 1954;**68**:1568–75

3. Friedman EA. Labor: Clinical Evaluation and Management, 2nd edn. New York: Appleton-Century-Crofts; 1978

4. NICE Guidelines. Intrapartum care: care of healthy women and their babies during childbirth. 2007. RCOG Press. Updated 2010 www.nice.org.uk/guidance/cg55

5. American College of Obstetricians and Gynecologists. ACOG Practice Bulletin Number 49, December 2003. Dystocia and augmentation of labor. Obstet Gynecol 2003;**106**:1445–53

6. American College of Obstetricians and Gynecologists. Obstetric Care Consensus No 1: Safe prevention of the primary cesarean delivery. Obstet Gynecol 2014;**123**:693–711

7. Zhang J, Landy HJ, Branch DW, *et al.* (Consortium on Safe Labor). Contemporary patterns of spontaneous labor with normal neonatal outcomes. Obstet Gynecol 2010;**116**:1281–7

8. Hendricks CH, Brenner WE, Kraus G. Normal cervical dilatation pattern in late pregnancy and labor. Am J Obstet Gynecol 1970;**106**:1065–82

9. Maghoma J, Buchmann EJ. Maternal and fetal risks associated with prolonged latent phase of labor. J Obstet Gynaecol 2002;**22**:16–19

10. Friedman EA, Neff RK. Labor and delivery: impact on offspring. PSG, Littleton, MA (1987)

11. Chelmow D, Kilpatrick SJ, Laros RK. Maternal and neonatal outcomes after prolonged latent phase. Obstet Gynecol 1993;**81**:486–91

12. Cheng YW, Shaffer BL, Bryant AS, Caughey AB. Length of the first stage of labor and associated perinatal outcomes in nulliparous women. J Obstet Gynaecol 2010;**116**:1127–35

13. Malone FD, Geary M, Chelmow D, *et al.* Prolonged labor in nulliparas: lesson from the active management of labor. Obstet Gynecol 1996;**88**:211–15

14. Gharoro EP, Enabudoso EJ. Labor management: an appraisal of the role of false labor and latent phase on the delivery mode. J Obstet Gynecol 2006;**26**:534–37

15. Jackson DB, Lang JM, Ecker J, Swartz WH, Heeren T. Impact of collaborative management and early admission in labor on method of delivery. J Obstet Gynecol Neonatal Nurs 2003;**32**:147–57

16. Bailit, JL, Dierker LR, Blanchard MH, Mercer BM. Outcome of women presenting in active versus latent phase of spontaneous labor. Obstet Gynecol, 2005;**105**:77–9

17. Holmes P, Oppenheimer LW, Wen SW. The relationship between cervical dilatation at initial presentation in labor and subsequent interventions. Br J Obstet Gynaecol 2001;**108**:1120–24

18. Hemminki E, Simukka R. The timing on hospital admission and progress of labor. Eur J Obstet Gynecol Reprod Biol 1986;**22**:85–94

19. Cunningham FG, Gant NF, Leveno KJ. Section V. Abnormal labor. In: Williams Obstetrics, 21st edn. New York: McGraw-Hill; 2001:425–67

20. American College of Obstetricians and Gynecologists. ACOG Practice Bulletin Number 49, December 2003. Dystocia and augmentation of labor. Obstet Gynecol 2003;**106**:1445–53

21. Neal JL, Lowe NK, Patrick TE, Cabbage LA, Corwin EJ. What is the slowest-yet-normal cervical dilation rate among nulliparous women with spontaneous labor onset? J Obstet Gynecol Neonatal Nurs 2010;**39**:361–9

22. Neal JL, Lowe NK, Ahijevych KL, *et al.* "Active labor" duration and dilation rates among low-risk, nulliparous women with spontaneous labor onset: a systematic review. J Midwifery Womens Health 2010;**55**:308–18

23. Perinatal Care in the Netherlands 2012 (in Dutch) Stichting Perinatale Registratie Nederland. www.peri natreg.nl

24. O'Driscoll K, Meagher D, Robson M. *Active Management of Labour*, 4th edn. London: Mosby; 2003

25. Robson M, Hartigan L, Murphy M. Methods of achieving and maintaining an appropriate caesarean section rate. Best Pract Res Clin Obstet Gynaecol 2013;**27**:297–308

26. Graseck A, Tuuli M, Roehl K, *et al.* Fetal descent in labor. Obstet Gynecol 2014;**123**:521–6

27. Sellheim H. Die Beziehungen des Geburtskanales und des Geburtsobjectes zur Geburtsmechanik. Leipzig: Thieme; 1906 (in German)

28. De Snoo K. Beknopt leerboek der verloskunde. Groningen: Wolters; 1910 (in Dutch)

Second-stage labor redefined

From the biological point of view, most aspects of human birth discussed so far can be compared with those seen in other higher mammalian species. The unique characteristic of human birth – not found in any other species – concerns second-stage labor and is an anatomical one: the internal and external rotation of the fetal head during the expulsion. Rotation is an adaptation to the curved birth tract that resulted from our upright posture.[1] Even apes have a more or less straight birth canal, and rotation of the fetal head does not occur in the birth of these higher primates.[2]

11.1 Passage through the osseous and soft parts

Successful completion of the wedging phase of first-stage labor and arrival at the natural and true expulsion stage (10.5) provide clinical proof of adequate pelvic capacity. The largest diameter of the fetal head has well passed the pelvic inlet, and the entire skull is now in the pelvis (Fig. 11.1). Apart from vanishingly rare cases with a selective pelvic outlet contraction, a safe vaginal birth is now a near-certainty. From this point forward, the woman has only to overpower the resistance of her pelvic soft tissues (Fig. 11.2), which admittedly requires enormous force in the first labor. Failure to accomplish a smooth and safe expulsion is a dynamic problem, not a mechanical disorder.

At the start of the true expulsion stage, the entire fetal head is already in the pelvis. Anatomical proportions no longer play a decisive role. Expulsion is a matter of force.

11.1.1 Pelvic adequacy

Proximal to the pelvic floor, the pelvic bone structure defines the pelvic capacity. At the pelvic floor, the birth canal curves 90° under the pubic bone. From this point forward, it is exclusively the soft tissue compartment of the vagina, pelvic floor, perineum, and vulva that bounds the birth tract (Fig. 11.2).

The normal position of the occiput at the onset of second-stage labor is in the transverse or oblique diameter (Fig. 11.1). The combined force of the uterus and abdominal muscles propels the fetal head further down and through the opening of the levator ani. At this deep point, which marks the pelvic floor, the rectangular curve of the birth canal provokes the internal rotation of the fetal head, followed by extension (deflexion).

11.1.2 Internal rotation and extension

Imagine trying to insert a flexible hose into a stiff pipe with a distant right angle. The hose will get stuck at the rectangular curve unless its end has been cut diagonally. When this is done, the outer cut end will automatically take the inside turn.[3,4] This same

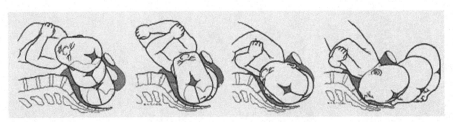

Figure 11.1 Descent and cardinal movements of the fetal head. The occiput turns into the anterior position at the pelvic floor, not earlier. Beyond this point, the only resistance left lies in the soft tissues. The head is born through extension (deflexion).

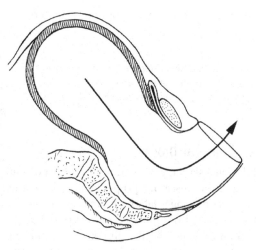

Figure 11.2 Transition of the osseous and soft part of the birth canal at the pelvic floor, where the axis of the birth canal (arrow) curves 90° as it passes under the pubic bone.

principle of plumber's physics applies to the asymmetrical fetal head.

> *The fetal head rotates to the anterior position on the pelvic floor at the intersection of the bony and soft tissue portions of the birth canal. The resistance during expulsion lies exclusively in the stretchy pelvic floor, vagina, perineum, and vulva.*

The fetal head has an eccentric outer pole – typically the occiput – and the birth tract makes a right angle at the pelvic floor. At this deep level, the propulsive forces and the direction of the soft birth canal impose the internal rotation (Fig. 11.1). Since the soft birth canal is oriented upward (in the view shown in Fig. 11.1), extension (deflexion) must occur before the head can pass through it. The expulsive forces push the head against the pelvic floor, forcing the head's extension (deflexion), which brings the base of the occiput into direct contact with the inferior margin of the pubic bone (Fig. 11.1). As the fetal head pushes on the soft division of the birth canal, the perineum begins to bulge visibly, and the anus becomes greatly stretched. With increasing distension of the vulva, the head is born by further extension.

The dynamics of expulsion

$$\text{Effective expulsion} = \frac{\text{Force of uterus and voluntary muscles}}{\text{Resistance of pelvic soft tissues}}$$

Because the above ratio is much more favorable in women who previously gave birth by the vaginal route (higher numerator, smaller denominator), the expulsion is significantly shorter in parous labor than in nulliparous labor. With expert conduct and care, multiparas hardly ever need assistance with forceps or vacuum (<1%, see Chapter 27).

11.1.3 Maternal position

In most hospitals, women are encouraged to deliver their babies in the supine position, which is actually quite unnatural. The supine position is so common now that caregivers and mothers alike do not recognize it for the intervention it is.

The most common positions for delivery cited in the anthropological literature are squatting, kneeling, and sitting.[2] Squatting during childbirth is common in cultures in which women spend considerable portions of their time in a squatting position while cooking, caring for infants, and conducting other activities.[5] In western societies, however, very few women have the stamina to remain in this position for the time usually required to deliver a child, and a specially designed pillow or birthing stool might be helpful. The supported squatting position might increase intra-abdominal pressure and allow a woman's expulsive efforts to work with gravity. Furthermore, this position orients the pelvic outlet more horizontally to facilitate easy extension, crowning, and expulsion.[6,7]

These claims were supported by a randomized controlled trial that showed squatting shortened second-stage labor as compared with the recumbent position and significantly reduced both instrumental delivery rates and perineal tears while infant outcomes were similar.[8]

> *There is no justification for requiring or actively encouraging a supine position in second-stage labor.*

Clearly, the best policy is to allow each woman to deliver her baby in a position in which she feels most comfortable. It should be noted that an epidural block seriously restricts her options in this regard.

11.1.4 Duration of expulsion

As long as the baby is fine, and the woman is making progress, there is no reason to intervene based on the passage of time alone. Besides, when the start of active pushing is properly timed – taking full advantage of the expulsion reflex – the second stage of labor is short. Half of all nulliparas (without an epidural) in our hospital deliver their babies spontaneously within 35 minutes and 95% within an hour. Expulsion in parous labors is even considerably shorter.

11.2 Pitfalls, obsolete tenets, and misconceptions

Some ideas and actions are so commonplace in conventional care that their disturbing effects on the natural course of labor and delivery are hardly ever recognized.

11.2.1 Wrong diagnosis

Although full dilatation often coincides with the initiation of the natural reflex to bear down, this is not always so. In that case, the fetal head is still at relatively high station and the active expulsion stage has – by definition – not yet begun.

Yet, many birth care professionals instruct the woman to start pushing in the absence of the natural expulsion reflex, just because the cervix no longer presents an obstacle. As the fetal head is still at high station, her unnatural and thus premature efforts to deliver her baby then become unnecessarily long and difficult. She is likely to waste her energy and resolve. The ensuing slow progress and progressive exhaustion – both physically and emotionally – may then lead to a failed expulsion that has to be resolved by instrumental delivery. Indeed, many vaginal operative deliveries are avoided when pushing is not forced until the natural expulsion reflex is activated (Chapter 27).

> Premature pushing before the natural expulsion reflex is activated leads to an unnecessarily long expulsion effort, exhaustion, and instrument-assisted delivery.

Clearly, as long as a woman feels no urge to push after reaching full dilatation, she is still in the first stage of labor and should not be encouraged to bear down at this point. Continued absence of the pushing reflex at full dilatation is a problem in the first stage of labor and must be treated accordingly. The first step in nulliparous labor is improving uterine force using oxytocin. If this fails to give the desired effect, a cesarean section is the only safe option (Chapters 17, 21, 22).

> Waiting for deep descent and the natural expulsion reflex to occur before the commencement of active pushing effectively reduces instrumental deliveries.

11.2.2 Epidural block

Epidural analgesia suppresses the natural expulsion reflex, thereby obfuscating proper diagnosis of the onset of second-stage labor. Premature pushing, topped by impaired voluntary muscle action, explains why an epidural lengthens the (ill-defined) expulsion stage substantially and why it leads to more instrumental deliveries (RR 1.42, 95% CI 1.28 to 1.57, 23 trials, 7935 women) as evidenced by the Cochrane review.[9]

Another meta-analysis showed an increased rate of spontaneous vaginal delivery in women with an epidural when pushing was delayed compared with immediate pushing at assessment of full dilatation (61.5% compared with 56.9%, pooled RR 1.09, 95% CI 1.03–1.15) but, obviously, operative delivery rates were high in both groups.[10]

> Epidural analgesia thwarts proper diagnosis and management of second-stage labor and is strongly associated with instrumental delivery.

11.2.3 Inaccuracy of pelvic planes

Traditionally, fetal descent is estimated with reference to imaginary pelvic planes. The mid-pelvic plane (0-station) is then regarded as the demarcation line between vaginal or abdominal operative delivery when second-stage labor fails to progress. However, the use of pelvic planes echoes an obsolete mechanistic view of birth and should be abandoned.

Station assignment is notoriously imprecise with a wide inter-observer variability.[11,12] Substantial molding and caput succedaneum aggravate the inaccuracy. The deepest part of the fetal head may appear to have passed 0-station while its largest diameter is still above the pelvic inlet. In such a case, a foolhardy attempt to deliver the baby by forceps or vacuum can be genuinely traumatic because the functional capacity of the pelvis is still uncertain, and the vagina and pelvic floor are not yet stretched. If rotation and extraction are undertaken, the obstetrician has to pull hard, often too hard, and practice shows that once an effort at instrumental extraction is begun it is very difficult to stop. In such a case, both mother and baby would have been much better off if the woman had not reached full dilatation at all.

> The use of pelvic planes to assess descent and to decide between vaginal or abdominal operative delivery is fraught with imprecision and should be abandoned.

11.2.4 Safe instrumental delivery

An absolute prerequisite for a safe instrumental vaginal delivery is full engagement of the fetal head, meaning that its largest diameter has passed the pelvic inlet and that the entire fetal skull is in the pelvis (Fig. 11.1). Station assignment is not reliable in this regard. Full engagement can only be reliably assessed by bimanual examination during a contraction interval. One hand softly grabs above the pubis and shakes gently. Whenever the exterior hand can palpate the fetal head or the probing fingers in the vagina feel any movement, the largest diameter has not yet passed the pelvic inlet. In that case, an instrumental delivery is unsafe for mother and child. In obese women, the same information can be obtained with a supra-pubic ultrasound trans-section made parallel to the pelvic inlet.[13]

> The deciding criterion for allowing delivery by instrumental traction is descent of the largest diameter of the fetal head past the pelvic inlet.

11.2.5 Confusing misnomers

The diagnosis "transverse arrest" should be discarded. It is a misnomer attributable to a lack of understanding of the natural process of descent and rotation during the course of normal expulsion. To orthodox obstetricians the term seems to imply a mechanical obstruction, which should be resolved by manual correction, rotational forceps, or mid-pelvic vacuum extraction.[14,15]

In reality, however, the fetal head is normally in the transverse or oblique diameter of the pelvis when entering the second stage of labor. Internal forward rotation takes place at the pelvic floor, not earlier

(Fig. 11.1). Failure to rotate should be interpreted as an expression of inadequate driving force, and this should be treated accordingly with oxytocin (Chapter 21). Transverse arrest is a problem in the dynamics, not the mechanics of birth; "it is not the cause of the delay but rather the result."[16]

> Internal rotation and subsequent extension of the fetal head are a matter of force. Failure of the cardinal movements to occur does not result in but results from protracted expulsion.

Sonographic studies have shown that two-thirds of all children born with occiput posterior were occiput anterior in first-stage labor.[17] So, from a physics perspective, the expression "faulty internal rotation" is also nonsense. Whenever the fetal head is not flexed, i.e. when the sinciput presents (referred to as "neutral," or "military" attitude) at the moment it reaches the transition of the osseous and soft birth canal, it is the large fontanel that rests in the pelvic axis. In such a position, the expulsive force coerces the fetal head to turn face toward the pubis and the head is born with occiput posterior. This is a physiological phenomenon when the fetal head presents in a sincipital attitude.[18,19]

> The term "faulty internal rotation" is a misnomer.

11.3 Promoting spontaneous delivery

Since the social conditions that gave rise to rickets were eradicated almost a century ago, nearly all women in the post-industrialized world now have a normally shaped pelvis. Therefore, once the true active expulsion stage is reached, mechanical feto-pelvic proportions no longer play any decisive role for the completion of birth. Once the expulsion reflex is activated by deep descent of the fetal head, anatomical obstruction is virtually excluded. Failure to progress in accurately defined second-stage labor is a dynamic birth disorder and has little to do with obstruction. This fact is proven time and again by parous mothers, who needed assistance with vacuum or forceps in their first labor, but subsequently give birth by their own strength to equally large or even larger babies.

> *If a baby can be safely delivered by instrumental traction, then it also, in principle, should have been possible by spontaneous propulsion, provided the woman had enough strength and determination left.*

No one will deny that spontaneous delivery is highly preferable to delivery by forceps or vacuum extractor. A spontaneous vaginal delivery significantly contributes to women's satisfaction with the birth experience and is much friendlier and safer for the baby as well.

Key to a successful expulsion is adequate driving force in proportion to the resistance of the pelvic soft tissues. The available power and resolve of the birthing woman depends greatly on the antecedent events. This emphasizes the importance of a smooth, short, and tolerable first stage of labor, in order to preserve sufficient strength for the mother to deliver the baby by her own efforts. The overall birth-plan, specifically designed to offer all laboring women the maximum chance of a spontaneous, safe, and rewarding delivery, is the subject of the third section.

References

1. Naaktgeboren C. The biology of childbirth. In: Chalmers I, Keirse MJNC, Enkin M, eds. Effective Care in Pregnancy and Childbirth, Vol. 2: Childbirth. Oxford: Oxford University Press; 1998

2. Rosenberg K, Trevathan W. Birth: obstetrics and human evolution. Br J Obstet Gynaecol 2002;**109**:1199–206

3. Sellheim H. Die Beziehungen des Geburtskanales und des Geburtsobjectes zur Geburtsmechanik. Leipzig: Thieme; 1906 (in German)

4. De Snoo K. Beknopt leerboek der verloskunde. Groningen: Wolters; 1910 (in Dutch)

5. Trevathan W. Human Birth: An Evolutionary Perspective. New York: Aldine de Gruyter; 1987

6. Russell JPG. Moulding of the pelvic outlet. J Obstet Gynaecol Br Commonw 1969;**76**:817–20

7. Ashford JI. Posture for labor and birth. In: Rothman BK, ed. Encyclopedia of Childbearing. Phoenix, AZ: Oryx Press 1993:313–35

8. Gardosi J, Hutson M, B-Lynch C. Randomised, controlled trial of squatting in the second stage of labour. Lancet 1989;**2**:74–7

9. Anim-Somuah MA, Smyth RM, Jones L. Epidural versus non-epidural or no analgesia in labour. Cochrane Database Syst Rev 2011

10. Tuuli MG, Frey HA, Odibo AO, Macones GA, Cahill AG. Immediate compared with delayed pushing in the second stage of labor: a systematic review and meta-analysis. Obstet Gynecol 2012;**120**:660–8

11. Dupuis O, Silveira R, Zentner A, et al. Birth simulator: reliability of transvaginal assessment of fetal head station as defined by the American College of Obstetricians and Gynecologists classification. Am J Obstet Gynecol 2005;**192**:868–874

12. Buchmann E, Libhaber E. Interobserver agreement in intra-partum estimation of fetal head station. Int J Gynaecol Obstet 2008;**101**:285–9

13. Youssef A, Maroni E, Ragusa A, et al. Fetal head–symphysis distance: a simple and reliable ultrasound index of fetal head station in labor. Ultrasound Obstet Gynecol 2013;**41**:419–24

14. Stitely ML, Gherman RB. Labor with abnormal presentation and position. Obstet Gynecol Clin N Am 2005;**32**:165–79

15. Cunningham FG, Leveno KJ, Bloom SL. Dystocia: abnormal labor and delivery. In: Williams Obstetrics, 22nd edn. New York: McGraw-Hill; 2005

16. O'Driscoll K, Meagher D, Robson M. Active Management of Labour, 4th edn. London: Mosby; 2003

17. Gardberg M, Laakkonen E, Salevaara M. Intrapartum sonography and persistent occiput posterior position; a study of 408 deliveries. Obstet Gynecol 1998;**91**:746–9

18. Pritchard JA, MacDonald PC, eds. Williams Obstetrics, 16th edn. New York: Appleton-Century-Crofts, 1980. Chapters 12 and 16

19. Stitely ML, Gherman RB. Labor with abnormal presentation and position. Obstet Gynecol Clin N Am 2005;**32**:165–79

Chapter 12

Leading principles

"We are all working to one end, some with knowledge and design, others without knowing what they do."
– Marcus Aurelius

The analysis of the ills and challenges in the world of childbirth left no stone unturned (Section 1). Close re-examination of the basic physiology of parturition debunked false dogmas and identified the critical, biological and psychological preconditions required for a safe and rewarding labor and delivery (Section 2). The most significant themes with the most important practical consequences were:

- The notion that labor is a parasympathetic process.
- The importance of personal attention and consistent care.
- The fundamental differences between nulliparous and parous labor.
- A sharp distinction between spontaneous labor and induction.
- Rejection of the ill-founded concept of latent labor.
- Brevity of physiological labor.

The foregoing discussions touched the very heart of childbirth, and implicitly provide the clue to structural improvements: a systematic and real evidence-based approach to labor and delivery, which will be explained in full detail in this section. Before we begin, though, full credit must be given to the original inventors of this method of care.

12.1 The origin

The practical approach explained in the following chapters is largely based on the pioneering work of Kieran O'Driscoll and co-workers.[1] These obstetricians highlighted their concern that too many women were experiencing traumatic deliveries after prolonged labor, suffering greatly because of exhaustion, confusion, and intoxication with analgesic drugs. Recognizing this physical and emotional stress,

they introduced a revolutionary concept of labor care aimed at the rehumanization of birth by intensively supportive care and proactive prevention of long labor.[2]

12.1.1 Conceptual birth care

As his method of care evolved through the 1970s and 1980s in the National Maternity Hospital in Dublin, O'Driscoll was the first obstetrician to recognize and teach that expert labor care, targeted at spontaneous, safe and rewarding delivery, consists of five strongly interdependent components:

1. Pre-labor education of all childbearing women;
2. Personal, one-on-one supportive care for all laboring women;
3. A clear strategy to prevent long labor;
4. Sound labor ward organization;
5. Constant audit of all procedures and outcomes.

With regard to the interventional component, O'Driscoll introduced a purely pragmatic and simple approach, founded on the empirical evidence that "effective uterine action" is the key to spontaneous delivery.[3] He and his co-workers convincingly demonstrated that effective labor can be ensured in nearly all cases, with a very high degree of safety, provided a consistent policy is applied with a small number of rules that can be precisely stated. O'Driscoll named his revolutionary concept the *active management of labor*, highly inspiring in nearly all aspects except for its name.

12.1.2 Misunderstandings and controversy

The name proved to be a source of cognitive dissonance, confusion, and controversy. In the traditional childbirth world, the word "active" is a dirty word, and from the midwife's point of view the natural process of birth should not and cannot be "managed".[4] Prejudice explains why O'Driscoll's original and challenging treatise was hardly read, but disputed all the same on the basis of second- or third-hand information. Orthodox caregivers tend to have closed minds on the subject of labor. Ill-informed detractors even ridiculed the active management as "aggressive management" or "active mismanagement."[5]

> It is prejudice and ignorance that defeated the "active management of labor."

Negative sentiments were most strongly reflected in midwifery publications. One author, for instance, writes: "the assumption that labor and delivery should progress within a medical framework detracts from the uniqueness of each woman's labor."[6] Although such a statement might arise from a genuine concern regarding women's autonomy, it more likely originates in the unfounded assumption that most women do not desire minor interventions to prevent long labor.[7] Another skeptic fulminates: "the active management reduces women to a birth machine" and "puts laboring women on the conveyor belt."[8] Such lampoons bear testimony to ignorance, are wide of the mark, and do great injustice to one of the greatest and most inspiring obstetricians ever. In reality, the integral concept of active management – if applied correctly in all its components – effectively restores the imbalance between natural childbirth and intervention. Readers familiar with the classic treatise by O'Driscoll know that the adjective "active" stands for *proactive* and "*active involvement*, to enhance the experience of childbirth for the normal healthy mother."[2] This goal should be fully endorsed by all right-minded birth care providers worldwide.

12.1.3 Distortion, perversion, confusion

O'Driscoll and co-workers explicitly warned that no single component of their approach can be safely omitted because, like a jigsaw puzzle, the pieces fit snugly together to form a composite picture. However, the truth of the matter is that most followers to date have only adopted the interventional component – early acceleration of slow labor – while neglecting all other critical elements.[9] These key features include adequate pre-labor education, continuous supportive care, a positive attitude and personal commitment of birth attendants, active involvement of consultant-obstetricians in the supervision of first-stage labor, and constant peer review of all procedures and outcomes. A stripped and perverted version simply does not work and may even result in contrary effects.[5,10,11]

In reality, the other supportive elements of care are far more important than the technical procedures, but they cannot be implemented unless early correction of dysfunctional labor is also performed. Misinterpretation became a cause of deep concern. The policy was designed specifically for first labors, and it is this essential characteristic that has been widely ignored. The name "active management" has now come to signify different aspects of what may be broadly described as labor management, including parous labor. Confusion intensified, both in practice and in the literature. Most studies claiming to evaluate the active management differed strongly in their individual components compared with the original concept and, consequently, results were inconclusive about the efficacy in reducing cesarean rates.[9–11] Discussions deviated far from the elementary points O'Driscoll made, and active management finally foundered. His important clinical lessons on how to improve women's childbirth experience fell virtually into oblivion, while his ideas are more relevant today than ever (Section 1). Evidently, in order to distinguish the basic ideas from the misinterpretations and to regain an understanding of the clear benefits, one needs to examine and comprehend the full original concept. The present book elaborates and complements the original ideas and provides the clinical evidence supporting this women-friendly approach to childbirth.

12.1.4 Need for a new name

By now, however, the term "active management" is severely misapplied and widely misused. Aggressive induction protocols, routine amniotomy, excessive use of oxytocin including during parous labor, epidural analgesia, and even operative delivery are actions frequently thought to be synonymous with "active management of labor." Such pervasive misunderstandings led us to the conclusion that the apostrophized name has worn out, proved to be counterproductive, and should be replaced. It was not until we ceased using the name "active management" that the midwives and doctors who work in or refer to our hospital started to listen to the rational arguments, gradually began to cooperate, and finally grew enthusiastic through experience.

12.2 Proactive support of labor

The original active management of labor was purely empirical and authority-based without references ("the Dublin experience").[2] Of course, such an apodictic foundation is no longer acceptable in the present era of evidence-based medicine. It is precisely the confusion and distortion of the original concept, as well as the scientific requirement of providing independent and solid clinical evidence, that justify the present publication.

12.2.1 Justification and rehabilitation

This book advocates the re-birth of the original ideas by showing the urgent need for reforms (Section 1), by demonstrating its natural scientific basis (Section 2), and by providing reliable clinical evidence (this section). It is an effort to rehabilitate the concept and revitalize the guiding mind-lines as a means of promoting spontaneous and safe delivery and enhancing women's labor experience.

Every component will be tested following the precepts of real evidence-based medicine (6.5). Many of O'Driscoll's sharp observations will be cited, paraphrased, or quoted verbatim as his vigorous prose was second to none and cannot be improved. Not to outdo the pioneering master, but to bypass prejudice and cognitive dissonance that might deter exactly those who would benefit most from reading this book, we have given this method of care a more cognitively consonant name: *proactive support of labor.*

12.3 Guiding mind-line

The leading proposition is that most women prefer to give birth by their own efforts and that they want to accomplish this feat in an acceptable manner that is safe for both their babies and themselves. Despite appearances to the contrary at some critical moments, only very few women want to exchange this personal achievement for an operative delivery from the outset. That is why care – in all its aspects – must be directed toward clear and positive guidance to enhance women's self-reliance and confidence. Childbirth is a tremendous challenge, and women should, therefore, begin their labor well-prepared and as mentally and physically fit as possible. Secondly, they should be positively supported and effectively coached throughout the arduous dilatation stage in order to reach the expulsion stage with

enough strength and determination to deliver their child by their own strength. To this end, prevention of long labor is critical.

This leading principle has numerous practical implications for pre-labor guidance and preparation, for intrapartum moral support, and in fact for all aspects of childbirth including education, professionals' working relations, and care organization. It leaves no aspect of childbirth untouched. Since the interplay of the various elements of high-quality care is seldom or never discussed in standard textbooks, we will emphasize time and again the critical importance of providing the whole package of care. All medical and non-medical aspects of high-quality care are inextricably entwined. The following paragraphs give a short synopsis of the essentials.

> **Proactive support of labor**
>
> *To be able to give birth spontaneously, women should begin labor in a fit condition and remain emotionally and physically fit through the dilatation stage, in order to reach the expulsion stage with enough reserves to deliver their child by their own efforts. Personal attention and prevention of long labor are crucial in this respect.*

12.4 Features and benchmarks

While conventional childbirth is culturally shaped and characterized by inconsistencies and lack of standards for the care of normal labor (Section 1), *proactive support of labor* represents a cohesive conceptual framework, universally applicable in any professional birth setting.

12.4.1 Purpose and target group

Promotion of spontaneous and rewarding childbirth by the enhancement of professional labor and delivery skills is the objective. The subject is confined strictly to healthy women carrying a single, term fetus in the cephalic presentation. These women represent the great majority of all pregnancies. The discussion should not be confused by the introduction of severe maternal diseases, hemorrhage, pre-labor fetal compromise, or obstetrical abnormalities, especially those that implicate the fetus as a cause of obstruction such as twins or breech and other malpresentations.

Proactive support is designed specifically for labors of prototypical healthy women, carrying a single, healthy and term fetus in the vertex presentation.

12.4.2 Focus on first labors

No plan for childbirth can possibly be successful unless it starts from the proposition that the first labor is fundamentally different from all subsequent births. The birth of the first child is one of the most profound experiences, for better or worse, in a woman's life. A smooth and gratifying first delivery virtually guarantees that there will be few or no problems in a subsequent birth. In contrast, a traumatic first experience is likely to repeat itself, and a first cesarean delivery heightens the chances of repeat surgery.

The distinction between nulliparous and parous labor is even far more fundamental than is commonly realized: dystocia is frequently observed in nulliparas and is primarily of dynamic origin (and not infrequently iatrogenic). In contrast, dystocia is rare in parous labors, but when it occurs it typically originates in birth obstruction (Chapter 13).

12.4.3 Natural scientific basis

The concept of *proactive support* is firmly rooted in natural science. All the following chapters should be read in constant conjunction with Section 2. Several important issues will be reiterated. This serves to translate the key points into different clinical contexts, and repetition serves educational purposes as well.

12.4.4 Overall birth-plan

Pregnant women see several caregivers for their antenatal and intrapartum care: nurses, birth educators, midwives, obstetricians, sonographers, residents, and interns, in random order. Modern obstetrics is teamwork. Hence, high-quality care has become impossible without a consistent, well-defined plan that all personnel cooperating in one practice should agree to and comply with. A central plan for the conduct and care of labor has nothing to do with artificial regimentation of the natural process of birth.[2] To guard pregnant women against inconsistencies in information and care is a matter of plain common sense and a mark of respect for women.

12.4.5 The "medical" component

Correct diagnosis is the most important item in the rational supervision of labor. This equally applies to the diagnosis of labor onset (Chapter 14) and the diagnosis of ineffective labor (Chapter 15). Detailed causal diagnostics (Chapter 21 and 22) further guides rational strategies for timely treatment of slow labor, before the situation needlessly worsens with exhaustion of both mother and her uterus. The well-defined concept of a "good childbirth experience" (Chapter 10) with prospective criteria for adequate progression is used to replace the utterly vague notion of "normal" labor that can only be defined in retrospect.

Early detection and timely correction of slow labor do not lead to more interventions. Rather, the exact opposite is the case.

12.4.6 Personal attention

Supportive care and safety of mother and child mean that women in labor should never be left alone. To this end, one-on-one companionship in labor is the central component of proactive support and the reason why well-trained nurses, possibly supplemented with certified doulas, are invaluable in providing this method of care (Chapter 16). Personal support also favors parasympathetic control, which is crucial for a smooth and safe birth. The idea of personal involvement also applies to the midwives and obstetricians who are ultimately responsible. These providers should not stay back-stage and run in only when full dilatation has occurred or in the event of an emergency. Every woman in labor should have a personal attendant to support her during the entire labor and delivery. Prevention of long labor has the additional advantage that shift changes for all care providers during any given labor are kept to a minimum. Personal commitment and continuity of staff are key to a rewarding childbirth experience for mothers and caregivers alike.

Personal attention, emotional support, and positive coaching are even more important than the medical policies, but these skills cannot be exerted to their maximum effect unless dysfunctional labor is corrected in time as well.

12.4.7 Coaching

Ideally, a birth attendant is primarily a coach who helps the pregnant woman to access her innate strength and navigate the discomforts of late pregnancy and the exertion of labor. This is in contrast to a doctor or paramedic who "treats" the patient. Thus, some essential components of being a good labor and delivery coach include:

- Properly preparing each woman for her forthcoming labor and delivery;
- Adherence to a simple and mutually consented birth-plan;
- Patiently awaiting the natural onset of labor;
- Providing continuous, personal care;
- Maintaining a positive, motivating attitude during pregnancy and the whole labor;
- Warding against demoralizing remarks and actions from all persons in attendance;
- Preserving safety and acting decisively.

In short, one must be as clear and consistent as possible while conveying the utmost respect for all birthing women and staff who support them.

> *A competent birth attendant is primarily a coach.*

12.4.8 Pre-labor preparation and promises

With the overall plan, any pregnant woman can now be well prepared for the forthcoming labor and can be given two firm guarantees: that she will not be in labor longer than 12 hours and that she will never be left without a midwife, a personal nurse, and/or a doula by her side at all times. These two affirmations completely change the face of women's expectations of labor. Taken together they are at the very heart of the matter, and in practice they are entirely dependent on each other.

> *All medical and non-medical aspects of high-quality care are inextricably entwined.*

Pre-labor education is best provided on an individual basis through consultation with nurses or midwives who have ongoing experience in the delivery ward (Chapter 18). Pre-labor preparation is aimed at reinforcement of women's confidence, and firm promises about labor support, short labor, and availability of effective pain relief should be made. Pre-labor preparation is relevant and effective only if promises made are kept. This means that all care-givers must comply with the central strategy in words and deeds. Modern birth care is teamwork, and teamwork necessitates strict adherence to agreements and shared protocols.

12.4.9 Coping with pain

The pain of labor and delivery puts women's emotional stability to the test. There is no pain and stress from everyday life that is comparable to the physical pains inflicted by the birth of a first child. However, since labor pain is fundamentally different from the pain of wounds or infections, the obstetrical approach must be radically different from the purely medical approach of using analgesic drugs or epidural block (Chapter 19). The best antidote to labor pain is intensive supportive care on a one-on-one basis, and accelerating a slow labor is far more constructive than the provision of medical pain relief alone. The potentially negative impact of medical pain relief on all other aspects of labor should be fully acknowledged (Chapter 20), and a good bedside manner requires an open appreciation of the many other methods for coping with the pain and discomfort of labor.

12.4.10 Restrictive use of induction

Induction of labor wreaks absolute havoc on the experience and outcome of labor. The duration of labor is artificially prolonged, physical and emotional stress both increase, there is a greater demand for analgesia, and operative delivery rates are inflated. What is more, long inductions lay disproportional claim on staff, affecting care for all other women and disrupting the delivery service as a whole. Induction accomplishes the exact opposite of that for which *proactive support of labor* strives. The use of induction should be restricted to strictly selected cases with a genuine medical indication (Chapter 23).

12.4.11 Safety for mother and child

What is good for mothers is mostly good for their babies. Both benefit from care directed toward reducing the possibility of maternal exhaustion, especially when this is typically followed by a potentially traumatic instrumental delivery. Conversely, both mother and child are needlessly harmed by an invasive artificial delivery performed on the basis of an incorrect interpretation of a fetal indication. The dictum "when in doubt, get it out" is all too often put into practice, but it represents an oversimplification of a complex set of problems. It is for this reason that we present a clear and physiological approach to the identification of the fetus truly at risk and the effective prevention of perinatal hypoxic brain injury and associated medico-legal litigation (Chapter 24).

12.4.12 Appropriate working relations

In the final analysis, it is the midwives and labor room nurses who will convert most recommendations into practice. But obstetricians will have to take the lead by creating the proper organization and allowing the conditions needed for nurses and midwives to do their job adequately. With a consistent birth-plan, nurses and midwives no longer remain powerless to influence the course of difficult labor, as the nurse-midwife is authorized to accelerate slow labor according to the strict guidelines (Chapter 17). She no longer suffers unfair criticism, because of the agreed protocols and constant back-up by expert medical staff. Redefinition of professional working relationships and the very existence of a central policy of care greatly enhance team spirit among nurses, midwives, and doctors – dynamics that are a prerequisite for excellent birth care.

12.4.13 Organization

The welfare of mothers and their babies should not depend on the time of the day that labor happens to occur. All women have the right to the same optimal birth care, 24 hours a day and 7 days a week. At the same time, care providers have the right to normal working hours and acceptable workloads. Suggestions for an organization uniting both interests are discussed in Chapter 25.

Poor organization can quickly unravel the best of intentions. In particular, one-on-one nursing throughout labor is often thought to be utopian because of a lack of financial and human resources. However, hospital managers should realize that a substantial reduction in cesarean sections translates into an equal reduction in post-operative care, freeing nurses to work in the delivery rooms. High-quality birth care and sound economics can surely complement one another. Furthermore, the organization should not be subject to territorial disputes between midwives and obstetricians. Mother-centered care should replace provider-centered care (Chapter 25).

12.4.14 Constant audit and quality control

The creation of high-quality care in childbirth is a continuously evolving process that must be maintained by a careful audit of all procedures and outcomes. Meaningful internal audit (at the hospital level) starts with a detailed assessment of all medical and non-medical aspects of care that should initiate modifications where necessary. Quality relates to outcomes, and outcomes guide processes.[12] Crucial components of an effective internal audit cycle will be discussed in detail (Chapter 26).

Meaningful external audit – i.e. benchmarking of intervention rates and outcomes between hospitals and across different birth settings – requires the use of a classification system based on comparable categories of pregnant women. The 10-groups classification, introduced by Robson *et al.*, is internationally recognized as the most appropriate system in this respect.[12] The intervention rates and outcomes in our practice will be presented in that way (Chapter 27). The results incontestably show that the policy framework of *proactive support of labor* reduces cesarean and instrumental delivery rates in a women-friendly fashion and that this method of care is completely safe for mothers and babies.

Proactive support of labor safely enhances women's childbirth experiences and strikes a new balance between optimal maternal and fetal outcomes.

References

1. O'Driscoll K, Jackson RJA, Gallagher JT. Prevention of prolonged labour. Br Med J 1969;2:477–80

2. O'Driscoll K, Meagher D, Robson M. Active Management of Labour, 4th edn. London: Mosby; 2003

3. O'Driscoll K, Stronge JM, Minogue M. Active management of labour. Br Med J 1973;3:135–7

4. Kaufman KJ. Effective control or effective care. Birth 1993;**20**:150–61

5. Olah KS, Gee H. The active mismanagement of labour. Br J Obstet Gynaecol 1996;**103**:729–31

6. Axten S. Is active management always necessary? Modern Midwife 1995;5:18–20

7. Pates JA, Satin AJ. Active management of labor. Obstet Gynecol Clin N Am 2005;**32**:221–30

8. Wagner M. Pursuing the Birth Machine: the Search for Appropriate Birth Technology, Sydney & London: ACE Graphics; 1994

9. Stratton JF. Active management of labour: Standards vary among institutions. Br Med J 1994;**309**:1015 author reply 1016–17

10. Thornton JG. Active management of labour; it does not reduce the rate of caesarean delivery. Br Med J 1996;**313**:378

11. Thornton JG. Active management of labour. Curr Opin Obstet Gynecol 1997;**9**:366–9

12. Robson M, Hartigan L, Murphy M. Methods of achieving and maintaining an appropriate caesarean section rate. Best Pract Res Clin Obstet and Gynaecol 2013;**27**:297–308

Nulliparous versus parous labor

13

Every discourse on the supervision of labor should begin with the fundamental distinction between the first and subsequent births. Strangely enough, leading textbooks and official guidelines hardly ever devote a separate chapter to this important issue. In mainstream practice the conduct of labor is troublingly confused because of misplaced extrapolation of nullipara-specific birth disorders to multiparas and vice versa. In reality, the duration of labor, the nature of labor disorders, and the impact of the birth experience differ so radically between the first and subsequent births that they justify the following striking statement made by O'Driscoll:

> *"Nulliparas and multiparas behave like different biological species in nearly all matters relating to labor and delivery."*[1]

13.1 Unique first experience

A woman may have several children but she becomes a mother only once. The crucial importance of the course and outcome of a woman's first childbirth cannot be overemphasized. The physical and emotional impact of the first experience determines a woman's expectation and attitude to all later births.

A woman with a positive first experience is unlikely to be worried about the next delivery, while the outlook of a woman with a negative birth experience is marred by fears of a repeat performance. The emotional trauma may have serious repercussions outside the narrow range of vision of midwifery and obstetrics as it can haunt a woman for the rest of her life (2.4.1). A traumatic first experience severely undermines mother–child bonding, may affect her marriage, and has occasionally so severely a scarring effect that the woman even decides against having a second child despite earlier plans of having a larger family.

Typically, the residual effect of a traumatic first delivery reveals itself during a pre-conception consultation or early in her second pregnancy in an urgent request for pre-labor commitment to epidural analgesia or even an elective cesarean section. Ironically, a prompt accession to such requests reinforces her fear about labor, for which there is no foundation in clinical practice. The sequence of events in first childbirth is generally not predictive of the course of later births.

> *In contrast to what most people and even care providers assume, a problematic first labor does not provide a prognostic sign for troubles in subsequent births. There is virtually no connection.*

13.2 Parity-specific features

Long, exhausting labor is a problem specific to first labor. In contrast, parous women do not suffer from dysfunctional labor to a significant extent, provided their parasympathetic condition – which is essential for normal birth – has not been destroyed beforehand by the emotional trauma of an ill-managed previous birth.

The message is all too clear: there is only one first birth experience, so invest the utmost in the care of first labor and few or no problems will be encountered in later births. Conversely, the damage inflicted by a low standard of care and attention the first time round is usually irreversible; birth care for multiparas then becomes a futile and never-ending game of catch-up from the start. All the good intentions in a later birth will founder if the woman was emotionally traumatized during her first labor and/or if her uterus was scarred by a previous cesarean section.

> *The greatest risk factor for long labor and related complications is nulliparity.*

13.2.1 Duration of labor

The most distinctive feature of first labor compared with all subsequent births is its duration: the first is the worst. More than any other objective measure, the length of a first labor determines the emotional and physical impact of childbirth. Apart from the susceptibility to lasting psycho-emotional trauma, first-time mothers face a significantly greater risk of sustaining physical injury to themselves and their babies than do parous women. This is directly related to the longer duration of the first labor per se and to the consequently higher rate of intrusive interventions including operative deliveries.

Duration is the key problem of first labors. By implication, prevention of long labor provides the solution for most problems encountered in first labors. Short labor is best accomplished by ensuring sufficient progress from the very start and expert care rests on this proposition. When openly asked, no single expectant woman wishes her forthcoming labor to last longer than 12 hours.

> *Duration is the main problem of first labors, predisposing to operative deliveries and trauma. Prevention of long first labor is key to the solution of most labor problems.*

13.2.2 Nulliparous dynamics versus multiparous mechanics

The difference between troublesome nulliparous labor and difficult parous labor is analogous to the fundamental distinction in physics between labor dynamics and birth mechanics (10.4). The progress disorders frequently found in first labors are nearly without exception primarily rooted in poor dynamics – inefficient and therefore ineffective uterine force in relation to the resistance of the birth tract – and should, therefore, be treated with oxytocin.

In contrast, occasional dystocia in multiparas typically originates in obstruction caused by fetal malposition or relative macrosomia. These rules of thumb may sound rather simple and dogmatic but are, nonetheless, extremely relevant for intelligent and safe practice.

> *The most common cause of labor protraction and arrest disorders in nulliparous labor is insufficient uterine force, whereas dystocia in multiparous labor usually results from mechanical obstruction.*

13.2.3 Fetal distress

The comparatively long duration of first labors presents significantly more risks for firstborns. Compression of the umbilical cord is the most frequent cause of fetal compromise during labor, and the ability of the fetus to bear these intermittent incidents depends strongly on the duration of labor (Chapter 24). The second hazard for the fetus is uterine hypertonia in the intervals between contractions, leading to fetal hypoxia (Chapter 8). This typically occurs when an already exhausted uterus is stimulated with oxytocin (too late), or when labor is being induced (often unnecessarily). The third fetal hazard during labor is intrauterine infection, and the chance of this increases strongly with the duration of labor. Clearly, short first labor benefits babies (Chapter 24).

13.2.4 Birth trauma

Firstborns suffer trauma by manipulation much more frequently than subsequent offspring. In fact, birth injuries to the child or mother can be discussed under one heading: both mainly result from instrumental interventions in first labors, in particular forced traction.[2] This observation underscores the importance of a proactive policy that reduces forceps or vacuum deliveries. Both mothers and babies benefit greatly.

> *The comparatively long duration of first births presents significantly more fetal risks. Firstborns are exposed more and longer to risks of hypoxia, perinatal infection, and traumatic birth injuries.*

13.2.5 Rupture of uterus

The ultimate obstetric trauma is rupture of the uterus. This potentially catastrophic complication is life-threatening to both mother and child and is specific to parous labor.[3,4] The most common cause is a cesarean scar, and the chance of uterine rupture rises significantly when labor is induced or injudiciously stimulated with oxytocin.[5] Clearly, the best way to prevent this obstetric calamity is to avoid cesarean section the first time round.

It should be noted, however, that uterine rupture may occur even in multiparas with an uneventful obstetric history who now experience obstructed labor, and the greater the parity of the woman the greater the vulnerability of her uterus to rupture.[3] In contrast, rupture of a nulliparous uterus is such an exceptional event in western obstetrics that for practical purposes it can be assumed not to occur. Judicious use of oxytocin in first labor does not cause rupture of the uterus even if used to prove or exclude birth obstruction (Chapters 21, 22). This immunity from uterine rupture is another fundamental feature of first labor that has important clinical implications.

> "The nulliparous uterus is rupture-proof; the parous uterus is rupture-prone." [1]

13.3 Specification of parity

The term multipara or parous labor, as it has been used thus far, pertains to a woman who has had a previous vaginal birth. As the classification of G2 P1 is also used for a woman with a cesarean section in her history, additional specification is required. However, current classification and common terminology like "elective", "selective", "primary", "secondary", "emergency", or "planned" cesarean delivery is utterly confusing and provides no relevant information whatsoever to guide safe labor supervision or mode of delivery in the next pregnancy.

13.3.1 Classification of previous cesarean

Much more meaningful is the distinction between a pre-labor and an intrapartum cesarean delivery in the obstetrical history. In the context of the dynamics and mechanics of labor, it will best serve a woman with a uterine scar to realize what phase her previous labor had reached. This information is generally missing in studies claiming to examine the risks and success rates of labor after a cesarean, thus diminishing their relevance.

> The only classification of cesareans with clinical relevance for the next childbirth is the distinction between pre-labor and intrapartum cesareans.

13.3.2 Labor with a uterine scar

Safety and success rate of labor with a uterine scar is partly dependent on the extent of cervical dilatation reached at the prior cesarean delivery.[6] A woman who had a previous pre-labor cesarean should be considered a nullipara in all aspects of labor, i.e.,

prone to dysfunctional labor, except for the important fact that she is now vulnerable to uterine rupture as well. This status seriously restricts the possibilities of effective and safe use of oxytocin in a first labor after cesarean, and the odds of a safe and successful VBAC are therefore relatively slim. This consequence is hardly ever given enough consideration when suggesting a pre-labor cesarean in first pregnancy, e.g. for a breech presentation.

In contrast, a woman who had a cesarean in well-advanced labor can now be regarded as a cervical and uterine multipara though a vaginal nullipara: the first stage of labor can be expected to progress satisfactorily; the second stage will be comparable with that of all first deliveries. With expert management, the odds of a safe vaginal birth after a previous intrapartum cesarean are relatively high.

13.4 Parity-based approaches

The fact that the nulliparous uterus is frequently inefficient but immune to rupture, added to the information that the parous uterus is generally very efficient but relatively prone to rupture, has significant consequences for diagnosis and treatment of dysfunctional labor.

> **Fundamental distinction between nulliparous and parous labors**
> The causes of protraction and the risks of treatment are very different. Expert labor management rests on this premise.

13.4.1 Prolonged labor in nulliparas: dynamics

The all too common expectant attitude to labor typically results in late treatment of slow labor and often not before definite arrest and signs of maternal exhaustion are manifest (Section 1). As the functional capacity of the pelvis has not yet been proven by an earlier birth, slow progress of first labor is then considered to point to fetopelvic disproportion. This "mechanistic" misconception combined with misplaced anxiety over potential uterine rupture partly explains the commonly late or half-hearted use of low-dose oxytocin in these circumstances. As time passes, however, the exhausted uterus gradually becomes insensitive to stimulation, thereby rendering the administration of oxytocin ineffective (8.5.4). As a result, progression remains insufficient despite the use of oxytocin. This observation is then misconstrued as confirmation that a mechanical obstruction exists, a classic example of circular reasoning in which the obstetrician figuratively bites his/her own tail, but the consequent pain is for the laboring woman.

The correct point of view and policy are exactly the opposite of this approach. Failure to progress in first labor should always be regarded as an expression of ineffective uterine force until fetopelvic disproportion has been proven by reaching at least 6 to 7 cm dilatation, accompanied by substantial molding, caput succedaneum formation, and extreme hyperflexion of the non-descending head (10.4.3 and Chapter 22). The diagnosis of birth obstruction in first labor usually requires timely and proper use of oxytocin. In fact, true mechanical dystocia occurs in less than 1% of all first labors (Chapter 27).

> Oxytocin treatment in secondarily protracted first labor – to prove or exclude birth obstruction – poses no threat to the welfare of mother or fetus. This is certainly not the case in secondary protraction of parous labors.

13.4.2 Protracted labor in multiparas: mechanics

The guiding thought and clinical approach in problematic parous labor are fundamentally different. The experienced uterus is by nature efficient and cervical resistance is low, making ineffective uterine action exceedingly rare in spontaneous parous labor. However, secondary arrest in the wedging phase (10.4.2) occasionally occurs and should cause one to be extremely alert, because secondary protraction of parous labor is strongly indicative of obstruction with potentially dangerous complications (Chapter 22).

> Secondary delay in parous labor is highly indicative of mechanical obstruction. Oxytocin treatment is not without danger.

In common practice, however, too many birth attendants assume that mechanical obstruction is unlikely in a parous woman, even if labor is secondarily slowing down, because the functional capacity of the woman's pelvis has been proven by a previous birth. Nothing could be further from the truth. Because the unscarred parous uterus is by nature

effective in labor, and because multiparas are relatively at risk of uterine rupture, the utmost restraint should be exercised when considering oxytocin in a secondary arrest in parous labor (Chapter 21). This is especially true if an epidural, which masks the symptoms of imminent uterine rupture, has been administered. In case of labor with a uterine scar, oxytocin treatment of secondary arrest should be considered as a uterine rupture challenge test and must be condemned as utterly irresponsible.

13.4.3 Correct mindset

One of the most fundamental truths in obstetrics is that the etiology of difficult labor differs radically between the first labor and following labors. This statement might sound rather dogmatic, but it is nevertheless crucial for the correct mindset whenever confronted with a problematic, protracted labor:

> **Rule of thumb**
> Difficult nulliparous labor → dynamic labor disorder.
> Difficult multiparous labor → mechanical labor disorder.

In the interest of clarity and completeness, we must mention the obvious exceptions to this rule. Dynamic disorders occasionally do occur in parous labor, but when this happens there are always clearly identifiable causes:

- *Induction.* A woman's fear of recurrence of the traumatic course and operative conclusion of her first labor often becomes a self-fulfilling prophecy when the empathetic doctor promises to attend the delivery personally – thereby arranging an elective induction. Such a policy is a common mistake, as the induction procedure in itself often causes a protracted or failed labor (Chapters 21, 23). Obstetricians would best serve the interests of a scared parous woman were they to dispel her fears with a simple but clear explanation of the differences between a first and a second birth, and wait for spontaneous labor to occur.
- *Hypertonic dystocia.* This separate clinical entity, characterized by disorganized, inefficient uterine contractions and fetal distress, is secondary to a different pathological process altogether, involving inflammatory cytokine production in the myometrium as a result of passage of

meconium, chorioamnionitis, or intrauterine bleeding (8.5.5). Of course, this particular form of dynamic dystocia with concomitant fetal compromise can occur in nulliparous and parous labors alike (Chapter 21).

- *Sympathetic arousal.* Primary ineffective parous labor originates in the prior obliteration of the parasympathetic control through anxiety and fear, mostly as a residual effect of the previous traumatic birth experience. This results in treating last year's problems, thus rendering the care after the fact and often in vain. Again, the lesson is all too clear:

Key point

Invest the utmost in the course and outcome of first labor and few or no problems will be encountered in the following birth. Conversely, irreversible damage may result from a protracted first labor in which the physical and emotional vulnerability of the woman was insufficiently appreciated.

References

1. O'Driscoll K, Meagher D, Robson M. Active Management of Labour, 4th edn. London: Mosby; 2003

2. Johnson JH, Figueroa R, Garry D, Elimian A, Maulik D. Immediate maternal and neonatal effects of forceps and vacuum-assisted deliveries. Obstet Gynecol 2004;**103**:513–18

3. Smith JF, Wax JR. Rupture of the unscarred uterus. UpToDate. Accessed October 2014

4. Lang CT, Landon MB. Uterine dehiscence and rupture after previous cesarean delivery. UpToDate. Accessed October 2014

5. Rossi AC1, Prefumo F. Pregnancy outcomes of induced labor in women with previous cesarean section: a systematic review and meta-analysis. *Arch Gynecol Obstet* 2014 September 2. [Epub ahead of print]

6. Abildgaard H, Ingerslev MD, Nickelsen C, Secher NJ. Cervical dilation at the time of cesarean section for dystocia – effect on subsequent trial of labor. Acta Obstet Gynecol Scand 2013;**92**:193–7

Diagnosis of labor

Correct diagnosis is the foundation of responsible medical care, and this universal truth most certainly applies to childbirth as well. Yet the expression "diagnosis of labor" sounds rather strange to many ears. A computer search in PubMed renders no hits. The subject is evaded in the literature, where only cases said to be "in established labor" (?) are included in the reports. Textbooks and guidelines hardly ever address the subject in detail and seldom formulate strict clinical criteria for diagnosing labor. Midwives and doctors seem to rely on their experience and intuitive skills. In practice, however, many births are attended by younger caregivers who make the decision of admission to the labor ward without clear instructions of how to assess labor.

These omissions illustrate the general failure to appreciate that the onset of labor may represent a genuine diagnostic problem. The consequences can be seen on a daily basis in many hospitals and other birth settings, although these problems are rarely recognized for what they are. If labor is diagnosed in error, inappropriate measurements and interventions are employed. Conversely, if a timely and appropriate diagnosis of labor is not made, primary ineffective labor is not recognized and timely treatment is withheld.

> **Clinical onset of labor**
>
> *When the diagnosis of labor is incorrect, all subsequent policies will inevitably be incorrect too, and a troublesome domino effect ensues. A matter of such consequence should not be left to the patient/client to decide.*

14.1 Professional responsibility

Most pregnant women go into labor without any significant warning, whereas some may perceive a gradual run-up as they notice the pre-labor transformation of their uterus due to Braxton Hicks contractions (8.3.1). A gradual progression to actual labor can last for a number of days, but normally allows the woman to go about her everyday tasks. A clear, blood-free cervical mucus plug may break free and there may be intermittent periods of mild contractions. Considering the possibility of such a gradual progression to actual labor, it could be argued that there is no balanced clinical definition – in a strictly academic sense – for the precise moment at which labor begins. This view is all very well, but it should not distract from the responsibility to provide clarity if a woman calls upon the professional because she thinks her labor has begun. The ability to pinpoint an early stage at which labor can confidently be established is essential for competent supervision and professional conduct and care.

> *The greatest majority of women come into effective labor without any significant warning.*

In conventional practice, it is commonly assumed that women unerringly recognize the onset of their labor by natural instinct. As soon as regular, painful contractions occur, the alleged latent phase of labor, as defined by Friedman, is assumed to have begun.[1] This fallacy underlies the customary practice that the key decision, which forms the basis for admission and subsequent management, is left to the mother. She declares herself in labor, with the result that it is she who stipulates care and becomes the responsible party for the course of events, including all interventions that might occur thereafter. This practice, which leaves the initiative in the hands of "laypersons", is a common but anomalous route without any parallel in regular healthcare.[2] Consider how bizarre it would be to hospitalize a woman who thinks she has a hernia and schedule her for surgery without first performing proper diagnostics. Clearly, the first step in providing professional care in labor is to confirm or reject the woman's self-diagnosis of labor.

The diagnosis of labor is a clinical diagnosis based on objective symptoms, where the full responsibility rests with the professional and not with the pregnant woman.

14.1.1 A firm clinical decision

Although it could be argued that the diagnosis of labor is fraught with all the difficulties of trying to categorize a continuous variable, mothers-to-be do not benefit from a semantic academic exercise. The care provider must be resolute when confronted with an agitated woman who declares labor to have begun. It is after all the professional who is responsible and not the woman. The declaration of "A" has certain consequences, such as the irrevocable "B" that follows and will direct the course of events. Clarity is essential, and this requires a firm decision based on objective diagnostic criteria. For the expectant woman this is the point of no return. The waiting is over, the physical and emotional challenge begins, and she will not rest until her baby lies in her arms.

"A clinical diagnosis must, of its nature, be prospective and a diagnosis of labor is, in effect, a positive decision to commit a woman to delivery." [2]

From the biophysical perspective, labor begins with the sudden formation of myometrial gap junctions, resulting in electrically orchestrated uterine contractions exerting force (8.4.1). In clinical terms this means that contractions are now rendering a verifiable effect on the cervix.

14.2 Objective clinical symptoms

Painful contractions – at intervals of 10 minutes or less – are essential but not decisive; they must be accompanied by additional symptoms. We adopted the diagnostic criteria pioneered by O'Driscoll whereby the only real proof of labor is pains supported by dilatation and thus, by definition, full effacement (9.1.4). Other criteria that justify a clinical diagnosis of labor include pains supported by a bloody show or pains with spontaneous rupture of membranes. These empirical criteria for the diagnosis of labor have been evaluated by numerous clinical investigators and have proved to be correct and very practical: they allow a firm clinical decision in nearly every case.[2–15]

Of course, one could ask for references to double-blinded studies, but such information does not exist since it is not feasible to blind a woman on whether she is in labor or not. Given these limitations, we feel confident of the vast clinical experience supporting the criteria for labor presented here. As is always the case in clinical decision-making, the gratuitous appeal for "evidence" from impossible randomized trials does not remove the need to draw conclusions from what we do know from careful daily observations.

14.2.1 Pains

Regular painful contractions are a prerequisite for the diagnosis of labor. Without them, labor simply does not exist. Unfortunately, it is a common belief that persistent painful contractions *alone* provide conclusive evidence of labor. Although this assumption may not seem unreasonable late in pregnancy, the subjective element of pain and discomfort caused by Braxton Hicks contractions might be highly underestimated, in particular when the threshold for pain is low. Periods with Braxton Hicks contractions may come and go in late pregnancy and are an early sign of pre-labor uterine transformation (8.3.1). The pain they cause cannot be distinguished from true labor pains because both are of uterine origin. To diagnose labor, it must be established that the contractions are genuine labor pains, meaning that they have a progressive effect on the cervix.

A diagnosis of labor based solely on regular, painful contractions is an elementary mistake.

14.2.2 Effacement and dilatation

The diagnosis of labor is simple if the woman has contractions less than 10 minutes apart, a fully effaced cervix, and a few centimeters' dilatation. An easy birth can be anticipated with confidence. About 80% of all nulliparas who self-diagnose labor indeed already present themselves with a completely effaced cervix, and labor can be unequivocally accepted on the basis of this additional symptom alone.[2,16] Considering the decisive importance of effacement and dilatation, it is imperative that the terms be used correctly: dilatation is the diameter of the external os of the fully effaced cervix (9.1.4).

Proof of labor

The transition from full effacement to dilatation is – in the presence of painful contractions – definitive, physical proof that labor has begun.

Diagnostic problems usually arise in nulliparas with a low pain threshold who believe themselves to be in labor but in whom the cervix is not yet fully effaced. Imprecise terminology may then lead to mistaken conclusions. Cervical accessibility may be wrongly interpreted as dilatation (9.1.3) and, consequently, labor may be accepted in error. This mistake can easily result in an unnecessarily long ordeal of exhaustion and suffering, with a cesarean delivery as the only exit strategy.

14.2.3 Bloody show

If the cervix is not yet fully effaced, a bloody show provides relevant information because it is an objective sign that contractions are rendering an effect on the cervix and, therefore, represents a symptom very suggestive of labor. A show is a spontaneous vaginal release of blood-stained cervical mucus as a result of uterine contractions. Spontaneous means that it is not the result of a vaginal examination probing the cervical canal. This would be an artifact, just as bloody discharge after amniotomy for induction is an artifact. Blood loss without contractions is not a show either, although it is an indication for admission – not to the labor and delivery unit but to the antenatal ward. In contrast, contractions that spontaneously coincide with a bloody show have an objective effect and consequently can be clinically regarded as an objective sign of labor.

Definition

A show is the spontaneous vaginal discharge of blood-stained mucus that results from uterine contractions.

Approximately 70% of all women who report themselves in labor have a bloody show.[2] This symptom can legitimately – for reasons of consistent and clear practice – serve as a determining sign that labor has begun, even when the cervix is not yet fully effaced. As labor might not be optimally effective in this latter condition, progress to full effacement and dilatation should be monitored closely and if necessary promptly accelerated.

14.2.4 Ruptured membranes

In about 30% of women who report with painful contractions the membranes have already ruptured spontaneously.[2] This symptom is an even stronger indicator of the onset of labor than is a bloody show. Clinically, the diagnosis of labor is assessed along with all the consequences it implies.

A woman with contractions and broken membranes is in labor.

A clinical dilemma may arise when the membranes have ruptured spontaneously but there are no uterine contractions. There is still – by definition – no question of labor. A vaginal examination is contraindicated because of the risk of introducing infection. That is why we wait – if necessary, as long as 24–48 hours – for painful contractions to start.

More than 70% of women with pre-labor rupture of membranes (PROM) go into labor within 24 hours, and more than 85% within 48 hours.[17] As soon as regular and painful contractions commence, there is every reason to declare the woman in labor. A vaginal examination is then not only justified but indicated. At this point, the only appropriate policy – if necessary with early oxytocin treatment – is directed to a delivery within 12 hours regardless of the cervical status at the onset of the contractions. Waiting longer to assess labor makes no sense, because the woman will not become more fit with the ongoing pains. A delay in the diagnosis of labor is even irresponsible, because uterine contractility might very well be an early sign of intrauterine infection in cases of PROM.[17] It is for this reason that the convenience-motivated practice of sedating women who cannot sleep because of uterine irritability is counterproductive and even dangerous once the membranes are ruptured.

By definition, a false start is an incorrect diagnosis once membranes are broken.

14.2.5 Immediate progress

The diagnosis of labor is problematic if painful contractions are supported by neither full effacement nor show, nor loss of amniotic fluid. An observation period of no more than one to two hours is then advisable, during which time legitimate doubts should be communicated. If progression toward complete effacement is established, labor should be confirmed and accepted. After two hours without any progress, however, the diagnosis of labor must be firmly rejected. Any blood loss following vaginal examination is most likely an artifact.

14.3 The objective diagnosis of labor

Clarity is the hallmark of the professional care provider. For this reason a clear, prospective decision must be made in every case and as soon as possible, within a maximal timeframe of two hours. In the legal world a distinction is made between direct and indirect or circumstantial evidence. The clinical world is no different. Pains with dilatation – and so by definition full effacement – are the only direct proof of labor. A bloody show and rupture of membranes are strong circumstantial evidence.

> **Clinical evidence of the onset of labor**
>
> *Basic prerequisite: Painful contractions at intervals of 10 minutes or less*
>
> *Highly suggestive: Bloody show or ruptured membranes*
>
> *Objective proof: Full effacement*

14.3.1 Pre-labor instructions

Doctors and midwives tend to be notoriously vague whenever women ask questions about the onset of labor. With these objective criteria, clarity can now finally be offered. All mothers-to-be are encouraged to contact their provider and come to the hospital at an early stage when contractions become painful – resembling strong menstrual cramping – and are accompanied by a show or leakage of fluid or, failing either of these, when the pains come at regular intervals of 10 minutes or less for an hour. The need for professional confirmation of their provisional diagnosis should be clearly explained. Pre-labor education in accordance with actual practice is crucial for women to be properly prepared for the challenge of the forthcoming birth (Chapter 18).

> *Pre-labor education must be clear and correspond with actual practice.*

14.3.2 Documentation

The doctor or midwife who is responsible for the admission to the labor ward should commit the evidence of labor to permanent record in simple and explicit terms: painful contractions, full effacement, a bloody show, and/or spontaneously ruptured membranes. A simple statement "in labor," without explicitly mentioning the grounds on which this conclusion is based, is not acceptable.

Detailed record-keeping ensures that the evidence remains available even when the person concerned is no longer on duty. The diagnosis of labor decides admission to the labor ward, and in planned home births it is also from that moment on that professional responsibility starts and the midwife should stay and sit with her client. The graphic representation of labor progression (partogram) also begins at this point, no sooner and no later (Chapter 15).

> *For management and meaningful audit purposes, the grounds on which the diagnosis of labor is made must be committed to permanent record in simple and explicit terms: contractions and full effacement, or a show, or spontaneously ruptured membranes.*

Accurate record-keeping with a partogram forces professional care providers to make an objective diagnosis of labor and subsequently compels them to undertake timely assessment of progression. Exact information is a prerequisite for a rational, responsible policy as well as for meaningful audit (Chapters 26 and 27) and scientific evaluation of the supervision of labor. Therefore:

- The grounds on which the diagnosis is made are committed to a permanent record including the name of the responsible care provider, thus assuring accountability for the diagnosis of labor and all procedures and interventions that might follow.
- A woman is not admitted to the labor room unless she meets the strict criteria for the diagnosis of labor.
- No intervention whatsoever is permitted until a firm diagnosis of labor is made.
- There is deliberately no space on the partogram to record the period at home before the professional made the positive diagnosis of labor (Chapter 15).
- The duration of labor is recorded as the interval between the moment the professional confirmed

the diagnosis of labor and the birth of the baby. This equals the time she is admitted in the labor room until the baby lies in her arms.

> The labor-record and partogram begin at the moment the care provider confirms labor, not before and not after.

14.4 Indecision

Expert care requires first and foremost insight on the part of the responsible provider. The situation must be crystal clear from the outset in order for that person to convey the necessary information with clarity to the woman and her supporters: either she is or she is not in labor; there is no in-between.

14.4.1 Evasion of responsibility

Unfortunately, many caregivers tenaciously hold to the idea of a latent phase in early labor, although its scientific basis is highly questionable (10.1). The concept is also of little clinical concern and even counterproductive. The common use of such equivocal terms as "an early start," "latent labor," or "active labor not established" actually evades responsibility. Were a distinction of a latent phase possible in practice, it would still create confusion. Latent labor refers to a period of painful contractions that are not yet true labor pains. Such uterine irritability can last from a few to many hours and even, intermittently, for several days.[16] Determining whether or not true labor will actually start is a matter of waiting. Braxton Hicks contractions are normal in late pregnancy and can come and go. Thus, the latent phase of labor is by definition a retrospective diagnosis and therefore has no relevance for the uncertain woman who thinks she might be in labor.

On the contrary, she needs prospective guidance and a clear answer whether labor has begun or not. A clinical diagnosis must, by nature, be prospective and a diagnosis of labor is a positive decision to commit a woman to delivery. Labor literally means work: from the moment labor commences, the woman will have to work until her baby is born. A birth attendant is a coach, and a good coach is as clear and as resolute as possible. As in the world of sports, where a coach cannot adequately assist a sportswoman without a clear determination of the beginning of the game, the onset of the endeavor of labor must be pinpointed

as clearly as possible. Recognition of a latent phase is counterproductive in this respect.

> Ninety percent of pregnant women go into labor without any significant prelude. The "latent phase" is the cover of the insecure and indecisive birth attendant in the other 10%.

14.4.2 Avoided diagnosis

Conventional teaching generally overlooks the significance of complete cervical effacement. Consequently, many providers fail to recognize the early but decisive symptoms of labor and, therefore, remain vague about the clinical onset of labor.

A 2014 ACOG consensus report even suggests "before 6 cm of dilation is achieved, standards of 'active phase' progress should not be applied" (sic!).[18] The implication of this fallacy is recognition of a "latent phase" up to 6 cm. One might just as well evade responsibility for the diagnosis of labor until the baby's head can be seen in the vulva. Moreover, this awkward "recommendation" leaves providers without any guidance over what to do with women who never reach 6 cm dilatation spontaneously. ACOG based this consensus statement on a mistaken extrapolation of a survey study by Zangh et al. in a large contemporary US population.[19] That much-cited study showed an accelerated dilatation rate after 6 cm. In reality, of course, the researchers misinterpreted the retraction phase of labor as "latent phase" and the wedging phase as the "active phase" of labor (10.4.2). Moreover, caregivers in the hospitals contributing to that study had failed to define the onset of labor. Clearly, a retrospective study like this with undefined and heterogeneous labor policies gives no guidance whatsoever for expert care in early labor. It rather endorses the evasion of a clear management of labor up to 6 cm dilatation. The circular reasoning in this and other studies was discussed in Chapter 10 (10.3).

> Current guidelines fail to give proper guidance for the management of early labor.

Fear of being deemed an inexpert provider by making a false diagnosis of labor is the unjust excuse made for communicating vague phrases after a first examination that reveals less than 3 cm dilatation.

However, in childbirth practice – as in most aspects of life – the biggest problems arise through avoided decisions, not through mistaken ones. "Soft and indecisive doctors make dirty wounds" is a Dutch proverb.

An evasive answer or a pseudo-diagnosis of "latent labor" is confusing and counter-informative for all concerned. Vague phrases serve only as excuses for the care provider to avoid a clear diagnosis of labor. In effect, such behavior places full responsibility on the pregnant woman, where it certainly does not belong. Chaos ensues because such indecision also delays the second crucial diagnosis – whether labor is effective or not – and thus may lead to withholding of treatment when it is clearly indicated. This neglect is the most frequent, most pervasive, and most underestimated mistake in the conduct and care of labor (Chapters 15, 21). When a clear diagnosis of labor is delayed, many uteri will fail to respond properly to oxytocin in a later stage (8.5.4) when dystocia will eventually be undeniable for even the most conservative of labor supervisors.

> "Most errors in the supervision of labor result from decisions being avoided rather than from decisions wrongly made." [2]

14.5 Errors in diagnosis

No matter how carefully the clinical diagnosis of labor is made, a small chance remains that the course of events will prove it to be incorrect. No clinical diagnostic method is foolproof. Rather, the aim is to reduce the number of errors to a minimum by maximizing objectivity. A mistake can be made either way: a woman's self-diagnosis of labor may be falsely rejected or falsely accepted.

14.5.1 False-negative diagnosis

A woman who is initially assessed as not being in labor may report a short time later with an advanced stage of labor. This happens only occasionally given the early state in which labor is recognized by the proposed criteria. Besides, such an initially false-negative diagnosis has no adverse effects for the woman, unless she lives far from the hospital and was sent home. In that case, admission to the antenatal ward should have eliminated the possible embarrassment of an unassisted delivery at home or in a car.

14.5.2 False-positive diagnosis

In contrast, a false-positive diagnosis that incorrectly declares the woman to be in labor has far more ominous consequences. She is wrongly admitted to, and retained in, the labor room and exposed to the expectations, pressures, and stresses of that environment. Now there is no way back. Inevitably, after many hours in pain in which no progress is made, the morale suffers, not only of the mother but also that of her partner and the attendant who ought to sit with her. The woman's motivation weakens rapidly as her physical and mental condition deteriorates. Analgesic drugs and ineffective oxytocin aggravate the problem until the situation reaches a point at which there is but one way out: cesarean section. The indication for the cesarean delivery is likely to be registered as "dystocia,"[20] whereas the truth of the matter is that this woman was not in labor. A critical review of the clinical history is frequently impossible, because the evidence of labor is mostly documented poorly, if at all.

> All too many women are submitted to cesarean section for the indication "dystocia" when a state of labor never existed.

The risk of a false-positive diagnosis is strongly limited by adherence to the proposed criteria but it can never be totally eliminated. Hence, the small chance that the next hour may prove the initial diagnosis wrong should always be kept in mind. This applies with particular force when the diagnosis of labor is based on contractions accompanied solely by a "bloody show" but unsupported by full effacement or ruptured membranes. Should the contractions subside, then a timely and decisive correction is necessary to re-route the woman from a dead-end track. Professional care requires that a mistake be not only recognized but also openly acknowledged so that the policy can be corrected in time – within one hour. The ability to do this is a mark of quality in professional care.

On the other hand, amniotomy is the recommended policy when the frequency or intensity of the contractions subsides after a certain diagnosis of labor is made based on pains supported by full effacement. Likewise, all efforts should be made to achieve a delivery within 12 hours when the diagnosis of labor is supported by spontaneous rupture of membranes. In that case, uterine stimulation must be started immediately – for the reasons explained above (14.2.4) – if progression fails, regardless of cervical status.

> *The maximum level of objectivity reduces the number of mistakes to a minimum.*

14.6 False start

About 10% of all nulliparas call their midwife or come to the hospital convinced that they are in labor only to find that they do not meet the objective criteria for labor: painful uterine contractions are not accompanied by full effacement and there is neither a bloody show nor leakage of amniotic fluid. This is called a false start.

> *A false start is when a woman believes herself to be in labor on the basis of painful contractions that are not supported by other, objective evidence of labor.*

14.6.1 Factors contributing to a false start

Because care providers often give cryptic answers when asked about how to determine when labor has begun, it is not surprising that inexperienced nulliparas sometimes make a mistake. Indeed, it is remarkable that 90% of first-time mothers-to-be correctly recognize the beginning of their labor. The real problem is for the remaining 10% with a false start.

Ironically, a false start frequently occurs late in the evening when the community-based midwife has just gone to bed and the youngest resident or intern is holding the fort at the hospital. Thus, the agitated woman and her insecure partner may receive vague and evasive answers. They begin to realize that the birth professional from whom they expected to receive clear answers cannot or will not establish whether labor has begun.

As a result, the woman loses trust not only in herself but also in the care provider. Furthermore, this vagueness stymies her partner, nurse, or doula, and no-one knows in which direction to guide and coach the woman. A distinctly uneasy atmosphere arises. Uncertainty increases anxiety, lowers the pain threshold, and sets off a vicious circle of anxiety, stress, and pain.

The thoughtless care provider will further strengthen any false anticipation by keeping the woman in the labor room and sweeping or stripping the membranes only to worsen the contractility and pain. Now there is a good chance that the presumptive labor will not progress while the important symptom of a show is rendered useless.

In the home situation, the most disastrous comment late in the evening is "call me if it gets any worse." That is typically coupled with a failure to check back until morning. A clear decision has been avoided and the woman may have reached the point of exhaustion before labor has even begun.

14.6.2 Management of a false start

The first step is to offer a clear explanation that labor has not yet begun. When the reasons for this conclusion are presented with clear arguments, using comprehensible language and with professional and convincing firmness, this information is generally well accepted. A woman must not remain in the labor ward any longer than is necessary to make a diagnosis, in other words, no more than one to two hours.

When the woman understands that her labor has not yet begun, and if she is at ease at that moment and does not live too far from the hospital, she can return home. If she remains anxious and feels insecure, it makes more sense for her to stay the night in the antenatal ward and possibly to be given a sleeping tablet. True sedation – an injection of pethidine combined with a powerful sedative – is necessary only when the agitated woman has lost her composure. In our experience fewer than 2% of all nulliparas need this drastic clinical treatment for a persistent false start.

> *A woman having a false start does not belong in the labor room.*

A woman who chooses to give birth at home and is now experiencing a false start should be approached similarly. Her midwife should suggest a shower or bath and the bed should be freshened up and rearranged. The woman's partner need not come home from work and the auxiliary maternity nurse should not be mobilized. Tranquility and confidence must be restored. A mild sedative might help. If the woman calls a few hours later, her midwife should promptly and personally see her again. Diagnoses via telephone are simply impossible and, therefore, unacceptable. If the woman is still not in labor, her uneasiness may reach such a state of agitation that admission to the hospital for clinical sedation becomes the most prudent course of action. In the final analysis, clients of community-based midwives can be competently treated with clinical sedation on a consultative basis. The woman can then return home well rested the following morning, transferred back to her trusted midwife, and later deliver her baby with her (Chapter 25). Prerequisite for this facility, fostering continuity in care, is that the philosophies of home practices and hospital must be on the same wavelength and that policies – from both sides – must be consistently executed. This can occur only if both professions share the same objective criteria for the diagnosis of labor.

A persistent false start is a serious clinical condition, requiring prompt and rigorous treatment.

14.6.3 Sedation versus pain relief

The fundamental distinction between sedation and pain relief must be made absolutely clear. Clinical sedation is the ultimate treatment of a tenacious false start. The aim is to break the vicious circle created by false anticipation of birth. Therefore, strong sedatives or narcotics should never be administered in the labor room but always on the antenatal ward: the patient must sleep.

Conversely, a woman who is truly in labor must keep her head clear and remain fit. A woman in labor should therefore never be sedated. If effective pain relief in labor is needed, epidural is the method of choice. Clearly an epidural block should never be given before a strict diagnosis of labor and thus a commitment to delivery is made (Chapter 20).

There is no place for sedative drugs in the labor room. A woman in labor must keep her head clear.

14.6.4 Preventing a false start

A critical review of false starts will show that most are directly or indirectly iatrogenic and thus preventable. At the last prenatal visit, false expectations are all too often created by the information that the woman's cervix is already "ripe". When the woman is tired of

being pregnant and wants to know when it will end, a vaginal examination will generally do more harm than good. If there is no medical indication, one should not do an internal examination!

False starts are often provider-caused and thus preventable.

Stripping the membranes in late pregnancy is an even worse procedure and in our view is utterly reprehensible. When performed as vigorously as it should be, it is very painful but mostly ineffective all the same.[21,22] In addition, sweeping the membranes raises false expectations, prompts uterine irritability, and invariably leads to artificial blood loss, rendering the symptom of bloody show useless.

Doctors have even more means to induce a false start. Along with the influx of diagnostic techniques has come an increase in iatrogenic anxiety and uncertainty (4.1 and 4.2). Under the pretext of "better safe than sorry," a decision for priming the cervix for induction with prostaglandins is then easily made. However, the general assumption "if it doesn't help you, it won't harm you" is absolutely invalid. In reality, cervical priming is the best gambit to a disastrous false start and all the related misery, agony, and despair.

Pre-labor stripping (sweeping the membranes) is a reprehensible procedure. Cervical priming with prostaglandins is an even more potent means for inducing a disastrous false start.

Emphasis on the "due date" is unwise from the outset. The pregnant woman directs her expectations toward this date, and if she goes past it the waiting becomes increasingly difficult. Therefore, we prefer to speak of the full-term period, which lasts until 42 weeks.

If the term pregnant woman is nonetheless tired of waiting, then offering explanations is much wiser than a vaginal examination to evaluate cervical ripeness. As soon as she understands the risks of a protracted and failed induction, and that labor and delivery will go much more easily – and thus more safely – when her uterus is ready for this process, even the most rigidly scheduled of pregnant women will summon the patience to wait for labor to begin spontaneously. Agreement on a "latest date of delivery," being the post-term date (41–42 weeks) on which labor will be induced, is a feasible and helpful strategy accepted by most women.[23]

> Instead of the routine assessment of "the due date," a pregnant woman is better given the "latest date of delivery."

14.7 Proactive support of labor

Offering true help and support during labor is possible only with absolute clarity of thought and action. Therefore, two early decisions must be made in every case:

1. Whether the woman is or is not in labor; and if she is
2. Whether labor is effective or not.

If caregivers considered these elementary questions every time when summoned with a client/patient experiencing contractions, and if providers took full responsibility for making firm decisions, the majority of protracted, traumatic, and failing labors ending in operative deliveries could be prevented. Any supposedly subtler or more nuanced approach as defended by many midwives and conventional obstetricians (who, by the way, hardly ever see a woman in the early stages of labor) actually leads to poor (non-) management, marred by vagueness and indecision. In contrast, a clear and consistent birth-plan involves strict rules that must be put into practice at all times:

> **Rules governing expert management of early labor**
> - No intervention whatsoever is permitted until a firm diagnosis of labor is made.
> - The responsible midwife or doctor presents the evidence of labor on permanent record in simple and explicit terms: pains, bloody show, ruptured membranes, full effacement.
> - From that moment on, a partogram is kept in all cases and labor must progress adequately.

References

1. Friedman EA. Labor: Clinical Evaluation and Management, 2nd edn. New York: Appleton-Century-Crofts; 1978

2. O'Driscoll K, Meagher D, Robson M. Active Management of Labour, 4th edn. London: Mosby; 2003

3. Turner M, Brassil M, Gordon H. Active management of labor associated with a decrease in the cesarean section rate in nulliparas. Obstet Gynecol 1988;**71**:150–4

4. Akoury H, Brodie G, Caddick R, *et al.* Active management of labor and operative delivery in nulliparous women. Am J Obstet Gynecol 1988;**158**:255–8

5. Boylan P, Frankowski R, Rountree R, *et al.* Effect of active management on the incidence of cesarean section for dystocia in nulliparas. Am J Perinatol 1991;**8**:373–9

6. Lopez-Zeno J, Peaceman A, Adashek JA, Socol ML. A controlled trial of a program for the active management of labor. N Engl J Med 1992;**326**:450–4

7. Frigoletto F, Lieberman E, Lang J, *et al.* A clinical trial of active management of labor. N Engl J Med 1995;**333**:745–50

8. Cammu H, van Eeckhout E. A randomised controlled trial of early versus delayed use of amniotomy and oxytocin infusion in nulliparous labour. Br J Obstet Gynaecol 1996;**103**:313–18

9. Fraser W, Vendittelli F, Krauss I, Breart G. Effects of early augmentation of labour with amniotomy and oxytocin in nulliparous women: a meta-analysis. Br J Obstet Gynaecol 1998;**105**:189–94

10. Fraser W, Marcoux S, Moutquin J, *et al.* Effect of early amniotomy on the risk of dystocia in nulliparous women. N Engl J Med 1993;**328**:1145–9

11. Boylan P, Parisi V. Effect of active management on latent phase labor. Am J Perinatol 1990;**7**:363–5

12. Masoli P, Picó V, Pellerano IB. Manejo activo del parto. Experiencia en el hospital Gustavo Fricke. Rev Chil Obstet Ginecol 1986;**51**:223–30

13. Vengadasalam D. Active management of labour: an approach to reducing the rising caesarean rate. Singapore J Obstet Gynecol 1986;**17**:33–6

14. Hogston P, Noble W. Active management of labor: the Portsmouth experience. J Obstet Gynaecol 1993;**13**:340–2

15. Impey L, Hobson J, O'Herlihy C. Graphic analysis of actively managed labor: prospective computation of labor progress in 500 consecutive nulliparous women in spontaneous labor at term. Am J Obstet Gynecol 2000;**183**:438–43

16. Hendricks CH, Brenner WE, Kraus G. Normal cervical dilatation pattern in late pregnancy and labor. Am J Obstet Gynecol 1970;**106**:1065–82

17. Scorza WE. Management of premature rupture of the fetal membranes at term. UpToDate. Accessed October 2014

18. American College of Obstetricians and Gynecologists. Obstetric Care Consensus No 1: Safe prevention of the

primary cesarean delivery. Obstet Gynecol 2014;**123**:693–711

19. Zhang J, Landy HJ, Branch DW, *et al.* (Consortium on Safe Labor.) Contemporary patterns of spontaneous labor with normal neonatal outcomes. Obstet Gynecol 2010;**116**:1281–7

20. Stewart PJ, Duhlberg C, Arnill AC, Elmslie T, Hall PF. Diagnosis of dystocia and management with cesarean section among primiparous women in Ottowa Carleton. Can Med Assoc J 1990;**142**:459–63

21. Wing DA. Induction of labor. UpToDate. Accessed October 2014

22. Boulvain M, Stan CM, Irion O. Membrane sweeping for induction of labour. Cochrane Database Syst Rev 2005 DOI: 10.1002/14651858. CD000451.pub2

23. Ayers S, Collenette A, Hollis B, Manyonda I. Feasibility study of a Latest Date of Delivery (LDD) system of managing pregnancy. J Psychosom Obstet Gynecol 2005;**26**:167–71

Chapter 15

Prevention of long labor

When a pregnant woman asks her care provider how long her forthcoming labor might last, she usually gets an evasive answer. Apparently, prospective norms for the duration of childbirth are not clearly set since "normal labor" is still widely considered as a characterization made in retrospect, when a baby has been born in good condition without medical interference, regardless of the time it took. However, a retrospective deduction does not positively inspire caregivers towards a sensible rationale for the conduct and care of labor in order to achieve the ultimate prize of spontaneous delivery. The word "normal" literally means remaining sufficiently within "norms", and such a classification should of course be prospective.

15.1 Duration of labor: definition

As explained previously (10.3), it remains elusive to determine a clear cut-off point for the "normal" duration of labor because of unsolvable methodological limitations. Instead, we therefore defined an upper boundary for the duration of labor and delivery that is acceptable in terms of safety for mother and child, and in terms of women's ability to endure the birth process: 12 hours. Labor duration determines, more than any other measurable factor, how taxing the birth will be, not only for the parturient but also for her partner, her baby, and the birth attendants who ought to care for all of them. In this context, it is imperative to have a clear understanding of what is meant by labor duration:

> **Definition**
>
> *The duration of labor is recorded as the number of hours from the moment the birth professional confirms the diagnosis of labor until the baby is born.*

For hospital births, the duration of labor equals the time a woman spends in the delivery unit, provided that no one is admitted unless she meets the strict criteria for the diagnosis of labor as defined in the previous chapter (14.3). On practical grounds, in the sense of policy of care, the third stage of labor is not included in this definition.

It is evident that every woman in whom labor is established has been in labor before arriving at the hospital or before the midwife's arrival at the home. However, to estimate the duration from such evidence is guesswork. It is pointless to speculate on the "latent" phase or the time the woman was in labor before she decided to call for professional help. Moreover, it has no relevance for the subsequent supervision of the labor. Instead, there are strong practical arguments in favor of the above definition:

- The woman decides for herself when she calls for her midwife or will go to the hospital.
- Professional responsibility begins only when a woman elects to place herself in a professional's care.
- The diagnosis of labor is the responsibility of the midwife or doctor.
- From the moment the professional declares a woman to be in labor she/he is fully responsible and accountable for the maximum duration of that labor.
- Duration of labor is now accurately recorded for purposes of comparison. Meaningful audit of procedures and outcomes requires accurate information.
- Most mothers tend to recall the duration of their labor in this manner.

The beneficial effects of this prospective working definition cannot be overestimated since failure to define what is clearly one of the most basic parameters of birth has been the major obstacle to improvements in the conduct and care of labor for many years.

15.2 Concept of good childbirth

A good childbirth experience is the ultimate goal to which all professionals concerned with labor and delivery should consciously aspire. Therefore, we should replace the retrospective notion of "natural" and "normal" as our criteria for good practice in midwifery and obstetrics with a prospective definition of a good childbirth.[1] This definition should be posted in a prominent position in every antenatal clinic and every delivery unit to serve as a clear statement of common purpose:

> **Prospective definition**
>
> *A good childbirth starts spontaneously and progresses at least 1 cm/h. The woman gives birth to her baby vaginally, by her own efforts, within 12 hours, and without harm to either party.*

This is not to say that induction, outlet instrumental delivery, or cesarean delivery should never be practiced, but rather that they should be practiced with the utmost discretion as the lesser of two evils.

Professionals, who are protective of the term "normal" birth, should take notice of the consensus statement on "normal birth" from the UK Maternity Care Working Party consisting of representatives from the Royal College of Midwives, the RCOG, and the UK National Childbirth Trust.[2] The task force does not exclude selective use of amniotomy and oxytocin in "normal" labor. Indeed, these measures should not be designated as "abnormal" as they are particularly taken to restore "normalcy" of labor.

Positively, the ability to restrict the duration of labor without extending the use of surgical intervention is the most important advantage of expert birth care nowadays. Labor and delivery need no longer be a slow and nightmarish agony.

15.3 Partogram

A visual record of progression is exceedingly elucidating and very useful for expert supervision of labor (Fig. 15.1). Simplicity is the key. The partogram, as designed by Philpott and modified by Hendricks and O'Driscoll, starts at the well-defined diagnosis of labor, and progress during the first stage of labor is measured exclusively in terms of dilatation. A cervix that is completely effaced is marked at 1 cm because the external os is always open to this extent. Dilatation

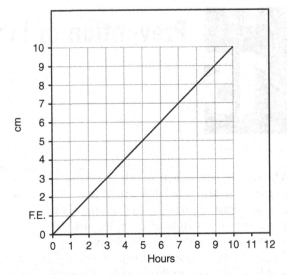

Figure 15.1 The partogram. FE = full effacement. No allowance is made for the time prior to the diagnosis of labor. The diagonal demarcates the lower boundary of acceptable progress.

in centimeters is plotted against time in hours with an *x*-to-*y* axis ratio of 1:1. The diagonal line is the boundary indicating the slowest rate of progress accepted. There is intentionally no space on the graph for the period prior to the point of labor confirmation or for births lasting longer than 12 hours. The partogram covers a period of 10 hours for the first stage and 2 hours for the second stage.

15.3.1 Simple, visual record

The partogram begins at the moment the diagnosis of labor is confirmed by the responsible care provider (14.2). The time prior to diagnosis is not taken into consideration: if the first examination reveals 4 centimeters dilatation, the partogram begins at 4 cm on the vertical axis, which corresponds with zero hour on the horizontal axis (Fig. 15.3). Such a finding does not mean, as is often suggested, that the woman was in labor long before record-keeping commenced; rather it should be viewed as a sign of effective labor.

The partogram is used as a prospective tool in all cases, not as an optional graph to be made in retrospect when arrest of labor is already final. Obligatory sticking to the partogram keeps the attention of care providers on the task at hand. Labor is considered effective when the graph remains on the left-hand side of the reference diagonal and is at least as steep

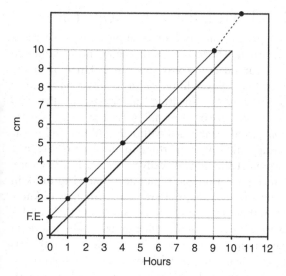

Figure 15.2 Example 1. Effective labor.

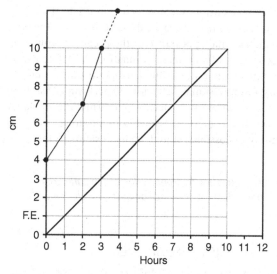

Figure 15.3 Example 2. Effective labor.

(Figs. 15.2 and 15.3). Deviations from the norm are instantly apparent (Chapter 21).

15.3.2 Preferential partogram design

The method of partographic representation strongly affects obstetric decision-making. The simpler it is the better it is. A study examining hypothetical situations plotted on different partogram designs showed that the one-on-one x-to-y axis ratio and the exclusion of a latent phase were associated with the fewest decisions to perform a cesarean section.[3] So the usage of partograms of commercially available electronic dossiers with asymmetrical x-to-y axis ratios should be discouraged.

We also advise against the use of the WHO partogram,[4] originally designed to assist labor management in third-world birth centers, or other partogram designs that are similarly crammed with minute details on station and position of the fetal head, contraction frequency, fetal heartbeat counts, etc. Such details usually distract from the sole purpose, which is to relate progress to passage of time. Furthermore, these partogram designs disregard a strict diagnosis of labor, recognizing a "latent phase" of labor that is allowed to last 12 hours before an "action-line" is passed. Clearly, the result defeats the purpose of keeping a partogram. The use of a variety of partogram designs explains why a meta-analysis fails to support evidence for the benefits of keeping a partogram.[5]

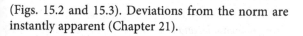

The partogram designed by the WHO neglects an objective diagnosis of labor, includes a latent phase of 12 hours, and should, therefore, not be used.

An interactive app with the preferential partogram design can be downloaded at www.apparent apps.com. This interactive app is available not only to professionals, but also to clients/patients. The partogram-app gives advice for the course of action, based on the principles of proactive support of labor. Use of the app by providers and parents-to-be promotes clarity and enhances good communication during labor.

15.4 Monitoring progress

Accurate assessment of the onset of labor and effective control of its duration within a timeframe of 12 hours represent the most important measures to avoid prolonged labor and related emotional trauma, instrumental delivery, and cesarean section. To reiterate, recognition of a latent phase of labor is counterproductive in this respect. Prospective keeping of the partogram in the proposed design forces the care provider to make two early decisions in every case:

- to establish labor; and if so,
- whether labor is effective or not.

The irony is that midwives often avoid these crucial early decisions, whereas many obstetricians, especially in smaller hospitals, conveniently delegate these to a nurse, who must then make these decisions on the basis of the external appearance of the pregnant woman in the absence of a vaginal examination (VE). Obligatory and prospective use of the partogram puts an end to this unprofessional behavior. Expert supervision of labor requires an objective confirmation of labor onset and regular assessments of progress, which is simply impossible without vaginal examinations.

> *"Close attention to progress during the early hours of labor is the best insurance against difficulties later."* [6]

15.4.1 Early assessments

Progress should be monitored at intervals of one hour, as 4 hours is much too long to wait to discover that labor has not advanced. Slow progress in the first 3 hours is a clear indication of ineffective labor, and corrective action should be taken without delay. As soon as dilatation has reached 3 cm, the frequency of VEs should be reduced to once every 2 hours.

The emphasis placed on early labor differs fundamentally from conventional practices when no worthwhile clinical decision is considered until a woman has been in labor for several hours and the threat of complications is imminent. "Such belated decision-making involves primarily the rescue of mothers and babies from potentially dangerous predicaments that develop over a protracted period of time in what were initially normal cases. No serious thought is given to prevention."[6]

15.5 Patient information and guidance

Practice must correspond with information given before labor (Chapter 19). In contrast to the usually half-hearted instructions, the pregnant woman is best encouraged to come to the hospital at an early stage as soon as she assumes her labor has begun. If she has been educated on the importance of the professional confirmation of her provisional diagnosis and the initial assessments of labor progression, then the provider must act accordingly. Pre-labor agreements that are not kept in the delivery room strongly undermine a woman's confidence, not only in the staff on duty but also in the labor department as a whole.

15.5.1 Prediction of the hour of birth

Intrapartum care and information must be clear and consistent. The use of mystifying medical jargon as a cloak for indecision or the utterance of inanities to the effect that "all is well" or "progress is as good as can be expected" each constitute "an intolerable affront to the intelligence of women."[6] A clear pattern of dilatation can be established within 2–3 hours, and linear extrapolation of the partogram enables the caregiver to predict the hour of delivery in nearly every case. "Since most women are not accustomed to think in terms of dilatation, but are merely anxious to know when their baby will be born, informing them of this expected arrival time – give or take 1 hour – is of paramount importance."[6] The knowledge that there is a predictable end in sight boosts morale, not only of the woman but also of the people involved in supporting and comforting her.

> **Boosting morale**
> *Communication must be exact, consistent, comprehensible, and motivating at all times. The expected time of delivery – give or take an hour – can be established in the early stages of labor and should be conveyed to every parturient within 3 hours after admission.*

15.5.2 Vaginal examinations: clarity versus "disruption"

Despite all these considerations, many caregivers feel disheartened with the proposed early assessments, claiming that nature must take its course and that VEs are unnecessarily interfering and burdensome for a woman. These caregivers should realize, however, that the proposed early examinations are done exclusively to evaluate dilatation and that these assessments are brief and minimally disruptive. Indeed, the orthodox ritual of checking the fetopelvic relationship by assessing the station and position of the fetal occiput at each VE is not only burdensome but is superfluous and counterproductive at this stage. During early first-stage labor, this routine can only provide irrelevant information of "unfavorable position" such as occiput posterior ("stargazer"), to the effect that the supervisor gets off on the wrong foot and imparts a discouraging note to the event. A pessimistic prognostic assessment tends to self-fulfillment by iatrogenic dynamic birth disorders (Chapter 21).

VEs in the retraction phase of labor (10.4.2) should focus solely on cervical effacement and dilatation and thus should be brief, minimally disruptive, hardly painful, and not too discomforting to the woman.

Regular assessments keep the woman posted on her progress. After each VE, the result is conveyed directly to her as it is plotted on the partogram in her presence. At that time, it is decided when the next evaluation will be, and that appointment should be kept strictly. Like a sportswoman's coach, a birth attendant simply cannot supervise and motivate a woman in labor without having a clear determination of its beginning, and certainly not without regular and timely evaluation of its progress.

A vaginal examination with the restricted purpose of assessing dilatation is brief and minimally disruptive.

Incidentally, when one applies the rules of *proactive support*, the total number of VEs – 3.7 times on average – is actually lower than in conventional practices where slow, long labors are tolerated.[7] As long as progress is satisfactory, labor is monitored exclusively by dilatation rate. Only when the wedging phase becomes manifest by a secondary slowing beyond 6 cm is there good reason to assess the station, position, and attitude of the fetal head, as well as the presence of caput succedaneum and molding. As long as dilatation progresses smoothly, however, these data are *de facto* irrelevant.

15.6 Timely corrective action

Early dilatation rate strongly determines the course of labor and predicts its outcome. Old studies from the pre-epidural era provide the best information. Cardozo *et al.*, for instance, reported in the 1980s that a normal cervimetric pattern resulted in a vaginal delivery rate of 98.4%, whereas primary dysfunctional labor that could be improved by oxytocin had a 93.8% incidence of vaginal delivery.[8] But if there was no improvement in the rate of cervical dilatation when oxytocin was administered, the vaginal delivery rate was only 22.7%. In an Israeli study on the predictive value of dilatation rates, more than 93% of nulliparas who dilated at a rate of ≥ 1 cm/h from the onset of labor succeeded in giving birth spontaneously, whereas more than 70% of more slowly dilating women ultimately had an operative delivery.[9]

Who can maintain that a tolerant attitude to slow labor is friendly to women? The passive approach of many caregivers appears to be based more on atavistic ideology and/or territorial interests (Section 1), than the preferences and needs of their clients/patients. When openly asked, no single pregnant woman wishes her forthcoming labor to last more than 12 hours.

Turning the tide of ever-increasing cesarean rates remains impossible as long as caregivers fail to recognize prospective criteria for adequate progress in early labor.

15.6.1 Amniotomy and oxytocin

Proactive support of labor does not medicalize birth, but rather ensures an acceptable course of the process. When dilatation proceeds well, the membranes are left intact. If progress is <1 cm/h, there is justifiable cause for artificial rupture of membranes. This applies to both home and hospital births. If amniotomy does not accelerate progress within 1–2 hours, or if, at any later stage, the rate of progress remains less than 1 cm/h, oxytocin should be started promptly (Chapter 17). At this precise time, a woman who is laboring at home should be transferred to the hospital without delay. The further a woman's course of labor deviates from the norm, the higher the associated chance of exhaustion, operative delivery, and emotional trauma.

It is high time to replace the ill-defined criterion "natural" or "normal" as a guiding principle in midwifery and obstetrics with the notion of a good childbirth experience.

It should be noted that the majority of women supervised according to these principles do not need oxytocin at all (Chapter 27). This policy does not lead to more frequent use of oxytocin but rather to better selection and more appropriate timing of it. In our Dutch secondary care practice, the use of oxytocin (31% of all labors, including inductions; see Chapter 27) matches the 50th percentile of the Dutch National Obstetric Registration for secondary care. Analysis of international figures reveals similar or even higher rates.

Critics – mostly unaware of the oxytocin treatment rate in mainstream childbirth (but often too late or for dubiously indicated inductions) – often argue that 30% of women receiving oxytocin is not normal. Such criticism is countered with the question of whether the current 50% rate of operative deliveries in first labors is normal.

Proactive support of labor does not mean more frequent use of oxytocin, but rather better timed.

If, after institution of timely measures, delivery is not imminent after 12 hours, a cesarean should be considered. In fact, prevention of emotional trauma is of even greater value than the avoidance of cesarean delivery. Supportive, proactive direction toward a spontaneous delivery within 12 hours is not aggressive but pre-emptive and above all friendly to the woman. When honestly informed about likely scenarios, women with initially slow labor invariably prefer a pre-emptive IV-line with oxytocin in their arm to a needle in their back, a vacuum-cup or forceps in their vagina, or a knife in their lower belly at a later stage. We have yet to meet the mother having just given birth after 6 or 10 hours, who complains that her labor was too short.

Labor should not be allowed to cross the partographic diagonal for more than two hours.

15.6.2 Mutual advantages

A major benefit of the proactive restriction of labor duration is that more than 80% of all nulliparas deliver within 8 hours, the duration of a care provider's duty shifts.[10,11] This facilitates personally committed care (Chapter 16). The length of labor should be regarded as an independent quality parameter, as long duration of labor strongly affects the attitude of professional staff. O'Driscoll and Meagher observed "[in conventional obstetrics]… a shared sense of impotence in the face of widespread physical suffering, and even moral degradation, frequently colors the attitude of nurses, midwives, and doctors from their early student days. As a result, many birth care providers either tend to avoid the delivery room as

much as possible, or tend to resort to excessive use of analgesia to alleviate otherwise intolerable personal stress."[6] Indeed, timely prevention of long labor completely changes the face of childbirth for all concerned.

Control of labor duration is as important for staff as it is for their clients/patients.

References

1. Robson M, Hartigan L, Murphy M. Methods of achieving and maintaining an appropriate caesarean section rate. Best Pract Res Clin Obstet Gynaecol 2013;**27**:297–308

2. Maternity Care Working Party. *Making Normal Birth a Reality: Image of a Normal Birth*; 2007; available at: www.appg-maternity.org.uk

3. Cartmill R, Thornton J. Effect of presentation of partogram information on obstetric decision-making. Lancet 1992;**339**:1520–2

4. World Health Organization partograph in management of labour. World Health Organization Maternal Health and Safe Motherhood Programme. Lancet 1994;**343**:1399–404

5. Lavender T, Hart A, Smyth R. Effect of partogram use on outcomes for women in spontaneous labour at term. Cochrane Database Syst Rev 2013

6. O'Driscoll K, Meagher D. Active Management of Labour, 4th edn. London: Mosby; 2003

7. Impey L, Boylan P. Active management of labour revisited. Br J Obstet Gynaecol 1999;**106**:183–7

8. Cardozo LD, Gibb DM, Studd JW, *et al.* Predictive value of cervimetric labour patterns in primigravidae. Br J Obstet Gynaecol 1982;**89**:33–8

9. Melmed H, Evans M. Predictive value of cervical dilatation rates, I. Primigravids. Obstet Gynecol 1976;**47**:1568–75

10. Hogston P, Noble W. Active management of labor: the Portsmouth experience. J Obstet Gynaecol 1993;**17**:340–2

11. Impey L, Hobson J, O'herlihy C. Graphic analysis of actively managed labor: prospective computation of labor progress in 500 consecutive nulliparous women in spontaneous labor at term. Am J Obstet Gynecol 2000;**183**:438–43

Chapter 16

Personal attention and support

Giving birth is a parasympathetic process, a physiological condition that requires a feeling of ease, quietude, comfort, confidence, and security. When these environmental conditions are not met, anxiety and fear inevitably trigger a stress response that inhibits uterine contractions and increases the likelihood of prolonged, dysfunctional labor (7.3.2). Parasympathetic dominance in labor is best promoted by a one-on-one female companion and the personal attention of a trustworthy professional who watches over the parturient's safety and ensures that labor progresses. This is a double-edged sword: the demanding requirements of non-stop presence, personal commitment, and continuous labor support are strongly correlated with a fixed limit on the maximum duration of labor, because neither is possible without the other. Work schedules exceeding 12 hours are unrealistic.

16.1 Lack of supportive care

Until 50–60 years ago, childbirth was primarily a woman's world, one in which women of all cultures were attended and supported by other women during labor and delivery. Over the past five to six decades, however, hospitals have replaced the familiar environment of home. Doctors have replaced midwives for low-risk births, and nursing staff have replaced female family members as supporters during birth. Childbirth in modern maternity centers currently subjects women to institutional routines, a lack of privacy, unfamiliar personnel, work shift changes, and other conditions as highlighted in Chapter 4 that inevitably undermine the parasympathetic process of birth. These conditions usually have an adverse effect on the physiological course of the labor process, increase the chances of obstetric excess, and set a vicious circle into being.

16.1.1 Discontinuous care

The ability of nurses and midwives to provide unbounded labor support is usually limited by their simultaneous responsibility for more than one laboring woman. Added to this, they may very well begin or end work shifts in the middle of a woman's labor, usually work in short-staffed institutions, and spend a large proportion of their time managing technology and keeping records (Chapter 4).

Continuous and personal supportive care during labor has become the exception rather than the rule.

16.1.2 Post-modern trends

Legitimate concerns about the "dehumanization" of women's birthing experience in the hospital have led to calls for a return to home births attended by independent midwives.[1–4] This post-modern trend presumes the superiority of autonomous midwifery care during normal labor, but the documented results of formal midwifery-centered childbirth practices in Holland argue against this proposition (5.3). Unlike the midwives of earlier times – who worked around the clock and stayed with their laboring clients from beginning to end – contemporary midwives have their own family life, disallowing duty shifts longer than 8 hours. Additional tasks for other "clients" further prevent them from providing continuous labor support at home or in alternative birth centers. As a result, periodic visits at intervals of 3 hours or more during the first stage of labor are now common practice in autonomous midwifery care. Evidently, this situation is far from ideal and is, in fact, irresponsible, as shown by the Dutch results (5.3). Clearly, advocates of home births should be cautioned not to replace obstetric excess by non-attendance.

Too many autonomous midwives no longer sit with their laboring clients throughout the entire birth process, nullifying the alleged superiority and safety of their care.

16.1.3 Birth environments

The key issue is not the location of birth – be it the hospital, a primary birth center, or at home – but rather what supports the best chance of a safe and rewarding delivery. Improvement of basic care can only be brought about through radical changes in both secondary and primary care and in the close cooperation between them (Chapter 25).

The prime necessity for rehumanizing childbirth is adequate and continuous support for women by women during all labors regardless of the place of birth. In addition, every effort should be made to ensure that a woman's birthing environment is non-stressful, empowering, communicative of respect, private, and not dictated by routines that may be experienced as harsh and add risk without discernible benefits. At the same time, fetal well-being must be monitored and adequate progress must be ensured. These obligatory assessments and measures might be experienced as disruptive, but the consequent potential stress is best counteracted by adequate pre-labor preparation (Chapter 18), personal commitment and continuity of care from the provider, as well as continuous support from a well-informed, female one-on-one companion in labor. The organizational implications of this system will be addressed in Chapter 25.

> Not the location of birth, but personal attention, commitment, continuous support, and a well-defined birth-plan are the key factors in rehumanizing childbirth and providing effective, safe, and rewarding birth care.

16.2 Personal attention and personal continuity

Paradoxically, the often-encountered tolerance of long labors by midwives wreaks havoc with this basic requirement of continual presence throughout the entire labor and delivery. The midwife attending a home birth should never leave her laboring client. To reiterate: if you are not there, you don't give care. If continuous attendance cannot be guaranteed, then home birth becomes irresponsible (5.3.3).

On the other hand, hospitals must take positive steps to prevent several members of staff from simultaneously attending the same parturient. Personal attention and continuity of care require that every woman in labor has face-to-face attendance by one midwife or one resident who is known to her by name.

The provider must appreciate that in every individual case giving birth is a unique life event for each woman, and a casual or impersonal approach is experienced as insensitive and is counterproductive. While a midwife or a resident may attend more than one laboring woman, the attention of the nurse is preferably confined to a single parturient. Nurses should be selected on the basis of supportive skills and should be trained to be sufficiently aware of the constant need for such skills. A woman's experience of labor depends largely on the quality of the relationship established with the nurse assigned to her personally.[5] Clearly, personal attention does *not* mean a group of nurses caring for an equivalent number of laboring women on a collective basis.

> In the labor and delivery unit, the nurse's attention should be confined to one parturient only.

16.2.1 Mutual dependency

In the final analysis, it is the labor room nurses and the midwives who should convert most recommendations into practice (Chapter 25). Although few consultants will dispute the importance of personal attention and continuous support, many continue only to pay lip service to the ideal while taking no interest in the implementation of a labor protocol that truly enables the frontline birth attendants to provide such intensive care.

By intentionally limiting the duration of labor to a maximum of 12 hours, the shift changes of the care providers during labor are kept to a minimum. When the rules of *proactive support of labor* are applied, 80% of all nulliparas give birth within the timeframe of one duty shift, and the disadvantage of the inevitable personal discontinuity in the other 20% is buffered by the knowledge that only one shift change will occur and that the succeeding care provider will follow exactly the same, consistent policy for the conduct and care of labor.

> Continuous personal attention and prevention of long labor are mutually dependent; neither one is feasible without the other.

Reliance on the endeavors of the personal nurse is no excuse for the midwife or doctor to stay "backstage" and to enter the room only on full dilatation or in the event of an emergency. The midwife and physician must also be actively involved and commit themselves to regular assessments of labor progress, the woman's physical and emotional status, and the well-being of the fetus. A redefinition of the responsibilities and proper working relations between nurses, midwives, and physicians is absolutely mandatory and will be addressed in Chapter 25.

16.3 Continuous support during labor

Women report that one of the most disturbing prospects of labor is the fear of being left alone, and unfortunately such fears of isolation are only too well founded in common childbirth practices.[1,6] Effective provisions must be made to resolve this situation. One-on-one companionship in labor forms the cornerstone of *proactive support of labor.*

> *A central feature of excellent care is the promise that the woman will not be left alone during her labor at any time.*

Mere physical presence is not enough. Supportive care involves eye contact, friendly touch, reassurance, encouragement, consistent information and advice, emotional support, words of praise, comfort measures, and advocacy, which means helping the woman articulate her wishes to the medical staff.[5] The one-on-one female companion in labor – the personal nurse (and/or certified doula) – carries out this important task.

16.3.1 Evidence for continuous support

Continuous support by women for women effectively reduces anxiety and fear and associated adverse effects during labor. The latest systematic Cochrane review[7] of the evidence on continuous support for women during childbirth clearly proves that women who experience one-on-one supportive care are:

- Less likely to have a cesarean section (RR = 0.78, 95% CI 0.67–0.91);
- Less likely to have a forceps or vacuum delivery (RR = 0.90, 95% CI 0.85–0.96);
- Less likely to report a negative birth experience (RR = 0.69, 95% CI 0.59–0.79);
- Less likely to need regional analgesia (RR = 0.93, 95% CI 0.88–0.99);
- More likely to have a spontaneous vaginal birth (RR = 1.08, 95% CI 1.04–1.12).

The meta-analysis did not detect any adverse effects and none are plausible. The effects of continuous support were consistently positive in all trials, but the degree of benefit varied among institutions owing to differences in standard practices. Institutions varied in policies as to whether routine electronic fetal monitoring was used, whether epidural analgesia was available 24/7, whether they allowed additional support people of the woman's own choosing to be present, and whether early use of labor acceleration was standard policy. Indeed, a clear labor management protocol is critical, and in fact the whole package of *proactive support of labor* achieves far more than the sum of its individual components (Chapter 27).

> *One-on-one supportive care during labor has been shown to confer important benefits without attendant risks (Evidence level A).*

The Cochrane review included both multiparas and nulliparas and, therefore, the beneficial effects of continuous labor support on first labor outcomes – the main group of interest – were probably diluted. Another meta-analysis specifically focused on first labors (four trials, $n = 1349$),[8] and all advantageous effects of continuous labor support were demonstrated to be far more pronounced, including a significant shortening of first labor:

> Beneficial effects of continuous labor support on first labors (Evidence level A):
> 1. Shortening of first labors by 2.8 hours on average (95% CI 2.2–3.4 hours);
> 2. Reduction of the need for labor augmentation; RR 0.44 (95% CI 0.4–0.7);
> 3. Doubling of the spontaneous delivery rate; RR 2.01 (95% CI 1.5–2.7);
> 4. Reduction of cesarean deliveries by half; RR 0.54 (95% CI 0.4–0.6);
> 5. Reduction of instrumental vaginal deliveries by half; RR 0.46 (95% CI 0.3–0.7).

16.3.2 Early support

The meta-analyses also provide evidence of a "dose–response" phenomenon. A strong and prolonged dose of continuous support is the most effective, and the benefits are strongest when one-on-one support begins in early labor. This is an important finding because it confirms and emphasizes the necessity of an early, clear-cut diagnosis of labor and early assessment of labor effectiveness as discussed in the previous two chapters.

16.3.3 One-on-one companion in labor

All trials included in the systematic reviews involved one-on-one support provided by experienced women who had given birth themselves or/and had received education and practiced as nurses, midwives, doulas, or childbirth educators. An additional finding of the Cochrane meta-analysis was that the effects of continuous support appear to vary by type of provider. The effects of continuous support are stronger when the provider is not a member of the staff and thus has no obligation to anyone other than the woman in labor. The reduction in operative births may be less when women receive support from nurses or midwives whose training, role, and/ or identity involve responsibilities that extend beyond labor support. Divided loyalties and duties in addition to labor support as well as the constraints of institutional policies and routines may all play a role. This emphasizes the need for reevaluation of all well-intended nursing rituals (4.1.2), which will undoubtedly show that many of these can be safely discarded, freeing nurses to focus on their primary task: supportive care.

> *Continuous labor support is most effective when it begins in early labor and when it is provided by a caregiver who has an exclusive focus on this task (Evidence level A).*

The hospital delivery unit should be designated an intensive care area, not with regard to high-tech equipment but rather with regard to intensive one-on-one nursing. But hospital managers advocating "lean" and "managed care" – and mostly unencumbered by insight into the essential requirements for high-quality childbirth – often preclude such a provision because of lack of funds. These hospital administrators should realize, however, that a substantial reduction in cesarean deliveries translates into an equally substantial reduction in postoperative care, thus freeing nurses to work in the delivery rooms. Good birth care and sound economics can surely complement one another (Chapter 25).

> *The hospital delivery unit should be designated an intensive care area, not with regard to high-tech equipment but rather with regard to intensive one-on-one nursing.*

In the authors' hospital, one-on-one nursing is practiced and all employees are trained in the principles of *proactive support of labor* aimed at a spontaneous delivery within 12 hours. With this overall policy, the highest spontaneous vaginal delivery rate for years in a row has been achieved in the national league tables, without any adverse effects on perinatal outcomes (Chapter 27). Admittedly, it is increasingly difficult to optimize nursing staff quotas, as is the case in most maternity centers where economists increasingly dictate the rules. This is another reason why specific attention should be given to the possibility of labor support by well-trained but non-institutional staff.

16.3.4 Doula services

Over the past decade, several initiatives to employ the services of women with special training in labor support have begun in some countries. This new member of the caregiver team is commonly known as a doula (δουλη is the Greek word for "female slave" or "handmaiden"). She may, however, also be called a labor companion, birth partner, labor support specialist, labor assistant, or birth buddy. In the model pioneered chiefly in middle-class circles in the USA and Canada, the mother selects her doula during pregnancy; they establish a personal relationship that is likely also to involve the woman's partner, and they discuss the mother's preferences and concerns before labor.[6]

The pregnant woman may have other priorities besides medical help, because she does not leave her work, community, life-experiences, and family responsibilities behind when she enters the hospital to give birth. Her doula has detailed knowledge of the particular circumstances and is, therefore, likely to be in a better position to provide personal care and comfort than unfamiliar hospital staff. The doula brings her experience and training, often to the level of certification, to the labor support role during childbirth and helps to improve morale and the woman's labor environment.

> *Continuous, personal attention and professional support during labor should be the norm rather than the exception.*

The doula and/or the personal labor room nurse rallies the mother's own powers and helps her cope with the natural pain and discomfort of labor and delivery. The evidence clearly dictates that there should be serious medical and political efforts not only to promote continuous support of all laboring women by a doula or nursing equivalent but also to provide resources for its universal implementation. In most places, a lot of improvements still need to be made.

16.3.5 Presence of partners and other people

No controlled trials have evaluated the effects of women's partners, family members, or friends as providers of labor support. Insights into the nature and value of such support have been gleaned from observational studies, but self-selection presents a major problem in the interpretation and the potential for making generalizations on the basis of the results of such studies.

In practice, hospitals vary greatly in the extent to which they permit people of the woman's own choosing in labor wards. It would be imprudent, though, to assume that the presence of several people will provide additional support. Family and friends such as husbands and partners may be there to share the experience rather than to provide support. When there are major tensions in the couple's relationship, practical and emotional support in labor by the partner may be difficult to provide or to accept.

Paradoxically, loving partners may feel powerless and suffer as much as their laboring woman who is experiencing pain and exertion. As a result, partners may unwittingly undermine the woman's ability to cope with labor and delivery. It should be noted that allowing fathers into the labor rooms coincides historically with the staggering increase in the use of epidural analgesia, other interventions, and operative delivery rates. Some husbands/partners are bad doulas indeed.

It would be unwise to rely exclusively on the supportive skills of expectant fathers, women's relatives, or friends.

Nevertheless, the presence of fathers in the labor room is now the norm, and many hospitals permit other lay people to be present as well. Indeed, where women have strong preferences for who should be with them at this time, these should be respected. Given the difficulties of generalizing, though, the proper policy must be one of sensitivity by the staff to the possible negative effects of the presence of certain fathers and relatives or friends. In some cases, a café around the corner might be a better place for them to wait, not only for the sake of the woman giving birth, but for the sake of everyone involved.

In the labor room, women have, generally speaking, far more to gain from the presence of a female companion who is not only sympathetic but also well-informed and therefore in a much better position to provide the type of firm support and guidance that are needed. However, effective support by nurses and/or doulas, in turn, is always strongly dependent on a clear and consistent conduct of labor by the midwife or doctor. In effect, continuous labor support cannot be implemented unless early correction of dysfunctional labor is performed as well. Contemporary childbirth is teamwork, and teamwork requires an overall, consistent birth-plan.

References

1. Osbourne A. A culture of fear: the midwifery perspective. *Midwifery Matters* Issue no. **100**, Spring 2004

2. Block J. *Pushed: The Painful Truth about Childbirth and Modern Maternity Care.* Cambridge, MA: Da Capo Press; 2007

3. Wagner M. *Born in the USA: How a Broken Maternity System Must Be Fixed to Put Women and Children First.* Berkeley, CA: University of California Press; 2007

4. Lake R, Epstein E. The Business of Being Born. A documentary film (2007) www.thebusinessofbeing born.com/about.htm

5. Hodnett ED. Pain and women's satisfaction with the experience of childbirth: a systematic review. *Am J Obstet Gynecol* 2002;**186**(Suppl.):160–72

6. Klaus M, Kennel JH, Klaus PH. *Doula Book; How a Trained Labor Companion Can Help You Have a Shorter, Easier, and Healthier Birth.* Cambridge, MA: Da Capo; 2002

7. Hodnett ED, Gates S, Hofmeyr J, Sakala C. Continuous support for women during childbirth. Cochrane Database Syst Rev 2013 July DOI: 10.1002/14651858. CD003766.pub5

8. Zhang J, Bernasko JW, Leybovich E, Fahs M, Hatch MC. Continuous labor support from labor attendant for primiparous women: a meta-analysis. *Obstet Gynecol* 1996;**88**:739–44

Amniotomy and oxytocin

Clinical practice with regard to acceleration of labor is often difficult to comprehend. In many maternity units, there is no protocol for the diagnosis and treatment of slow labor, and each doctor seems to have fixed preferences for which there is no factual basis. In effect, some obstetricians criticize midwives or residents for rupturing the membranes – especially late in the evening – whereas others criticize those who dare to consult them for slow labor when the membranes are still intact. Timing and dosage of oxytocin treatment also vary widely. While some obstetricians forbid any measures in the "latent phase of labor," others order the administration of oxytocin without prior amniotomy. One consultant may feel that a solution with 2.5 IU of oxytocin best accelerates labor, whereas another may prefer to use 5 IU and yet another 10 IU in the syringe. To complicate matters even further, some doctors use all three doses consecutively on the same woman. No wonder residents and nurses may become utterly confused. In such capricious circumstances, mistakes are bound to happen. Clearly, high-quality care demands an overall plan and explicit rules for the timing of amniotomy and the execution of oxytocin treatment, and criticism should be directed toward those who do not comply.

17.1 Controversies about amniotomy

Although artificial rupture of the membranes is among the most commonly performed procedures in obstetrics, there is a lack of reliable data on this issue. The literature is confusing because amniotomy cannot be studied in isolation. Action taken in one direction is likely to have repercussions in another, and such information is generally missing from publications on this subject.

17.1.1 Routine versus selective amniotomy

By the time a diagnosis of labor is made, spontaneous rupture of the fetal membranes has already occurred in

30% of women (14.2.4). Management of the 70% who begin labor with intact membranes is controversial. Some providers artificially rupture the fetal membranes on a routine basis to check for meconium and to place a scalp electrode. Others, on principle, attempt to preserve the membranes as long as possible.

Evidence-based medicine has not provided the answer, as it depends on interpretation of the literature. A 2013 Cochrane systematic review of 15 RCTs, comparing the outcome of women managed with routine amniotomy versus those in whom preservation of intact membranes was planned, yielded contradictory results.[1] Although routine amniotomy at labor onset (definition?) did not result in a significant reduction in the average duration of labor, this procedure did reduce the need for oxytocin treatment in a later stage (RR 0.72, 95% CI 0.54–0.96). Routine amniotomy also significantly reduced the risk of "dysfunctional labor" (RR 0.60, 95% CI 0.44–0.82). However, there was a trend toward a higher cesarean delivery rate (RR 1.27, 95% CI 0.99–1.63) after routine early amniotomy.

As so often in meta-analyses, interpretation is problematic. A severe limitation of the source studies was the lack of information or inconsistency in the timing of amniotomy with respect to cervical dilatation. In 20 to 60% of women assigned to the control groups, the membranes were artificially ruptured at some later stage "if indicated" though not further specified. The reviewers speculated that the trend to more cesarean deliveries might result from amniotomy-related abnormalities as detected by cardiotocography (CTG), or early recognition of meconium, thus lowering the threshold for operative delivery. Another explanation might be clinical suspicion of infection when long labor is still tolerated after routine amniotomy at labor onset. As always, a meta-analysis cannot be stronger than the studies that contribute to it. Despite or because of the lack of information on the total package of care in the studies reviewed, the Cochrane reviewers concluded that amniotomy should not be used routinely as part of standard labor management and care.

This viewpoint is in accordance with the principles of *proactive support of labor* that any intervention should be performed only when indicated, but when indicated, action should be definite. Amniotomy should be reserved for women with abnormally slow progress of labor or when there is any doubt about fetal status. Abnormal progress must, of course, be defined. This diagnosis should be made during the course of labor whenever dilatation is less than 1 cm/h (15.6).

> *The policy of routine amniotomy at labor onset should be abandoned.*

17.1.2 Indication for amniotomy

Naturally, there are women in whom labor will accelerate spontaneously after an initially slow onset. However, birth attendants do not possess a crystal ball; with that same chance, expectancy might very well result in an overly long labor and related agony. In this context, we remind readers that the mean duration of the "latent phase" as defined by Friedman was 8.6 hours (+2 SD 20.6 hours) for first labor and that the range was 1 to 44 hours, with a maximum of 20 hours still accepted as statistically "normal" (sic).[2] The fallacy of the recent ACOG consensus statement "before 6 cm of dilatation is achieved, standards of 'active phase' progress should not be applied"[3] was debunked in Chapter 14. Clearly, it is better to dismiss the concept of the latent phase altogether (Chapter 10).

There is no doubt that timely amniotomy can convert slow labor to normal progression. To assure a delivery within 12 hours, prospective criteria for progress are needed, and early diagnosis and prompt treatment of slow labor are mandatory. For this reason, we rupture the membranes whenever progress is less than 1 cm/h at any stage, even at 1 cm dilatation. As the diagnosis of labor itself, amniotomy embodies a firm commitment to delivery. There is no way back, and policies must be clear and must be followed.

> *The membranes should be ruptured whenever labor progress is less than 1 cm/h, even if dilatation is only 1 cm (= fully effaced cervix).*

There is no justification for postponing amniotomy when labor is slow. Neither the fetus nor the mother benefits from a long labor. Furthermore, amniotomy provides valuable information on the possible causative involvement of meconium (8.5.5) whenever (early) labor is slow.

These considerations equally apply to home births. There is no valid reason to forbid midwives to rupture the membranes at home if early labor is too slow. On the contrary, criticism should be reserved for those who do not. An unengaged fetal head is the only contraindication for amniotomy at home, but this situation at labor onset is in itself reason enough for immediate transfer to the hospital.

17.1.3 Safety of amniotomy

A variety of hazards related to amniotomy has been postulated but never substantiated. It has been suggested that increased pressure differences around the fetal skull, combined with a reduction in amniotic fluid, predispose to fetal skull deformity, an increased incidence of decelerations in fetal heart rate, and fetal distress. However, the studies intended to show these effects were subject to considerable selection bias and do not permit any reliable conclusions. Only one prospective, randomized study identified increased mild and moderate umbilical cord compression patterns on the CTG as a result of amniotomy, but no serious problems were found and the rate of cesarean delivery for fetal distress was unaffected.[4] Surveillance of the fetus during birth will be extensively addressed in Chapter 24.

A floating fetal head is the only contraindication for amniotomy, and cesarean delivery is the only safe option. When the fetal head is in the pelvic inlet but is unstable, care should be taken to avoid dislodging it when rupturing the membranes. An assistant who applies fundal and superpubic pressure will eliminate the risk of cord prolapse. If there is additional polyhydramnios, it might be prudent to use a small gauge needle, rather than a hook, to puncture the fetal membranes, and to perform the procedure in the operating room.[5] This "controlled amniotomy" minimizes the risk of gushing amniotic fluid and permits emergency cesarean delivery in the event of a cord prolapse. The need for these precautions, however, is exceptional.

Intrapartum amniotomy does not increase the need for narcotic or epidural analgesia or the risk of maternal infection. Two Cochrane meta-analyses found no significant effects of amniotomy for standard indicators of maternal or neonatal morbidity.[1,6]

It can be safely concluded that artificial rupture of membranes (AROM) for acceleration of slow labor is a safe and effective procedure, provided the fetal head is engaged and amniotomy is employed as a component of an overall plan. Additional measures to restrict the duration of labor effectively prevent the development of intra-uterine infection.

> *Amniotomy performed to accelerate slow labor is a safe and effective procedure (Evidence level A).*

17.2 Judicious use of oxytocin

Misconceptions about the risks and benefits of oxytocin stubbornly persist in the minds of many providers because of adverse experiences with oxytocin used for induction. Added to that, oxytocin in spontaneous but slow labor is often started too late and at too low a dosage. The literature is similarly blurred and marred by misinterpretations and inaccuracies. Many recommendations in official guidelines are rooted in shallow soil.

17.2.1 Misunderstandings

- Firstly, many studies confuse acceleration with induction. Even the most influential American textbook *Williams Obstetrics* (2005) casually states "there is only a semantic difference between labor induction and augmentation," whereas nothing could be further from the truth. The fundamental distinction between induction and acceleration needs constant reiteration.
- Secondly, randomized trials comparing early and delayed oxytocin treatment failed to detect effects on cesarean rates.[4] However, these studies only started in the alleged "active stage" of labor, so they actually compared late with very late acceleration. In truth, the greatest benefits of oxytocin are often achieved at an earlier stage. Again, the concept of the latent phase should be abandoned (10.1).
- Thirdly, use of oxytocin cannot be examined in isolation. Lack of information of concomitant measures thwarts the interpretation of the reported randomized trials.
- Fourthly, in most publications the problem of the exhausted uterus after an inordinate delay (8.5.4)

is underappreciated, neglected, or plainly unknown to the authors.
- Finally, and most importantly, most if not all studies and guidelines on labor protraction fail to recognize the fundamentally different causes in nulliparous and parous labor. In fact, oxytocin is safe and effective in the former, but may be hazardous in the latter.

> *The literature on the use of oxytocin in labor is blurred and marred by inaccuracies. Many recommendations, even in formal guidelines, are in part founded on quicksand.*

17.2.2 Basic considerations

- Oxytocin is a powerful uterine stimulant, provided that the myometrium has been transformed, in other words that there are sufficient CAPs (contraction associated proteins) present (8.3.2). This explains why oxytocin is highly effective in accelerating spontaneous labor and why it acts unpredictably in labor induction.
- Slow progress in early labor points to an incomplete operating system that still can be established rapidly by oxytocin. The explanation for the effectiveness of amniotomy and oxytocin in speeding up early labor is an accelerated completion of the myometrial gap junction system, improving the electrical orchestration and recruiting the maximum number of myometrial cells for contractile action (8.4.1).
- A prerequisite for effective acceleration of spontaneous labor is either spontaneous or artificial rupture of the membranes. Amniotomy reduces the need for oxytocin, and so-called "dry" stimulation is ineffective and not rooted in any logical framework. Once the diagnosis of labor is established, a point of no return has been reached; if progress is slow, the first step is amniotomy.
- Oxytocin increases PGE_2 and intracellular calcium concentration in the myometrium, thereby increasing uterine force (Chapter 8). This explains its ability to correct protraction and arrest disorders in both the first and second stages of labor (Chapter 21).
- Oxytocin improves both the efficiency and frequency of uterine contractions resulting in

enhanced force per contraction and more cumulative force per unit time.

- Appropriate timing is crucial. Prolonged labor results in accumulation of lactic acid in the uterus, as well as myometrial desensitization through a loss of oxytocin-binding sites. The effect of oxytocin in these circumstances may be decreased responsiveness, or, paradoxically, uterine tetanic spasms may occur, each of which is a feature of stimulating an exhausted, refractory uterus, loaded with lactic acid (8.5.4).
- It cannot be overemphasized that the proposed protocol for the use of oxytocin must be restricted to term nulliparas with a single cephalic fetus and a reassuring fetal status.
- Misapplication of the method to other, wholly unsuitable categories of patients has given rise to reports of obstetric disasters, such as fetal acidemia, trauma, complicated breech delivery, or uterine rupture in parous women, including those laboring after previous cesarean delivery.

17.3 Effectiveness and safety

Early amniotomy and oxytocin, in appropriate doses, is so effective at accelerating slow labor that the diagnosis of labor must be seriously doubted if these measures fail to produce the desired response. This is commonplace in practices where the woman's self-diagnosis of labor is taken for granted (Chapter 14).

17.3.1 Prevention of long labor

The sole purpose of accelerating slow progress in spontaneous labor is prevention of prolonged labor. The evidence shows that early correction of slow spontaneous labor is highly effective in this regard, in particular in first labors.

The latest Cochrane review included 11 RCTs that enrolled women who were in spontaneous labor and randomly allocated them to amniotomy and oxytocin if slow progress ensued or to (undefined) expectant management.[4] Of note is that the meta-analysis did not factor in parity, a reprehensible omission that dilutes the effects in nulliparous labors. Nevertheless, the review evidenced that early acceleration – as an isolated intervention – shortens labor (–1.11 hours, 95% CI –1.82 to –0.41) and reduces the risk of cesarean delivery (RR 0.87, 95% CI 0.77–0.99).[4]

The positive effects are much more pronounced in first labors and if early acceleration is used as a component of an overall plan. An Oxford study, for instance, analyzed a cohort of 500 actively managed nulliparas.[7] The mean cervical dilatation at admission was 1.7 cm, and the mean duration of labor was 6.1 hours; all but 2.8% were delivered within 12 hours, and the cesarean rate was only 5.4%. Two RCTs testing the "active management" in nulliparas also showed highly significant reductions in the incidence of labor lasting >12 hours: from 19% to 5% and from 26% to 9%.[8,9] The latest Cochrane review (2013) evidenced significantly fewer labors lasting more than 12 hours and a lower cesarean delivery rate in the active management group (RR 0.77, 95% CI 0.63 to 0.94).[10]

Reduction in the incidence of prolonged labor is an independent outcome parameter of paramount importance, since prolonged labor is strongly associated with a traumatizing childbirth experience. Elimination of negative birth experiences without resorting to operative delivery is the main objective of expert care.

Early correction of slow labor is highly effective in the prevention of long labor (Evidence level A) and related traumatizing birth experiences.

17.3.2 Safety

The octapeptide oxytocin is one of the most specific therapeutic agents there is and has no side effects, aside from its intrinsic antidiuretic effect. Danger of water intoxication arises only after IV administration of high doses along with excessive salt-free fluid loads.[11] If used correctly, water intoxication cannot occur. However, a good therapeutic agent is as safe as the one who applies it. Danger hides not in the agent but in users who do not follow a protocol that provides a highly effective series of safeguards (Table 17.1).

When the responsibility for execution of labor acceleration is left to residents, midwives, or nurses, the rules must be explicit and rigidly enforced. Oxytocin should always be administered intravenously. To avoid bolus administration, the infusion should be inserted into the main intravenous line close to the venipuncture site.

A fixed, standard concentration must be used at all times and preferably administered by an electronically

Table 17.1 Rules governing the safe use of oxytocin

1. Use only in nulliparous women with a single fetus in the cephalic presentation
2. Start of labor is spontaneous
3. Membranes are ruptured and the amniotic fluid is clear
4. The fetus is in good condition
5. Oxytocin is started on time
6. A standard concentration is used at all times
7. The only variable is the infusion rate
8. Direct and continuous nursing supervision is mandatory
9. Nurses/midwives may increase the dosage to a pre-fixed maximum of 40 mU/min

Table 17.2 Safe and effective dosage schedule for oxytocin

- A standard concentration of 5 IU in 50 ml balanced salt solution is used at all times
- IV pump starts with 3 ml/h = 5 mU/min
- The dose is titrated to its effect (dose increments of 3 ml/h at intervals of 15 minutes
- Tachysystole (>6 contractions per 15 minutes) is reason to decrease the dose by half
- The maximum dose is 24 ml/h = 40 mU/min
- Evidence of fetal distress is the only absolute bar to oxytocin treatment

The evidence supports a high-dose oxytocin regimen (Evidence level A).

safeguarded IV pump. The only variable is the infusion rate. However, lack of sophisticated infusion equipment is not an excuse for delay in oxytocin treatment, because a simple infusion gravity feed may perform equally well, provided a personal nurse carefully monitors it. This is an issue of great practical importance in third-world hospitals where infusion pumps may not be available.

17.3.3 Dosage scheme

Oxytocin is administered incrementally to titrate dose to effect because it is not possible to predict a woman's response to a particular dosage.[12] Many obstetric units still use low-dose oxytocin, although the evidence strongly supports the higher-dose regimens.[13]

The 2013 Cochrane review evaluated randomized studies that compared high-dose oxytocin (arbitrarily defined as 4 mU per minute or more) with lower doses. The use of the high dosage was associated with a significant reduction in the length of labor (mean difference –3.50 hours; 95% CI –6.38 to –0.62) and cesarean rates (RR 0.62; 95% CI 0.44–0.86). The high-dose regimens also reduced the need for instrumental deliveries: spontaneous birth rate was significantly higher (RR 1.35; 95% CI 1.13–1.62) while no effects were observed on maternal or perinatal morbidities.[13]

These studies highlight the importance of *how* oxytocin is used, not simply *whether* oxytocin is used. In many a practice, however, oxytocin is still used in a dose so low that 20 hours would be needed to reach the average target dose intended to ensure delivery within 12 hours. Indeed, the evidence suggests that the customary low-dose regimens actually contribute to the high intrapartum cesarean rates in many hospitals.[14]

The purpose is to restore adequate progression within 1 to 2 hours. The evidence-based benefits favor a high-dose oxytocin regimen, with incremental increases at short intervals. It is for this reason that we recommend the protocol shown in Table 17.2.

This regimen is safe and can be delegated without reservation to an adequately trained nurse or midwife who stays at the bedside and monitors the frequency of contractions.[15] Following this step-by-step protocol, progress of labor is almost invariably restored within one hour, and the maximum dose allowed is attained at the shortest possible time: 75 minutes. This regimen is safe and effective only when the rules are rigidly enforced.

Birth attendants should not reduce the rate of infusion simply because the mother complains of pain, which is to be expected. Questioning the established infusion rate is a common manifestation of a low level of confidence in the system and usually derives from lack of knowledge and imprecise instructions. Suggestions that women regard oxytocin with suspicion and decline acceleration because of the pain result from serious misunderstandings originating in centers where, paradoxically, induction rates are high.

The protocol-directed administration of oxytocin can be left to the responsibility of an adequately trained nurse or midwife.

17.3.4 Oxytocin and pain

Every birth attendant who has worked in a hospital is familiar with the so-called "oxytocin contractions" characterized by a rapid increase in intrauterine pressure followed by a sharp peak and a rapid decrease on the monitor. It is common to hear statements that these contractions are more painful than others. This is probably true. However, people forget that such sharply peaked oxytocin contractions are, without exception, specific to induction. In contrast to induction, labor acceleration normalizes contractions, including the normal, intrinsic pain, and there is no reason to assume that these contractions should be any more painful. It is important to note that because oxytocin in spontaneous labor shortens the birth process, there is, in fact, a decreased need for pain relief measures (Chapters 19, 20).

Prevention of long labors reduces the need for medical pain relief measures.

17.3.5 Duration of oxytocin treatment

There are no reliable data to recommend a maximum duration for oxytocin administration to treat dysfunctional labor. The ACOG[16] "2-hour rule" to define failed augmentation should be abandoned.[3,12,17] In fact, the most important issue is early timing to avoid an exhausted uterus that has gradually become unresponsive to oxytocin.

For these reasons, we do not use fixed time restraints for oxytocin administration. On the other hand, we never allow labor to transgress the partographic reference-line for more than 2 hours.

If progress remains inadequate despite high-dose oxytocin, the woman is offered a cesarean delivery. If dystocia has been treated in time and with the proper dose, continuing oxytocin treatment makes no sense. Such a prolonged but ineffective treatment is unduly harsh and even needlessly traumatizing for the laboring woman. An inescapable cesarean delivery is best performed on time.

Most complications of cesarean delivery relate directly to the pre-cesarean length of labor. Therefore, cesarean delivery is suggested to every woman for whom an easy vaginal delivery is not near at hand after 12 hours of labor. A delivery within 12 hours constitutes the guiding principle of expert labor care. Despite these seemingly extreme measures, overall cesarean rates for dystocia are effectively kept low (Chapter 27).

Table 17.3 Causes of poor response to oxytocin

- Error in diagnosis of labor (or induction)
- Intact membranes
- Delay in oxytocin
- Inadequate dose in the infusion pump
- Appropriate dose but hesitant, half-hearted use

By design, cesarean delivery is offered whenever an easy vaginal delivery is not near at hand after 12 hours of adequately supported labor.

17.3.6 Poor response

Provided the inclusion criteria (Table 17.1) and other preconditions (Table 17.2) are met, oxytocin will invariably increase both the frequency and force of the contractions. Poor response to oxytocin results from inexpert labor management (Table 17.3).

17.4 Maternal and fetal surveillance

The goal of using oxytocin is rapid correction of ineffective labor while avoiding hyperstimulation that might compromise the fetus. Thus, progression in dilatation is the only parameter by which to evaluate the effect of oxytocin (9.3), and a doubtful fetal status is the only indication to decrease or discontinue the infusion.

Therefore, the personal nurse evaluates both uterine action and fetal heart rate on a regular basis. Oxytocin should be halved or discontinued if contractions persist as more than seven in a 15-minute period, if they last longer than 60 seconds, or if the fetal status is disconcerting. No special equipment is needed for these assessments. Fetal condition can be monitored as in any labor (Chapter 24) and the bedside nurse can easily assess the frequency and duration of contractions with her hand on the woman's abdomen, which, by the way, enhances personal involvement and attention in labor. Intrauterine pressure catheters are not needed and are preferably not used (9.3.2).

Safeguards

Oxytocin must be halved or discontinued if contractions occur more frequently than seven times in a 15-minute period, if they last longer than 60 seconds, or if fetal status becomes doubtful.

17.4.1 No pressure catheters

Intrauterine gauges might be helpful in extremely obese patients, but there is no evidence to demonstrate any improvement in perinatal outcome attributable to the routine use of intrauterine pressure measurements.[18,19] On the contrary, intrauterine pressure monitoring is usually counterproductive, because it easily becomes a technical substitute for personal nursing attention and care. Moreover, intrauterine pressure catheters are an unnecessary annoyance, are not without complications, are a source of infection, and are expensive.

17.4.2 Hyperstimulation

Oxytocin improves the efficiency of uterine contractions, resulting in more force per contraction (8.4.1). Oxytocin also increases the frequency of contractions, thereby enhancing uterine force per unit time as well.

The term tachysystole is used to distinguish hyperstimulation without corresponding fetal heart rate abnormalities from hypertonia in the intervals between contractions that may endanger the fetus. The former certainly occurs on occasion, but the latter is hardly ever seen when the above-mentioned inclusion criteria for use of oxytocin are met, and the protocol is strictly followed.

Tachysystole (seven or more contractions per 15 minutes) is in fact innocent and easily managed.[20–22] Immediate discontinuance of oxytocin almost instantly decreases the frequency of contractions, as the half-life of intravenous oxytocin is only 1–6 minutes.[11] Oxytocin might be resumed at half the latest dose if needed. In our experience, hyperstimulation is never an unmanageable problem, nor was it found to be a real problem in any of the previously discussed studies.

When the protocol is followed, uterine tachysystole is easily managed. Hyperstimulation resulting in fetal distress is specific to induction or to unduly delayed augmentation. It is not related to timely use of oxytocin in spontaneous labor.

17.4.3 Fetal intolerance

A healthy fetus is well-equipped to tolerate the stress of uterine contractions (8.7), unless accidents such as umbilical cord compression occur (Chapter 24). Cord compression happens equally frequently with or without oxytocin. The impact of such accidents on fetal well-being is the same in both cases. Since the purpose of oxytocin is to enhance labor, it inevitably contributes to the normal chance of fetal distress. Oxytocin does not, however, increase the risk of fetal hypoxia. The meta-analyses and structured reviews fail to detect any adverse effects on fetal outcomes.[12,13]

Fetal intolerance is a compelling reason to refrain from oxytocin.

Inability to give oxytocin in slow labor because of fetal distress is a straightforward indication for cesarean delivery. It should be noted, however, that dose-effect titration is problematic only after an excessive delay causing lactic acid accumulation in the myometrium and loss of oxytocin-receptors (Chapter 8). The only cases seen in our hospital are women who are transferred by autonomous midwives after an inordinate tolerance of slow labor at home.

Hypertonic dystocia is a completely different clinical entity (8.5.5). In this case the cells of the myometrium are randomly excited by chorioamnionitis, meconium, or intrauterine blood to the extent that the coordination and hence the efficiency and effectiveness of contractions are lost. This can lead to a hazardous and vicious circle involving dysfunctional labor and fetal distress. An experienced obstetrician should, of course, directly and personally supervise such a risky labor. If the fetus does not tolerate the uterine powers required for normal progress, a prompt cesarean is the only rational option. As always, policies must be clear and action must be resolute.

Hypertonic dystocia is a separate clinical entity altogether and unrelated to oxytocin.

17.5 Solving territorial disputes

In countries with healthcare systems that include the possibility of selected home births, the issue of acceleration of labor needs special agreements. Midwives attending home births are not allowed by law to administer oxytocin until after the birth of the baby. That is why women whose labor progresses unsatisfactorily need to be transferred to the hospital without delay. However, labor can be accelerated, without any rational objection, on a consultative outpatient basis. By having progression normalized, the woman can remain under the care and responsibility of her chosen and trusted midwife. The stipulation for this continuity in care is mutual trust and respect between community-based midwives and obstetricians, as well as a legal contract defining the responsibility and legal accountability of each (Chapter 25).

Furthermore, community-based midwives and hospital-bound obstetricians must be in absolute agreement regarding the criteria for adequate progression and adhere to the same time-specific indications for acceleration. A midwife who transfers a woman to the hospital far too late should not be surprised if the obstetrician – in an effort to catch up after the fact and confronted with a by now exhausted woman with a depleted, refractory uterus – takes over the subsequent care of the woman.

On the other hand, the midwife must be able to trust that on transferring the parturient to the hospital in due time the woman will remain under her continuing care and responsibility (Chapter 26). The obstetrician who first waits a couple of hours before drawing any conclusions, or worse yet, orders sedatives and does not see the woman until the following morning, undermines the necessary continuity of care and does nothing to generate trust in and respect for hospital care.

Clinical acceleration of slow labor can be provided, without any rational objection, on a consultative basis for midwife-led labors, promoting continuity in care.

17.6 Rules for other patients

It must be stressed that the rules for labor augmentation as outlined above apply only to healthy, term nulliparous women with a single fetus in good condition and in the vertex position. Oxytocin should be administered to other patients only under the direct supervision of an experienced obstetrician and heeding the following considerations:

- Although the basic principles of expert labor management are universally valid, the protocol cannot be automatically applied to breech or twin births.
- When the fetus is in the breech position, oxytocin can be used safely in spontaneous early labor (retraction phase). However, from 5 cm dilatation onward, oxytocin must be discontinued. During the wedging phase of a breech birth, oxytocin is not without risk, as secondary protraction might be the first sign of unfavorable fetopelvic proportions with dire consequences for the after-coming head. In case of a secondary protraction in a breech delivery, the strict rule applies: resort to a cesarean.

- In a multiple pregnancy, the uterus is under greater strain than in a singleton pregnancy and therefore might react less predictably.
- Dysfunctional labor is uncommon in parous women. After critical analysis, inefficient contractions only occur in multiparas who are induced, who are incorrectly declared in labor, who are negatively conditioned by a traumatizing previous birth, or whose labor is compromised by intrauterine meconium, blood, or pus (Chapter 13).
- Occasional secondary protraction and arrest disorder in parous labor is highly suggestive of relatively unfavorable fetopelvic proportions or absolute obstruction (Chapters 14 and 22). Use of oxytocin in such circumstances increases the risk of both maternal and fetal trauma, and in the case of a uterine scar, even uterine rupture.
- Late augmentation of parous labor should, therefore, only be allowed in the rare cases that obstruction can be explicitly ruled out (Chapter 21). Reassurance about such conditions must be definitively demonstrated by absence of molding, absence of substantial caput succedaneum, absence of extreme hyperflexion, and the absence of malposition of the fetal head. Augmentation of parous labor must always be explicitly and personally approved and supervised by the consultant on duty, and shoulder dystocia should be anticipated.

There is a grave obligation on the part of the obstetrician in charge to ensure that fetal obstruction has been excluded before oxytocin in parous labor is authorized.

References

1. Smyth RM, Markham C, Dowswell T. Amniotomy for shortening spontaneous labour. Cochrane Database Syst Rev 2013
2. Friedman, EA, ed. Labor Clinical Evaluation and Management, 2nd edn. New York: Appleton-Century – Crofts, 1978

3. American College of Obstetricians and Gynecologists. Obstetric Care Consensus No 1: Safe prevention of the primary cesarean delivery. Obstet Gynecol 2014;**123**:693–711

4. Garite TJ, Porto M, Carlson NJ, Rumney PJ, Reimbold PA. The influence of elective amniotomy on fetal heart rate patterns and the course of labor in term patients: a randomized study. Am J Obstet Gynecol 1993;**168**:1827–32

5. Funai EF, Norwitz ER. Management of normal labor and delivery. UpToDate. Accessed November 2014

6. Wei S, Wo BL, Qi HP, *et al.* Early amniotomy and early oxytocin for prevention of, or therapy for, delay in first stage spontaneous labour compared with routine care. Cochrane Database Syst Rev 2013

7. Impey L, Hobson J, O'herlihy C. Graphic analysis of actively managed labor: prospective computation of labor progress in 500 consecutive nulliparous women in spontaneous labor at term. Am J Obstet Gynecol 2000;**183**:438–43

8. Lopez-Zeno J, Peaceman A, Adashek JA, Socol ML. A controlled trial of a program of active management of labour. N Engl J Med 1992;**326**:450–4

9. Frigoletto F, Lieberman E, Lang JM, *et al.* A clinical trial of active management of labor. N Engl J Med 1995;**333**:745–50

10. Brown HC, Paranjothy S, Dowswell T, Thomas J. Package of care for active management in labour for reducing caesarean section rates in low-risk women. Cochrane Database Syst Rev 2013

11. Oxytocin: Drug information. UpToDate. Accessed October 2014

12. Ehsanipoor RM, Satin MR. Overview of normal labor and protraction and arrest disorders. UpToDate. Accessed November 2014

13. Kenyon S, Tokumasu H, Dowswell T, *et al.* High-dose versus low-dose oxytocin for augmentation of delayed labour. Cochrane Database Syst Rev 2013

14. Kotaska AJ, Klein MC, Liston RM. Epidural analgesia associated with low-dose oxytocin augmentation increases cesarean births: a critical look at the external validity of randomized trials. Am J Obstet Gynecol 2006;**194**; 809–14

15. Clayworth S. The nurse's role during oxytocin administration. MCN Am J Matern Child Nurs 2000;**25**:80–4

16. Dystocia and augmentation of labor. ACOG practice bulletin no 49. Obstet Gynecol 2003;**102**:1445–54; and *Int J Gynecol Obstet* 2004;**49**:315–24

17. NICE Guidelines. Intrapartum care: care of healthy women and their babies during childbirth. RCOG Press; 2007. Updated 2010 www.nice.org.uk/guidance/cg55

18. Chua S, Kurup A, Alkumaran S, Ratnam SS. Augmentation of labor: does internal tocography result in better obstetric outcome than external tocography? Obstet Gynecol 1990;**76**:164–7

19. Lucidi RS, Chez RA, Creasy RK. The clinical use of intrauterine pressure catheters. J Matern Fetal Med 2001;**10**:420–2

20. Heuser CC, Knight S, Esplin MS, *et al.* Tachysystole in term labor: incidence, risk factors, outcomes, and effect on fetal heart tracings. Am J Obstet Gynecol 2013;**209**:32.e1–6. Epub 2013 Apr 6

21. Frey H, Meister M, Kleweis S, Stuart J. Discussion: 'Tachysystole in term labor'. Am J Obstet Gynecol 2013;**209**:e6–7

22. Stewart RD, Bleich AT, Lo JY, *et al.* Defining uterine tachysystole: how much is too much? Am J Obstet Gynecol 2012;**207**:290.e1–6

18

Pre-labor preparation

Although women's expectations and involvement in decision-making are critical to their childbirth experience, many obstetricians and midwives still neglect pre-labor preparation as a topic of real interest. Providers rather appear to rely on the assumption that everything will turn out okay and – should this prove not to be the case – that there are but a few problems that cannot be handled with pain medication or cesarean section. Women's preparation for birth is generally left to antenatal classes conducted by self-employed birth educators or institutional physiotherapists. These teachers, however, are mostly far removed from actual childbirth practice. Left to themselves, professional status and job satisfaction suffer greatly. As a result, some birth educators even appear to be in open conflict with childbirth practitioners because they have developed little or no common ground. It is difficult to imagine how lessons in such circumstances could be reassuring to childbearing women.

18.1 Confusing antenatal classes

The widespread popularity of antenatal classes attests to the desire of expectant parents for childbirth education and training programs for labor coping strategies.[1,2] Despite the best of intentions, these classes may be counterproductive because certain expectations about labor support facilities may be roused that are unmet at labor and delivery. Classes vary widely in content, ranging from psycho-prophylaxis to yoga, from the use of birth balls to specific breathing and pushing techniques, from reflexology to aromatherapy, and so forth.[3] At birth, however, labor room staff frequently turn a blind eye and a deaf ear to what women were taught previously by "outsiders," and then the discrepancy between expectations and practice inevitably spoils women's childbirth experiences.

> *A mismatch between lessons and practice strongly undermines women's satisfaction with childbirth.*

Independent antenatal classes organized by official health agencies or coordinated by consumer groups equally suffer from a loss of credibility when birth educators are unable to state the labor management policy at the hospital and the available support facilities. Information provided in institutional classes will be more in line with actual practice, but antenatal classes in poorly organized centers may be worse than none at all because women are often left even more apprehensive than before. Institutional staff who cannot agree on a common policy of labor management represent the main impediment to improved standards of care. In such circumstances, class information may raise more questions than will be answered. Clearly, pre-labor preparation is of paramount importance, but this can only be effective when antenatal educators and birth care providers concur with and comply with a clear overall birth-plan.

> *Only when all care providers comply with a consistent birth-plan can clear and honest information and instructions be given and firm promises be made.*

Parous women prejudiced by adverse previous experiences tend to have closed minds on the subject of labor. They often set the wrong tone in classes with mixed parity. Group attention is then readily distracted by horror stories about individual bad experiences (elsewhere) and will inevitably be directed toward medical complications and artificial deliveries. For obvious reasons we prefer individual birth education and preferably through nursing consultation where ample time is taken for information on labor and delivery. Visits to the childbirth educators can be easily incorporated in antenatal clinics.

18.2 Purpose and practice

The main objective of pre-labor preparation is to define the woman's own role in childbirth and to offer her tools to fulfill it.[4] In order to enhance her sense of self-efficacy and confidence in her ability to cope, each childbearing woman must be able to rely on the promise that all efforts and help will be directed to a safe and rewarding delivery within a reasonable time.

18.2.1 Pre-labor education and training

A distinction should be made between the provision of information and training facilities: information on the labor management strategy – and how women themselves play a crucial role in achieving the prize of spontaneous delivery – is preferably given at the individual level. General training programs to teach women how to cope with the exertion and pain of first-stage labor, and how to reinforce the natural expulsive forces at the second stage, are suitable for group training.

18.2.2 Mutual responsibilities

It could easily be overlooked that getting pregnant is primarily a woman's own responsibility, and so is giving birth. Thus, a serious obligation rests on all expectant mothers to be well-prepared for the forthcoming birth. Nulliparas especially should take full advantage of the educational service on offer, which must be readily available and relevant in content. It is much too late to begin education in the labor and delivery room.

> *Pregnant women should be made aware that childbirth is primarily their responsibility.*

On the other hand, if more than lip service is to be paid to the proposition that education is an essential component of a center with pretensions of high-quality care, providers must cease to regard such facilities as optional extras. All doctors and midwives should subscribe to the importance of women's preparation for labor and delivery, and should be aware of its content. They should actively encourage their patients/clients, as well as the partners, to use the educational services.

> *All care providers should acknowledge the importance of pre-labor education, which should be readily available and relevant in content.*

18.3 Personal education

Above all, what is taught must be seen to correspond with actual practice. Therefore, explicit information on the forthcoming birth is best provided by a labor room nurse or midwife who has ongoing practical experience in the maternity center where the woman will give birth. No teacher should be engaged exclusively in this area because this, inevitably, leads to a condition of isolation, which is one of the main reasons why birth educators are virtually ignored by those in positions of greatest influence, the doctors.[4]

> *Childbirth education is best provided on an individual basis by labor room nurses or midwives who have ongoing experience in the delivery unit in question.*

18.3.1 Individual educational service

Institutional labor room nurses and/or midwives are in the best position to explain the process of birth and the actual care the woman can count on. Being directly involved in birth attendance in the unit in question, they know exactly what they are talking about. No two pregnant women are the same, and personal consultation enables birth educators to tailor their information to the individual in understandable language, trying to help each woman to overcome her personal fears and to answer her specific questions. They explain the available provisions for labor support and pain relief methods (Chapters 19 and 20). The woman's preferences and wishes are put on record, knowing that labor room staff will honor these, but unrealistic expectations are adjusted to match real practice. The keynote is mutual confidence and the unstinted message is: "We take you seriously."

> *Pre-labor education must correspond with actual practice.*

In our hospital, all pregnant women visit the institutional birth educator several times during pregnancy, starting at 12 weeks. Much more time is allotted for these consultations than the usually short visits to the doctor or midwife. The first consultation focuses on general health advice. The emotional shifts of pregnancy may be explored, and issues of sexuality and relationship with the spouse or partner may be discussed as well. Social and psychological problems need to be detected and professional help arranged if needed.

Education in late pregnancy is focused primarily on labor and delivery but may be expanded with information on breast-feeding and smooth postpartum adjustment to new motherhood. These consultations allow unique opportunities to provide a favorable image of the entire childbirth service to the consumers. Most importantly, a meaningful informed consent is obtained for the overall birth-plan, including epidural analgesia if effective pain relief should be needed. Informed consent sought during the throes of labor is meaningless both in medical and legal terms.

> *Personal one-on-one counseling allows meaningful informed consent with the labor management protocol, including additional measures that might be needed such as epidural analgesia.*

18.4 Relevant content

The guiding principle for adequate pre-labor preparation is to convince each woman that she has nothing to fear and that she is perfectly capable of giving birth by her own efforts. A motivating spirit is consciously nurtured, not only by the birth educators but also by all personnel, including doctors, midwives, nurses, residents, sonographers, secretaries, and other administrators. Negative psychology (4.2) must be rigidly avoided.

18.4.1 Pre-labor information

Our birth educators aim to provide accurate and reliable information about labor and delivery and the experiences that women will undergo or encounter. The elementary mechanisms of the natural birth process are clearly explained. A sharp distinction is made between induction of labor and treatment of abnormally slow progress after labor has begun spontaneously. The due date is established as a subsidiary item to avoid the pregnant woman directing her expectations toward this date. Instead, we emphasize the full term period and give the date of the latest day of delivery at 42 weeks (14.6.4).

Adequate information includes the relationship of late pregnancy symptoms such as Braxton Hicks contractions to underlying pre-labor processes (8.3). Suggestions for ways of alleviating these symptoms are given, as well as clear instructions as to when the pregnant woman should contact her care provider (14.3.1). The subjective symptoms of the onset of labor are explicitly explained as well as the need for professional confirmation of her provisional diagnosis of labor (14.1).

Each woman is taught the principles of the birth-plan, including the importance of early assessments and early measures to ensure adequate progress (15.4). The use of the partogram (15.3) is explained and how it is utilized to predict the time of delivery (15.5.1). Women are advised to check out the website and the partogram-app, serving as ancillary information and helpful tools.[5,6]

18.4.2 Promises and reassurances

Pain is discussed openly, but a positive sense of self-reliance is consciously nurtured. This is possible only if pre-labor information is accompanied by three firm promises:

1. That she will be supported by a personal, well-informed and sympathetic nurse;
2. That labor will not be allowed to last more than 12 hours (and it takes 6 hours on average);
3. That epidural analgesia will be available as soon as she should really need it.

The first two guarantees alone completely change the face of women's expectations. Taken together they are at the very heart of the matter and in practice they are entirely dependent on each other.

In some cases, epidural analgesia has an invaluable contribution to make to the care of first labor, but prior commitments should not be given (Chapter 20). Instant availability is key, of course, but a pre-labor commitment to provide an epidural tacitly confirms the idea that the pain will be unbearable and unwittingly encourages a negative and passive attitude to childbirth.[4]

> *The subject of pain in childbirth should never be discussed as a separate problem in isolation from all other relevant aspects of labor support and labor management.*

The three promises – which both the woman and the educator know will be honored at the critical moment – positively increase the pain threshold of most women and reduce the need for medical pain alleviation measures. Frank and honest information, including firm assurances, hugely change the outlook of all pregnant women in our practice. Our childbirth educators have yet to meet the first woman who fundamentally disagrees with the offered plan and who refuses to sign the informed pre-labor consent.

18.4.3 Parous rehabilitation

All nulliparas are encouraged to visit the birth educator several times during their pregnancy. The importance of this service for parous women depends on their obstetric history. If a woman previously gave birth vaginally to a child in good condition, she is likely to be confident about the course and outcome of the forthcoming birth. Even if she underwent an instrument-assisted delivery, a smooth labor and spontaneous delivery are now a near-certainty (Chapter 13).

If, in contrast, her first labor was a traumatic experience (elsewhere), pre-labor education will be primarily an exercise in rehabilitation. The fundamental difference between the first and the next birth should be clearly explained. The main purpose is to convince her that her second labor will not be comparable in any way with her first. While her first labor might have needed acceleration, perhaps an epidural, or even an instrument-assisted delivery, the second birth can confidently be expected to proceed smoothly and to be concluded by herself. Uncritical pre-labor commitment to epidural analgesia or a cesarean delivery – to solve a problem that will not occur – undermines the woman's self-confidence even further, no matter how grateful she may appear to be.[4]

18.5 Pre-labor training groups

All educators in our hospital are acquainted with the antenatal training courses on offer in the proximate neighborhood. They restrict their recommendations to those courses that are geared to the institutional provisions and that do not interfere with the principles and practice of *proactive support of labor*. The recommended group training programs – often including partners – attempt to impart skills for coping with the natural pain of labor and may include yoga, psycho-prophylaxis, mind–body techniques, and other labor coping techniques. Mutual feedback between the independent but affiliated trainers and the institutional educators and practitioners is taken care of on a regular basis so as to prevent mismatches between training programs and actual practice.

18.6 Standard debriefing

Ideally, all women revisit the educators 6 weeks after delivery to evaluate their experience. Without exception, women appreciate this opportunity to show their baby and to share their satisfaction or discontent with the care received throughout labor. This debriefing procedure provides invaluable information for internal audit (Chapter 26) and personal feedback to individual caregivers.

> Continual evaluation of women's satisfaction with their childbirth experiences is the very foundation of the system.

References

1. Lothian JA. Preparation for labor and childbirth. UpToDate. Accessed October 2014
2. Gagnon AJ, Sandall J. Individual or group antenatal education for childbirth or parenthood, or both. Cochrane Database Syst Rev 2007
3. Simkin, PT, Klein MC. Nonpharmacological approaches to management of labor pain. UpToDate. Accessed November 2014
4. O'Driscoll K, Meagher D, Robson M. *Active Management of Labour*, 4th edn. London: Mosby; 2003
5. Website: www.keepingbirthnormal.com
6. Partogram-app, available at: www.apparentapps.com

Chapter 19

Affective dimensions of labor pain

A significant feature of customary birth care is the emphasis placed on the physical element of pain and its relief. Many birth professionals seem to operate from the belief that the most important contribution providers can make to the comfort of women in labor is to ensure that their pain is relieved by epidural analgesia or opioid drugs.[1] As a result, only a minority of women in western countries currently give birth without pain medication. The overall effect, however, is far from impressive, even in the short-term sense of immediate consumer satisfaction, because the affective dimensions of pain in childbirth are readily ignored.

19.1 The nature of labor pain

Giving birth is the only physiological process in nature that causes pain, and the reasons for this have been "explained" with philosophical and religious arguments. Even so, the biological functions of pain in childbirth are clear: endorphins promote effective and mutual mother–child bonding (7.2). Most women instinctively feel that pain in childbirth is part of life and are justifiably proud of their achievement. Being a link in procreation since the origin of humankind, women know that they are responsible for the continued existence of the human species. Moreover, birth increases their pain threshold for the rest of their lives to an unparalleled level; if men had to endure birth pain, humankind would have become extinct long ago.

Clearly, the natural pain of labor is fundamentally different from pain associated with surgical wounds or other forms of injury. Accordingly, birth attendants' attitude to pain should be fundamentally different from that of a strictly medical approach. Use of epidural analgesia or opioid drugs is the easiest solution for doctors, but is largely unsatisfactory in its effects. Effectively easing the strain and pain of childbirth requires an overall birth-plan, characterized by clarity, prevention of long labor, and above all

empathic, respectful, personal, and continuously supportive care.

> *Pain in childbirth requires a fundamentally different approach from that of standard medicine, which is the use of drugs.*

19.1.1 Insecurity, anxiety, and pain

It is not the pain of labor that traumatizes women, but rather the lack of personal care in modern maternity centers, the feeling of not being heard, or the fear of being abandoned in so vulnerable a state (4.3.1). Fear and anxiety are strongly associated with increased pain perception during labor and modify pain through psychological and physiological mechanisms.[2] When a woman in labor is insufficiently prepared and supported she may experience a mounting sense of frustration because she feels herself to be a helpless victim of powerful forces of nature that she cannot actively influence. Swept along on a tide of events that she may not fully comprehend, she may lose self control, *a fortiori* when progress is slow and no one can or will tell her when her ordeal is likely to come to an end. Meanwhile, various birth attendants come and go, while for her the problem of protraction seems to begin all over again.[1] Inconsistent and discontinuous care only works to exacerbate the insecurity and anxiety, and fear of the unknown aggravates the pain. The inevitable stress response further undermines uterine efficiency and thus progress, and a vicious cycle ensues. A state of panic may develop that very well may trigger a lifelong post-traumatic stress syndrome (2.4.1). Clearly, large amounts of opioid drugs or an epidural block are not the first choice of prevention.

> *Nothing is more demoralizing and traumatizing than enduring intense pain with no end in sight.*

19.1.2 The physical element of pain in labor

That there is a physical element in the discomfort and pain of labor is beyond question and should never be denied. Giving birth is not a bodily pleasure, rather a challenge. Most women are willing to accept pain in childbirth but they do not wish the pains to over-whelm them.

The character of labor pains is a visceral cramp resembling intense dysmenorrhea, with which most women are at least somewhat familiar. Contractions last about a minute – within which the pain is intense for around 30 seconds – followed by a rest period in which the pain ceases completely. The pains recur every 3 minutes, somewhat less frequently at the beginning and more frequently toward the end. This amounts to 10 minutes of intense pain per hour and translates into less than one hour of intense pain during the course of a first labor of average duration (6 hours) and a max-imum of one hour and a half for a dilatational period of 10 hours. If prepared properly and as long as clarity and adequate labor support are maintained, the majority of women will manage without medication. The ability to restrict labor duration is crucial in this regard, since the time exposed to the stress, discomfort, and pain is the dominant element in the problem of labor pain.

> Labor duration is one of the key problems with regard to labor pain.

Pain in labor is essentially a problem of the first stage, with pain (nociceptive) stimuli arising from mechanical distension of the cervix and lower uterine segment.[3] Although the nociceptive stimuli are even more prevalent during the second stage of labor – because her pelvic floor, pelvic ligaments, vagina, and vulva are now being stretched – a woman is generally better able to cope because she now regains control of her situation. She senses that the conclusion of birth is near and that it can be accelerated by her own efforts. In this "active stage" of birth (10.5.3), the tremendous physical exertions required in pushing generally dis-tract her attention from the sensation of pain.

19.2 Spectrum of behavioral responses

Owing to the subjective element of discomfort and pain, women's individual reactions to labor vary enormously.[4] Hence, the full spectrum of emotional behavior can be observed in every busy delivery unit every single day. Nonetheless, a standard sequence of reactions progressing with variable velocity can be outlined.

A woman initially reacts with startled surprise (labor has finally begun), followed by conscious efforts to cope with the contractions. This increasingly requires concentration, which becomes more difficult the stronger and the more frequent the contractions become. In time, she tends to withdraw completely from contact with her surroundings during the con-tractions, keeping her eyes tightly closed in extreme concentration.

Up to this point, there are no insurmountable problems. As time passes, however, her reaction to the pains further intensifies. The woman may become agitated and restive. She may even react unreasonably to the well-meaning efforts at comfort and advice from her partner and birth attendants. Finally, after what for her is an excessively long period of pain, she can no longer concentrate during the pains and, what is worse, she can no longer relax during the contrac-tion intervals, let alone recover. Now, the intensity of the pains, and above all the duration of labor, threaten to unhinge her into violent and unmanageable beha-vior. She can become truly panicked and reach the point of life-long traumatization. "This scenario, where a woman continues to react long after a con-traction is over, should never be allowed to develop, because once contact is lost it is hard to reestablish."[1] Permanent loss of women's faculty for real commu-nication during labor is most often the product of inadequate preparation, lack of personal support, and inept labor management, in which no one is paying attention to the simple fact that the duration of first-stage labor exceeds the woman's stamina for endurance.

> The scenario of a woman continuing to react to pain between contractions – so that she cannot recover and becomes non-coachable – must be avoided at all times.

Again, simple reliance on epidural block or sys-temic opioids for pain relief is not the most appro-priate policy. Personal supportive care and timely correction of slow labor are usually far more construc-tive. A great easing of the throes of labor occurs as the impasse of ineffective labor is overcome and nor-mal progress is established, despite the fact that contractions are now much stronger. An additional benefit of early oxytocin treatment is the ability to predict the approximate hour of delivery and this is of paramount importance to the morale of all participants in the birth process. At the same time, this approach shows much more respect for the woman because it allows her to retain her dignity, mobility, and full control over her body and promotes her giving birth by her own efforts.

Proactive support of labor

The clear policy and prior assurances are in themselves half the work required to avoid pain medication and to achieve a spontaneous and non-traumatic birth.

19.3 Affective dimensions

Pain relief and satisfaction with the birth experience are not the same thing, although many doctors tend to equate them. Several systematic reviews suggest that pain and pain relief do not play major roles in women's satisfaction with their childbirth experience, unless expectations regarding either are not met.[5–7] When women themselves evaluate their labor and delivery, four factors prove to be of predominant importance:

Evidence-based contributors to women's childbirth satisfaction

1. The amount of support a woman receives from caregivers
2. The quality of her relationship with her caregivers
3. Her involvement with decision-making
4. Her personal expectations

(Hodnett)[5]

The structured reviews clearly show that the usual standardized and limited approach to labor pain management is often unsatisfactory for many women. Modifiable factors to enhance their labor experience include labor duration and adherence to a well-informed and consented birth-plan, as well as environmental conditions. Care and resources available to women as they look toward their birthing experiences and during the time of labor and birth will determine whether the sensory intensity of pain is experienced in a fundamentally negative or positive manner.[2]

Most women want to deliver their babies by their own efforts in full mental awareness. They do not wish to be deprived of that sense of achievement by intoxication with opioid drugs. Neither does an epidural catheter meet the needs of many women. Commitment to epidural analgesia presents a strange paradox in a society that celebrates individuals who endure great pain and distress in pursuit of mountain peaks or completion of a marathon race. The many women in our hospital/birth center who wish to avoid opioid drugs or epidural analgesia are neither misinformed nor martyrs. On the contrary, they are well prepared and know exactly what to expect during childbirth (Chapter 18). Consequently, they put trust in themselves and in the staff who care for them.

Pain should be viewed as only one component of the totality of the woman's labor and birth experience.

19.3.1 Environmental conditions

The complexity and individuality of the labor experience challenges providers in our unit to create and protect a birthing environment that promotes a woman's sense of self-efficacy and confidence in her ability to cope. To this end, a broad spectrum of non-pharmacological and pharmacological approaches to pain relief is incorporated in practice. Key is one-on-one companionship in labor (Chapter 16).

The nursing staff have been selected intentionally for their capability to communicate empathy and kindness, and for their skills in reassuring and encouraging distressed women. Appropriate equipment is available, including massage showers, areas where women can walk, side rails along the walls to lean on, rocking and straight chairs, birth balls, stools, and other positioning aids, rolling IV poles, and telemetry units. The nurses are trained in the safe and appropriate use of the birth bed to support a variety of positions. Importantly, the midwives and doctors are also knowledgeable and open-minded to assist with births in sitting or squatting positions. Added to that, of course, effective medical pain relief is instantly available should the need arrive (next chapter).

The effect of pain and pain relief on women's satisfaction with the birth experience is neither as obvious, nor as powerful as the effect of personal, supportive care and the adherence to a consented birth-plan.

References

1. O'Driscoll K, Meagher D, Robson M. Active Management of Labour, 4th edn. London: Mosby; 2003

2. Lowe NK. The nature of labor pain. Am J Obstet Gynecol 2002;**186**:16–24

3. Rowlands S, Permezel M. Physiology of pain in labour. Baillieres Clin Obstet Gynaecol 1998;**12**:347–62

4. Lowe NK. Individual variation in childbirth pain. J Psychosom Obstet Gynaecol 1987;**7**:183–92

5. Hodnett ED. Pain and women's satisfaction with the experience of childbirth: a systematic review. Am J Obstet Gynecol 2002;**186**:160–72

6. Jones L, Othman M, Dowswell T, et al. Pain management for women in labour: an overview of systematic reviews. Cochrane Database Syst Rev 2012

7. Lally JE, Murtagh MJ, Macphail S, Thomson R. More in hope than expectation: a systematic review of women's expectations and experience of pain relief in labour. BMC Med 2008;**6**:7

Pain relief re-examined

The ideal technique for medical pain relief in labor does not exist. Opioids seem to be the best systemic drugs available, but the amount of analgesia that can be achieved is directly proportional to unpleasant side effects such as orthostatic hypotension, dizziness, nausea, and – worst of all – loss of mental acuity. In addition, opioids rapidly cross the placenta and may cause neonatal sedation and neonatal respiratory depression. Epidural analgesia is far more effective and allows the woman to be awake and aware while the baby is alert at birth. Besides these obvious advantages, however, epidural block also involves several co-interventions and unintended effects on the course and outcome of labor. No good cause is served by pretending otherwise.

Various aspects of the use of epidural analgesia deserve far more serious attention than they usually get.

20.1 Epidural pain management

Although the overall policy of *proactive support* effectively reduces requests for pain relief, some women, for a variety of reasons, will desire or need, and subsequently experience, great benefits from epidural analgesia. This technique affords complete relief of labor pain in all but a few cases.

20.1.1 Popularity

Because epidural analgesia hugely changes the degree of medical intervention and maternal–fetal surveillance required, this technique has garnered both advocates and opponents of its use. As a consequence, rates vary widely and may come close to 100% in some hospitals. It is, however, mainly doctors who do not spend much time in the labor rooms themselves who advance the strongest arguments in favor of epidural analgesia in childbirth.[1] In some institutes, anesthesiologists have managed to gain access to prenatal classes where they preach the wonders of epidural block and usually say little or nothing about the possible adverse effects on the course and outcome of labor.

The question remains whether high rates of epidural analgesia are based on women's preferences or rather on the advantages of caregiver convenience, as epidural may easily serve as a substitute for intensive personal labor support.

Twenty-four-hour access to epidural service is imperative for any hospital with pretensions of providing high-quality care, but high rates of its use may actually reflect low standards of labor support.

20.1.2 Effectiveness of epidural block

Although none of the numerous epidural studies has assessed its impact on childbirth satisfaction or any other psychological outcome, the benefits are self-evident in selected cases. Few sights are more impressive than the instant relief of maternal distress that follows a successful epidural block. Unfortunately, this does not always occur. There are connective-tissue bands that may form septa within the lumbar epidural space.[2] Such septae may explain cases of unanesthetized windows or unilateral areas despite proper epidural placement.[3] A failed block occurs in 5 to 15%, and women should be told that this might happen.[4] Overall, 85–95% of women rate their pain relief as good to excellent.[4] Conversely, in 5–15%, epidural analgesia proves inadequate. A mismatch between prior expectations of pain-free labor and the disappointing effect may further hamper feasible labor coaching and precipitate requests for cesarean delivery as a result.

Epidural analgesia is generally very effective in the alleviation of pain, but there are several underestimated drawbacks as well.

20.1.3 Potential hazards

Placing an epidural block is a highly invasive procedure, entering the space around the dura mater surrounding the spinal cord. Owing to the pregnant woman's altered anatomical state, her restlessness during contractions, and the pregnancy-related swelling of the epidural venous plexus, the procedure can be technically challenging, especially in obese women. The most common complication involves accidental entry of the cerebrospinal space, which is estimated to occur in 2% of all epidural punctures.[5] The resultant leakage of cerebrospinal fluid results in severe, often incapacitating headache that may last for several days. This usually requires a second puncture after delivery to apply a blood patch to stop the leakage. However, if the initial spinal tap is not recognized, spinal injection of the anesthetic agent in the amount meant for epidural analgesia results in acute and profound depression of vital functions: circulatory collapse and respiratory arrest.[5] Even though this life-threatening complication is exceptional and can (should) be effectively prevented by the standard use of small test doses, the very possibility of such a calamity necessitates the stand-by presence of resuscitation and ventilation facilities. Inevitably, because of these precautions, the setting and atmosphere of epidural placement are highly medical, which some women may experience as a disruption of the intimate birthing surrounding.

Epidural makes labor much more technology-intensive than it needs to be.

A rare consequence of epidural analgesia – though very disappointing for the mother – is the increased chance of getting general anesthesia should super-emergency cesarean delivery be indicated for acute and severe fetal distress. The epidural top-up time needed for painless surgery takes way too long while not a few anesthetists refuse – rightly or wrongly – to administer a rapidly acting spinal block when an epidural catheter is in situ. Women should be informed about this well in advance of labor (Chapter 18).

20.1.4 Direct adverse effects

An effect inherent in the epidural technique is vasodilatation from sympathetic blockade and decreased cardiac output, resulting in maternal hypotension and reduced utero-placental blood flow, which may compromise fetal well-being. In the supine position, hypotension is compounded by obstructed venous return from uterine compression of the abdominal great veins. Even in the absence of hypotension measured in the arm, utero-placental blood flow may still be significantly reduced.[3] Despite precautions with IV fluid preloads, maternal hypotension is the most common complication of epidural analgesia, severe enough to require treatment with vasopressors in one-third of women.[6]

Maternal hypotension and related placental blood flow impairment occur in 30% of patients receiving an epidural block.

Other inadvertent effects such as voiding difficulties, nausea, pruritus, and shivering are common, but they are usually mild and only infrequently necessitate treatment.[6,7]

Far more worrying is the three-fold increased risk of intrapartum maternal fever of at least 38 °C related to epidural analgesia (RR = 3.34; 95% CI 2.63–4.23).[6,7] Fever occurs in 10–34% of all women with epidural.[8] The mechanism remains unclear. As the epidural origin cannot be distinguished from beginning intrauterine infection, newborns are usually admitted to the neonatal ward for observation and treatment with antibiotics as a precaution, but in retrospect mostly unnecessarily. Apart from undue parental worries and fears, baby and mother are separated for the first days after birth, which undermines smooth mother–child bonding. In the great majority of cases, sepsis evaluation turns out to be negative, so the intrapartum fever was simply attributable to epidural analgesia. The iatrogenic damage has been done, though.

Epidural increases the incidence of maternal fever and the likelihood of neonatal sepsis evaluation and antibiotic treatment.

Despite the advent of low-dose epidurals, the extent of impaired motor ability remains a cause for concern. An estimated 20% of women decline to stand up and complain of dizziness or sensation of motor weakness, despite normal blood pressure and motor ability tests.[4] For this reason, the appropriateness of the term "light" epidural is called into question.[6] The term "walking" epidural is also misleading and should be avoided because evidence shows that a large proportion of women (34–85%) who receive what has been called a "light" or "walking" epidural do not spend much time out of bed at all.[6] Possible reasons for this finding include that the motor block interferes with ability and stability, and that opiates given by the epidural route may contribute to drowsiness and fatigue. Furthermore, women are confined to bed by tubes and cords connecting them to various devices, and nurses have other responsibilities and are not available to assist with ambulation. Finally, caregivers may simply discourage ambulation as anesthesia protocols in many labor and delivery units prohibit women from getting out of bed because of safety issues and liability concerns. Women should be informed of this.

20.1.5 Indirect adverse effects

Several outstanding systematic reviews on epidural analgesia have been published, using varying study inclusion criteria for meta-analysis and addressing various co-interventions and unintended outcome variables.[4–7] The evidence is consistent about the following adverse outcomes:

- Epidural analgesia prolongs the first stage of labor.
- Epidural analgesia increases the need for oxytocin.
- Epidural analgesia turns natural labor into a fully medicalized event.
- Epidural analgesia prolongs the second stage of labor.
- Epidural analgesia increases instrumental delivery rates.
- Epidural analgesia increases third- and fourth-degree perineal lacerations.

Epidural analgesia decreases the likelihood of spontaneous vaginal delivery (Evidence level A).

Epidural block increases the odds of vacuum or forceps delivery (RR 1.42, 95% CI 1.28–1.57)[7], but there is still an ongoing debate over whether epidural analgesia affects cesarean section rates. Many studies have noted an association with an increased likelihood of cesarean delivery, but results are heavily practice-based. The crux of the discussion is whether the differences in cesarean rates observed are due to the epidural itself or to other differences between women who receive epidural analgesia and women who do not. A critical look at the external validity of the randomized trials suggests that cesarean rates for failure to progress need not be increased by epidural analgesia, provided labor is enhanced in time with appropriately high doses of oxytocin (17.3.3).[9,10]

20.1.6 Prejudicing nursing labor support

An important issue that has attracted much less attention so far than it should have is the impact of epidural analgesia on nursing and caregiving procedures. Use of epidural involves a complex cascade of technical nursing duties. It is typically recommended that maternal blood pressure be frequently assessed, as often as every 2–5 minutes during the first 30 minutes and every 15 minutes thereafter with stabilization, and then frequently continued throughout the remainder of labor. IV fluid loads must be adjusted to blood pressure readings. Continuous electronic fetal monitoring is another standard component of intrapartum care with epidurals. Normal supportive care may be severely jeopardized when nurses are immersed in these technical activities.

In maternity centers with high epidural rates, the ability to provide high-quality nursing care for all women, including those who do not choose epidural analgesia, becomes a major concern. Nurse work-sampling studies in centers with high epidural rates revealed that actual labor support activities were minimal compared with the time spent on other unit-level activities.[11–13] Continuous and supportive nursing care enhances a woman's sense of control and satisfaction with her childbirth experience and is implicated in decreased cesarean delivery rates (16.3.1). It seems, unfortunately, that many hospitals have already reached the point at which the labor support role must be rediscovered, and that nurses and other birth attendants must be newly trained in this important task.

Use of epidural analgesia involves a complex cascade of technical monitoring duties, increasing the workloads of nurses and midwives and distracting their attention from their labor support role.

20.1.7 Epidural and parous labors

The fundamental distinction between nulliparous labor and parous labor is the continuous red thread through the pages of this book, and this issue is of particular importance in the context of epidural analgesia.

High use of epidural analgesia in parous women stems from the mistaken belief that a valid comparison can be drawn between the first and a subsequent labor.[1] A woman who has had an unpleasant first experience, during which she may or may not have had epidural analgesia, frequently seeks a prior commitment on the next occasion because she fears that the prolongation of labor is likely to be repeated. However, there are no grounds for this assumption. Her doctor would serve her interests much more were she/he to address her fears with a clear explanation of the differences between a first and second birth (Chapter 13).

What is more, there is a gray area between anesthetics and obstetrics into which not a few disasters of childbirth fall. Especially if her first labor ended with a cesarean delivery, epidural block acts to increase the risk of a ruptured uterus because pain has an important warning function in this regard. Indeed, liberal use of epidural analgesia in parous women has emerged as an important factor in the late recognition of this calamity, and related medical negligence litigation effectively slashed the number of labors with a cesarean scar.[14]

> *Epidural analgesia in parous labor should be approached with specific reservations, in particular when the uterus is scarred by a previous cesarean section.*

20.1.8 Selective use

Clearly, there is an urgent need to redefine a joint nursing/midwifery and medical approach to epidural analgesia, heeding the following considerations:

- Epidural analgesia has an invaluable contribution to make to nulliparous labor, but…
- The relative contribution to labor in parous women is much less.
- Epidural service must be available 24/7, but:
- The indication should be individually assessed.
- A pre-labor commitment to epidural analgesia should not be made.
- An epidural should never be given before the diagnosis of labor is made.
- An epidural should never be used as a substitute for supportive care.
- An epidural should never serve as a substitute for corrective action if labor is slow.
- An epidural should never be used as a cover for prolonged labor.

A readily available epidural service is a prerequisite to high-quality maternity care, but so is individualization of its use. The fundamental objection against a pre-labor commitment to an epidural is that a promise prior to the event confirms a tacit premise that the pain of labor will be an intolerable experience. The truth is, however, that the pain experience in a first labor can scarcely be foretold, perhaps least of all by the inexperienced nullipara herself. The second reason for an expectant approach to an epidural is the fact that the duration of the first labor cannot be predicted.

> *Epidural analgesia should not be used or offered on a routine basis.*

Occasionally, epidural is given too late, just because a woman's doctor made the promise, and she now insists. This may happen when she comes to the hospital with her cervix already close to full dilatation. The result is that the beneficial effects in the apparently short first stage are more than offset by the adverse effects in the second stage of labor, the beginning of which is fully obscured by epidural analgesia (10.5).

Clearly, case selection and timing are critical. In some maternity centers an epidural is given too early, even before labor is diagnosed correctly. The result may be that, after much confusion, a cesarean is eventually performed on a woman who was not in labor. This consideration should preclude the use of epidural during priming/induction with prostaglandins before a firm commitment to delivery is established.

20.1.9 Improper use

Epidural analgesia is often improperly used as a palliative measure when labor is prolonged, as if duration of labor in itself were not important provided the mother suffers no pain. This is a serious misconception. Numerous risks increase with prolonged labor, including fetal distress, cesarean delivery, infection, meconium aspiration, instrumental delivery, maternal and perinatal birth injuries, post-partumhemorrhage, and so forth. Moreover, an epidural does not prevent the uterus from exhaustion after an extended duration of labor, leading to a refractory uterus resistant to oxytocin, or to the uterus reacting with hypertonia between contractions, which further compromises fetal well-being (Chapter 8).

Epidural analgesia is pain management, not a therapeutic treatment for labor disorders. There is only one exception: cervical edema in a panicked woman who bears down prematurely long before full dilatation has been reached (Chapter 21).

> Epidural analgesia is pain relief, not therapy for a prolonged labor.

20.1.10 Case selection for epidural

Pain management should always be individualized and discussed in the context of all other aspects of labor care and modalities of pain relief. Subject to the above reservations, there are three broad categories of women who derive the most benefit from epidural analgesia:

1. Nulliparas who are so disturbed at the very prospect of labor that they are already unduly upset at the point of admission. Their number should be limited thanks to adequate pre-labor preparation (Chapter 18).
2. Nulliparas who, despite an initial appearance of composure, become unduly upset soon afterward. Their number should be limited thanks to the high level of nursing support (Chapter 16).
3. Nulliparas who are transferred too late from home, in an attempt to retrieve their battered composure. Their number is closely related to the duration of labor as tolerated by independent midwives (Chapter 25).

Clearly, good maternity care requires an overall plan and mutual respect between doctors, midwives, and nurses. Doctors in particular should admit that the standards of care in labor are determined almost entirely by the efforts of well-motivated nurses and midwives. An obstetrician who appears critical of a nurse/midwife simply because occasionally a woman complains during a post-delivery visit that she had not had timely and adequate pain relief, strongly undermines the team spirit between caregivers, with detrimental overall consequences. O'Driscoll observed: "Doctors are seldom present to witness the particular circumstances, and it is all too easy to pose as being more humane, after the event. No personal commitment is required for this mode of behavior."[1]

20.1.11 Informed consent

Women's preferences and choices should be honored. That is to presume that the above information about the trade-offs of epidural analgesia has been provided without any pressure for or against. Antenatal visits to the birth educator (18.3) ensure that each woman as she approaches childbirth has access to all relevant information and becomes familiar with all policies, including epidural analgesia if needed. Giving information once labor has already started is much too late to acquire valid informed consent, which the anesthetist will justifiably demand when summoned to place the epidural catheter. Women should be informed well in advance and have access to this information again during labor, as part of an open and respectful informed consent process oriented toward women rather than toward professional liability concerns.

> Women should be informed about all pros and cons of epidural analgesia, well in advance of childbirth.

20.2 Systemic opioids in labor

In many maternity units, parenteral (intravenous or intramuscular) opioids are still used, either as first-line pain medication – that may preclude or precede epidural – or as an inferior alternative for epidural analgesia in settings where epidural service is not 24/7 available. A distinction should be made between long- and short-acting opiates.

20.2.1 Ban on long-acting opioids

The analgesic effect of long-acting opioids such as pethidine (INN) or meperidine (USAN) is very poor. These drugs act primarily by inducing somnolence, rather than producing analgesia per se, and should, therefore, not be used anymore in labor.[15–19] O'Driscoll and Meagher articulated the concomitant effects – in most publications euphemistically described as nausea and sedation:

> Some women suffer from intractable nausea and vomiting, sufficient to turn childbirth into a miserable experience. Some become profoundly depressed, introspective, and so overwhelmed with self-pity that they lapse eventually into a state of stupor, from which they are roused only by contractions, to make aimless protests and demand more and more drugs, until… a vicious circle is established. Some become

disorientated and so confused that they are unable to cooperate with their attendants, especially during the second stage of labor, when cooperation is essential if spontaneous delivery is to be achieved… In practice, many women in labor are deeply intoxicated… and likely to suffer from a hangover [and sometimes even partial retrograde amnesia], a most undesirable sequel to such a joyous occasion as the birth of a child. All these adverse effects may follow even a small dose of pethidine given to a person who has had no previous exposure to hard drugs.[1]

A woman in labor has to keep her head clear. The only remaining indication for the use of long-acting opioids concerns women presenting with a persistent false start (14.6.3). To potentiate the sedative effect and to mitigate the nausea, pethidine (meperidine) is best combined with an antihistamine such as promethazine or hydroxyzine.[15] This sedative cocktail should never be given in the labor ward, but exclusively in the antenatal ward: a woman in distress but not in labor must sleep! (Chapter 14).

It is imperative that the diagnosis of labor be rejected on good grounds before the woman is transferred to the antenatal ward, lest sedation imposes risks on the baby should it be born soon after. Meperidine, or pethidine, crosses the placenta and builds up in the baby because the half-life (15–23 hours) in the fetus is considerably longer than the half-life in the mother (3–6 hours).[20,21] This may lead to serious neonatal hypoventilation and other effects such as decreased neonatal alertness, lower neurobehavioral scores, and inhibition of the sucking reflex.[15]

Admittedly, these undesirable neonatal effects can be reversed by naloxone (a specific opiate antagonist), but the effects of pethidine last significantly longer than the naloxone reversal, which has been shown to be transient.[22] Consequently, there is serious potential to miss hazardous hypoventilation a few hours after birth when the naloxone has worn off. Several cases of early (near) sudden neonatal deaths due to pethidine-related respiratory depression have been reported.[15,23]

> The use of long-acting opiates such as pethidine (INN) or meperidine (USAN) is ineffective, involves serious neonatal risks, and causes more maternal discomfort than it relieves. These drugs should not be used any more in the labor and delivery room.

20.2.2 PCA with short-acting remifentanil

Whenever epidural analgesia is not an option – because of a medical contraindication or fear of the needle in the back – remifentanil is the only reasonable alternative.[24,25] This ultra-short-acting opioid is optimally delivered with an intravenous patient-controlled analgesia (PCA) regimen. Women self-dose the drug by controlling the infusion pump, which allows top-ups with lockout times to prevent overdose.

Remifentanil is a μ-opioid-receptor agonist with the advantage of rapid onset (30 to 60 seconds, with peak-effect at 2.5 minutes) and short wear-off time.[26] Although remifentanil crosses the placenta too, it does not cause neonatal depression because it is rapidly metabolized by non-specific plasma and tissue esterases. Remifentanil does, however, reduce fetal heart rate beat-to-beat variability, simulating a non-reassuring fetal status.[27] This may inadvertently lower the threshold for cesarean delivery. Both the maternal and fetal effects disappear within 10 minutes after discontinuing the infusion.[27]

The analgesic effect of remifentanil is far superior to pethidine (meperidine) but does not match that of epidural block.[24,25,28] Gradual diminution of the analgesic effect due to desensitization of the μ-receptors presents an occasional problem when administration time exceeds a period of 4 hours. The sedative and nauseating effects match those of all opioids, but the respiratory depressant effect is the most troublesome and mandates direct respiratory supervision by the nurse or continuous pulse oximetry, as well as stand-by facilities for oxygen supplementation and mask ventilation.[26,29]

As all opiates, remifentanil also aggravates the already increased gastric acid secretion and decreased gastrointestinal motility during labor. This imposes an increased risk of regurgitation and pulmonary aspiration in the unforeseen event of general anesthesia that is occasionally needed for a super-emergency cesarean delivery, manual removal of the placenta, surgical repair of fourth-degree lacerations, and so on.

> PCA with remifentanil is an effective method of pain relief in labor, but less effective than epidural analgesia. In terms of effect-to-risk ratio, it is no real competitor for an epidural block.

20.3 Paramedical techniques

Many alternatives are tried to provide some pain relief for women who wish to avoid an epidural or opioid drugs. These methods include, for example, nitrous oxygen inhalation, transcutaneous electrical nerve stimulation (TENS), sterile water injections in the skin of the lower back, acupuncture, and hypnosis.[17,30,31]

In particular in nations of the former British Empire, nitrous oxide is still used on a frequent basis. Perhaps the popularity there has to do with the example set by Queen Victoria, who gave birth to her children while inhaling analgesic gas, more than 150 years ago. Contemporary systematic reviews, however, found few fair or good-quality studies and no clear, quantitative, objective evidence of its analgesic efficacy for the effective relief of labor pain.[19] Women inhaling nitrous oxide are, however, more likely to experience vomiting, nausea, and dizziness.

TENS has been subjected to more controlled trials than any of the other modalities of non-invasive pain relief, but the results remain inconclusive.[32] There is no good evidence either that intra- or subcutaneous sterile water injection in the skin overlying the sacrum has objectively beneficial effects, and the same holds for acupuncture and hypnosis.[33] Suggestive evidence cited by advocates of these methods is mainly limited to single trials, and variability in the outcome measures hinders evaluations and comparisons of the efficacy and effectiveness of these methods.[17]

Most importantly, all studies and meta-analyses on these methods ignored the consensus among anesthesiological pain experts on meaningful outcome standards.[34] Reductions in pain should be reported as a percentage of the pain intensity assessed by a 0 to 10 numerical rating scale. Pain reductions of –50% indicate relevant benefit, whereas reductions of –10% may reflect an effect that is statistically significant, but clinically entirely irrelevant.[34]

There is no good evidence to claim any clinically relevant analgesic effect from inhaling nitrous oxide, nor from any of the non-pharmacological methods.

It is not to be expected that any of the paramedical methods of pain relief will pass this test of clinical significance. Advocates' claims of "evidence-based" beneficial effects in relieving pain exemplify the fact that nothing is as easy to misinterpret and abuse as statistics. The same critique applies to studies supporting bathing, touch and massage, mind–body techniques, maternal movement and position changes, counter-pressure or superficial heat and cold applied to the low back, biofeedback with attention focusing and distraction, music, white noise, aromatherapy, herbal medicines, homeopathy, and so on.

That is not to say, though, that these methods are useless. Whereas purely medical approaches are primarily directed at eliminating pain, these non-pharmacologic methods are mainly directed at "prevention of suffering."[30] Without a doubt, susceptible women may benefit from a placebo effect. The overall benefit, however, to accrue from these methods is most likely the personal attention involved in their application. Therefore, our birth indicators answer specific questions about these methods neutrally, and they openly discuss the feasibility of women's wishes (18.3.1). The only non-pharmacological method with a proven beneficial effect on women's labor experience is personal and supportive care on a one-to-one basis (16.3).

The best non-pharmacological method to help women cope with the pains of labor is continuous personal nursing attention and support.

Personal attention enhances the parasympathetic condition required for a smooth, safe, and rewarding labor and delivery. After implementation of the provisions and allowances needed, the dominant contemporary problem of dysfunctional labor can be revisited with new eyes and approached in a rational manner. The next two chapters will discuss the differential causal diagnostics that should guide expert care.

References

1. O'Driscoll K, Meagher D, Robson M. Active Management of Labour, 4th edn. New York: Mosby; 2003

2. Blomberg RG, Olsson SS. The lumbar epidural space in patients examined with epiduroscopy. Anesth Analg 1998;**68**:157–60

3. Althaus J, Wax J. Analgesia and anesthesia in labor. Obstet Gynecol Clin N Am 2005;**32**:231–44

4. Lieberman E, O'Donoghue C. Unintended effects of epidural analgesia during labor: A systematic review. Am J Obstet Gynecol 2002;**186**:31–68

5. Grant GJ. Adverse effects of neuraxial analgesia and anesthesia for obstetrics. UpToDate. Accessed November 2014

6. Mayberry LJ, Clemmens D, De A. Epidural analgesia side-effects, co-interventions, and care of women during childbirth: A systematic review. Am J Obstet Gynecol 2002;186:81–93

7. Anim-Somuah M, Smyth RM, Jones L. Epidural versus non-epidural or no analgesia in labour. Cochrane Database Syst Rev 2011

8. Chen KT. Intrapartum fever. UpToDate. Accessed November 2014

9. Impey L, MacQuillan K, Robson MS. Epidural analgesia need not increase operative delivery rates. Am J Obstet Gynecol 2000;182:358–63

10. Kotaska AJ, Klein MC, Liston RM. Epidural analgesia associated with low-dose oxytocin augmentation increases cesarean births: A critical look at the external validity of randomized trials. Am J Obstet Gynecol 2006;194:809–14

11. Cagnon AJ, Waghorn K. Supportive care by maternity nurses: a work sampling study in an intrapartum unit. Birth 1996;23:1–6

12. McNiven P, Hodnett E, O'Brian-Pallas LL. Supporting women in labor: a work sampling of the activities of labor and delivery nurses. Birth 1992;19:3–9

13. Gale J, Fothergill-Bourbonnais F, Chamberlain M. Measuring nursing support during childbirth. MCN Am J Matern Child Nurs 2001;26:264–71

14. Ophir E, Odeh M, Hirsch Y, Bornstein J. Uterine rupture during trial of labor: Controversy of induction's methods. Obstet Gynecol Surv 2012;67:734–45

15. Bricker L, Lavender T. Parenteral opioids for labor pain relief: A systematic review. *Am J Obstet Gynecol* 2002;186:94–109

16. Ullman R, Smith LA, Burns E, Mori R, Dowswell T. Parenteral opioids for maternal pain relief in labour. Cochrane Database Syst Rev 2010

17. Jones L, Othman M, Dowswell T, et al. Pain management for women in labour: an overview of systematic reviews. Cochrane Database Syst Rev 2012

18. Olofsson C, Ekblom A, Ekman-Ordeburg G, et al. Lack of analgesic effect of systemically administered morphine or pethidine on labour pain. Br J Obstet Gynaecol 1996;103:968–72

19. Grant GJ. Pharmacologic management of pain during labor and delivery. UpToDate. Accessed November 2014

20. Box D, Cochran D. Safe reduction in the administration of naloxone to newborn infants. Royal College of Paediatricians and Child Health, Fourth

Spring Meeting, York, UK, April 10–13, 2000. Arch Dis Child 82(Suppl 1):A312000

21. Caldwell J, Wakile LA, Notarianni LJ, et al. Maternal and neonatal disposition of pethidine in childbirth – a study using quantitative gas chromatography–mass spectrometry. Life Sci 1978;22:589–96

22. Rooth G, Lysikiewicz A, Huch R, Huch A. Some effects of maternal pethidine administration on the newborn. Br J Obstet Gynaecol 1983;90:28–33

23. Chamberlain G, Wraight A, Steer P. Pain and Its Relief in Childbirth. The results of a National Survey Conducted by the National Birthday Trust. Edinburgh: Churchill Livingstone; 1993

24. Liu ZQ, Chen XB, Li HB, Qiu MT, Duan T. A comparison of remifentanil parturient-controlled intravenous analgesia with epidural analgesia: a meta-analysis of randomized controlled trials. Anesth Analg 2014;118:598–603

25. Schnabel A, Hahn N, Broscheit J, et al. Remifentanil for labour analgesia: a meta-analysis of randomised controlled trials. Eur J Anaesthesiol 2012;29:177–85

26. Babenco HD, Conard PF, Gross JB. The pharmacodynamic effect of a remifentanil bolus on ventilatory control. Anesthesiology 2000;92(2):393–8

27. Kan RE, Hughes SC, Rosen MA, et al. Intravenous remifentanil: placental transfer, maternal and neonatal effects. Anesthesiology 1998;88(6):1467–74

28. Stocki D, Matot I, Einav S, et al. A randomized controlled trial of the efficacy and respiratory effects of patient-controlled intravenous remifentanil analgesia and patient-controlled epidural analgesia in laboring women. Anesth Analg 2014;118:589–97

29. Hawkins JL, Beaty BR. Update on obstetric anesthesia practices in the US. Anesthesiology 1999;91:A1060

30. Simkin, PT, Klein MC. Nonpharmacological approaches to management of labor pain. UpToDate. Accessed November 2014

31. Klomp T, van Poppel M, Jones L, et al. Inhaled analgesia for pain management in labour. Cochrane Database Syst Rev 2012

32. Dowswell T, Bedwell C, Lavender T, Neilson JP. Transcutaneous electrical nerve stimulation (TENS) for pain relief in labour. Cochrane Database Syst Rev 2009

33. Derry S, Straube S, Moore RA, Hancock H, Collins SL. Intracutaneous or subcutaneous sterile water injection compared with blinded controls for pain management in labour. Cochrane Database Syst Rev 2012

34. Dworkin RH, Turk DC, Wyrwich KW, et al. Interpreting the clinical importance of treatment outcomes in chronic pain clinical trials: IMMPACT recommendations. Consensus Statement. J Pain 2008;9:105–21

Chapter 21

Dynamic dystocia unraveled

Dystocia, or dysfunctional labor, is the most frequent indication for operative delivery reported in obstetric databases (2.1.1). However, this classification does not offer any clues for improving obstetric care, so the main purpose of these databases is defeated. Dystocia is not a diagnosis, but a symptom and a common pathway of a wide variety of problems encountered in labor. Failure to unravel this set of birth disorders is one of the major shortcomings in current obstetric training and practice. Interventions should be based on a diagnosis rather than a symptom. Only a causal diagnosis allows for pre-emptive measures and rational treatment. Diagnosis is the most important single factor guiding expert labor care, and critical for meaningful audit of procedures and outcomes.

> *Dystocia is a symptom, not a diagnosis. Only detailed causal diagnostics gives guidance to preventive measures and rational treatment.*

Adequate handling of dystocia requires insight in cause and effect. This, in turn, requires a thorough understanding of the dynamics and mechanics of labor and delivery as explored in Section 2. The present chapter focuses on the spectrum of dynamic labor disorders. This group represents nearly 99% of the labors with inadequate progress. One of the many outstanding lessons we have learned from O'Driscoll is that ensuring adequate uterine force not only shortens labor but also has the elucidating effect of isolating mechanical dystocia, or obstructed labor, as a separate clinical entity that is far less prevalent than generally assumed (Chapter 22).

21.1 The spectrum of dynamic labor disorders

Dynamic labor disorders may arise at various times during labor as distinct clinical types with distinct pathophysiological causes (Table 21.1). Each type,

however, always has one common feature, and that is inefficient force. This is proven time and again by the fact that progress of labor can – almost without exception – be restored with amniotomy and oxytocin, provided these measures are taken in time before the myometrium itself has become exhausted (refractory uterus).

> *Dystocia is heterogeneous in its manifestation and causation. Cause and effect need to be explored if progress in handling dysfunctional labor is to be made.*

Primary ineffective labor corresponds with a disorder in the retraction phase, whereas secondary protraction corresponds to a disorder in the wedging phase or in the expulsion stage (Chapter 10). A refractory uterus and hypertonic dystocia are two separate and clearly distinct clinical entities with specific consequences within the syndrome of dynamic dystocia (Table 21.1).

21.2 Primary ineffective labor

Typically, dysfunctional labor presents as a persistent pattern of slow dilatation from the very onset (Fig. 21.1). It is the most common yet least appreciated complication of first labors. Slow progress is almost exclusively confined to nulliparas in whom the cervix is dilated less than 3 cm at the onset of labor. What many professionals typically take for "latent labor" is in reality primary ineffective labor. The fallacious concept of the latent phase (10.1) explains why this condition is often not recognized as a true labor disorder. This leads to inept (non-)management in slow early labor whereby treatment is started too late and only after the fact. If not treated properly, such a prolonged early labor is strongly associated with adverse labor outcomes.[1–10]

Slow progress in the retraction phase is a purely dynamic problem that originates in suboptimal

Table 21.1 Distinct entities within the spectrum of dystocia

Clinical manifestation	Causal diagnosis	Pathophysiological etiology
1. Primary ineffective labor	– Insufficient uterine force in relation to cervical resistance	– Suboptimal uterine transformation/ activation – Adrenergic stress response
2. Secondary protraction or arrest	– Inadequate wedging action	– Insufficient uterine force to effect descent – **Obstruction** (Chapter 22)
3. No pushing reflex at full dilatation	– Insufficient descent upon full dilatation	– See secondary arrest
4. Arrested expulsion	– Lack of descent, rotation and/ or extension	– Insufficient uterine force – Maternal exhaustion – Pushing too early – Ineffective pushing technique
5. Refractory uterus	– Failure to respond to oxytocin	– Induction – Loss of oxytocin receptors – Exhausted, acidified uterus
6. Hypertonic dystocia	– Disorganized contractions – Insufficient interval uterine relaxation – Fetal distress	– Inflammatory cytokine production provoked by intrauterine meconium, blood, or pus

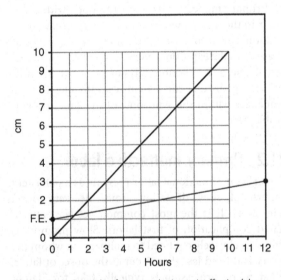

Figure 21.1 Example of untreated primary ineffective labor.

transformation of the myometrium and/or the cervix, with insufficient uterine force in relation to the cervical resistance as a result (8.5). When judged only by the painfulness and the manual assessment of uterine tone, the uterus appears to contract vigorously, but the contractions are insufficiently coordinated (inefficient) and, therefore, fail to exert effective force (9.3).

Undoubtedly, an adrenergic stress response also plays a role in many cases (7.3.2). This explains why primary dysfunctional labor occurs more frequently since hospitals have replaced the trusted environment of a woman's home.

> *Primary ineffective labor presents as a persistent pattern of slow dilatation from the very onset. This common problem is specific to first labor.*

It is crucial to appreciate that primary ineffective labor is specific to first labors. It hardly ever occurs in multiparas, except as an iatrogenic effect of induction (owing to absent or incomplete pre-labor cervical and myometrial transformation) or as a residual result of inadequate support at the first birth (emotional trauma → adrenergic stress response). Primary ineffective labor is a purely dynamic problem and has nothing to do with unfavorable fetopelvic proportions or fetal obstruction (Chapters 10, 22).

21.2.1 Prevalent non-management

Failure to confirm an early diagnosis of labor results in failure to recognize primary ineffective labor (Chapter 14). Hesitant and insecure birth attendants do not dare to declare a woman who has regular contractions and a fully effaced cervix to be in labor. Such muddling indecision circumvents diagnosis, and blocks rational conduct. Other care providers, who rightly accept labor, are reluctant to rupture the membranes in the "latent phase" and use loose, inaccurate criteria for normal labor such as painful and "strong" contractions on palpation instead of progress. This misapprehension leaves them one step behind from the outset if labor is too slow. Traditional midwives trust nature as long as possible and some primarily resort to herbal tea, foot massage, and the bathtub when labor gets tough. Such dilly-dallying is typically paired with refraining from "disruptive" vaginal examinations, let alone rupturing the membranes. At first glance, all this seems woman-friendly but it is a waste of time and energy. Four hours or more is much too long to discover that labor has hardly progressed. At the end of the day, the mother pays with a cesarean or instrumental delivery. The alleged maximum chance for a "natural" birth, thanks to endless patience, actually denies a woman a fair chance of a spontaneous (unassisted) delivery. Early diagnosis and prompt treatment are far more constructive and preventive.

> *Primary ineffective labor is by far the most frequent and most underrated complication of first childbirth. It should be resolved with early diagnosis and prompt treatment.*

21.2.2 Early recognition and correction

Slow progress should lead to early diagnosis and prompt treatment, long before a woman begins drifting toward prolonged labor and exhaustion. The uterus and cervix of a woman in labor are so predictably responsive to amniotomy (Fig. 21.2) and oxytocin (Fig. 21.3) that, whenever the rate of dilatation does not accelerate sharply after such treatment, the diagnosis of labor is almost certainly wrong. O'Driscoll drily observed: "Such cases are commonplace in practices where little attention is paid to the diagnosis of labor."[11]

Enhancement of slow early labor is safe and effective (Chapter 17). Amniotomy elicits the production and release of PGE_2 in the cervix and the myometrium. In many cases, this measure alone will normalize labor (Fig. 21.2) and, if not, additional oxytocin will almost certainly accomplish this (Fig. 21.3). The moment labor begins spontaneously, oxytocin receptors are widespread and the binding of oxytocin to

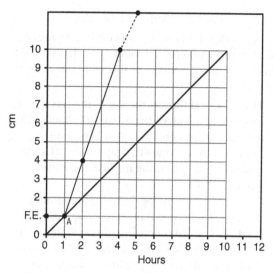

Figure 21.2 Example of early treatment with amniotomy (A).

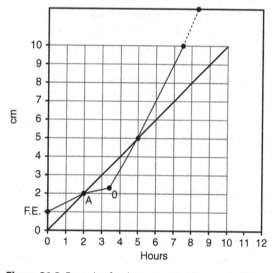

Figure 21.3 Example of early treatment with oxytocin (O).

those receptors enhances the production and release of PGE_2 in the myometrium – precisely where it must act. In sluggish early labor, the formation of the uterine conduction system is not yet adequate or complete (Chapter 8), but oxytocin quickly overcomes this. Inefficient contractions are greatly improved by oxytocin through quick completion of the formation of the myometrial gap junctions. Now the contractions become electrically orchestrated and thus efficient (Chapter 8). The effect is an adequate dilatation rate (Fig. 21.3).

21.2.3 Proactive support of labor

Good practice is, of course, not confined to measures for early correction of slow labor. The plan should be directed to the prevention of this common problem. Therefore:

- The biological transformation of the cervix and myometrium is given the maximum chance. Thus, the spontaneous onset of labor is patiently awaited. Labor is induced only on the relatively rare occasion of a strong medical necessity (Chapter 23).
- "Black worm psychology" (4.2) undermining confidence and provoking stress responses is carefully avoided. Therefore, discouraging terms such as "trial of labor" are never used (4.2.2), and a confident attitude and positive motivation is nurtured.
- All women are well prepared for labor, and policies are consistent and rigidly enforced.
- Every effort is made to ensure that the birth environment is non-stressful, and routine measures that add stress and risks without clear benefits are avoided.
- Personal attention and continuous support are guaranteed for the entirety of labor.

> Expert care in childbirth implies much more than just acceleration of early-presenting slow progress.

Empathy is crucial, but the caregiver cannot simply and meekly share a woman's ordeal. Indeed, clinical vigilance and measures to assure "normality" of the birth process are equally important. That is why:

- The diagnosis of labor is objectively verified and the caregiver pledges that the mother-to-be will hold her baby in her arms within 12 hours.
- The utmost clarity is offered. Nothing is as demoralizing for a woman in labor as ongoing pains without a useful effect and no end in sight. Thus, regular assessments of progress are made and the expected time of delivery is communicated.
- Inadequate progress of less than 1 cm/h is restored within 1 or at the most 2 hours in order to avoid unnecessary exhaustion of both the mother and her uterus.
- The first measure is amniotomy. If adequate progress is not achieved within one hour, oxytocin therapy is started.

- As long as these measures are taken in time, nulliparas almost invariably respond with a spectacular improvement in labor.
- These policies do not lead to more interventions. Rather, the exact opposite is achieved.

21.3 Secondary protraction and arrest

Much less frequently – in about 10% of first labors – dilatation slows down after having smoothly attained the initial 6–8 centimeters. Secondary protraction or arrest disorder is readily and instantly evident when a partogram is kept (Fig. 21.4).

The underlying pathophysiological problem is inadequate wedging action (10.4.1). The fundamental causes are inefficient uterine force or relatively unfavorable fetopelvic proportions, or a combination of those. Secondary arrest is indeed suggestive of fetal obstruction, but insufficient uterine force is still the most likely cause in first labors. This is proven time and again through the restoration of progress by oxytocin (Fig. 21.5), provided adequate doses are used and in good time to avoid uterine exhaustion.

> The most common cause of secondary protraction and arrest disorders in nulliparous labor is insufficient uterine force, whereas in multiparous labor it is mechanical obstruction caused by malposition or macrosomia.

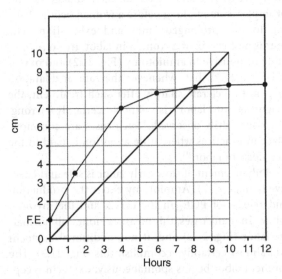

Figure 21.4 Untreated secondary protraction and arrest.

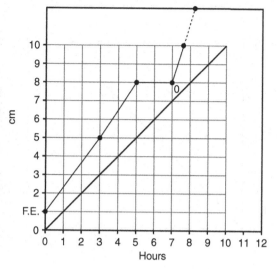

Figure 21.5 Successful treatment (nulliparous labor). O = oxytocin.

A systematic approach to the understanding and treatment of secondary arrest has long been inhibited by the mechanistic view of childbirth (3.3). This view maintains the misconception that oxytocin treatment may result in serious injury to both mother and child whenever there is the faintest possibility of cephalopelvic disproportion. As O'Driscoll put it: "As cephalopelvic disproportion can never, strictly speaking, be wholly excluded until labor has come to a successful conclusion, this caveat effectively ensures that oxytocin is not used to its potential effect for fear of dire consequences."[11] As labor cannot be brought to a successful conclusion without improving uterine force, this gives rise to a classic therapeutic deadlock and overdiagnosis of cephalopelvic disproportion (Chapter 22).

> *In most cases, secondary arrest is a dynamic birth disorder and must be treated as such with amniotomy and oxytocin. There is one overriding reservation: multiparity.*

21.3.1 Expert approach to secondary arrest

At all times, a clear distinction must be maintained between first and parous labor. As a rule, strong uterine action is the key to normality. But the parous uterus is by nature efficient in this regard, with much less cervical resistance to overcome. Secondary arrest in parous labor is, therefore, highly indicative of anatomical obstruction. The causes are either persistent malposition of the fetal head or a child substantially bigger than the previous one. Uterine contractions usually remain vigorous, whereas occasional decline of uterine action should first of all be regarded as a sign of a physiological protection mechanism preventing the lower segment of the uterus from dangerous overstretching. As obstruction carries a risk of uterine rupture, oxytocin in parous labors is allowed only in exceptional cases when obstruction has explicitly been ruled out on the basis of the following compulsory assessments:

- There is no caput succedaneum.
- There is no molding.
- There is no extreme hyperflexion.
- Malposition of the fetal head has been excluded.

> **Multiparas**
>
> *Secondary protraction of parous labor is a mechanical problem until proven otherwise. Parous labor should, therefore, be treated with oxytocin under strict reservations and special precautions only.*

In contrast, the possibility of a mechanical obstruction is not considered in first labors before uterine force is optimized by the judicious use of oxytocin (Chapter 17). In most cases enhancement of uterine force results in molding and caput succedaneum formation, which enhances lock and impact of the fetal head on the dilatational ring. This restores the wedging action and thus progress (Fig. 21.5). In addition, optimized uterine force may correct a possible asynclitism, and the additional hyperflexion of the fetal head will also afford an easier descent (10.4.3).

> **Nulliparas**
>
> *Secondary protraction in first labor should not be ascribed to cephalopelvic disparity until oxytocin has been given for a restricted period to ensure forceful contractions.*

It is important to remember that the force of contractions poses no threat to the fetus, and that nulliparas are virtually immune for uterine rupture. It is only when progress fails to respond to these measures that we resort to a cesarean section (Fig. 21.6).

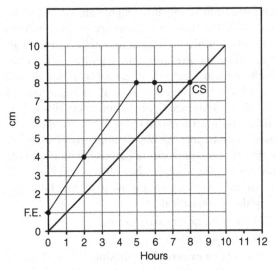

Figure 21.6 Secondary arrest of first labor due to mechanical obstruction. O = oxytocin; CS = cesarean section.

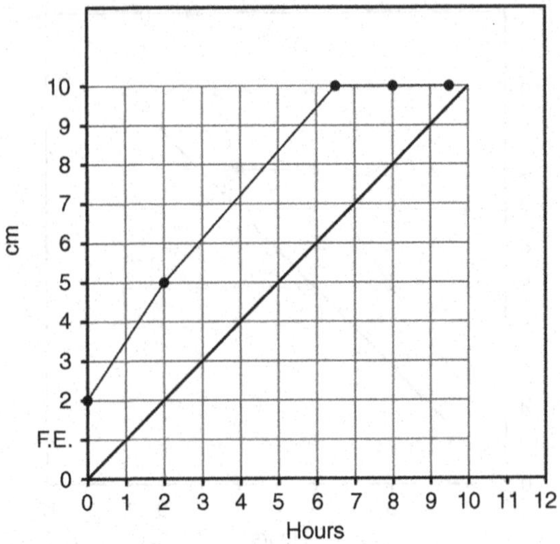

Figure 21.7 Untreated secondary arrest at full dilatation.

21.3.2 Cervical edema versus maximal cervical relaxation

In some cases, secondary arrest coincides with or may result from cervical edema. This cervical thickening is typically asymmetrical and localized in the anterior lip of the cervix.[12] This may occur with 'back labor', in ill-prepared and uncoachable women, or in a protracted, insufficiently supported labor. When a woman is panicked, she may start pushing long before her cervix attains full dilatation and the natural bearing down reflex is activated. Her attempt to speed up her labor has the opposite effect. It is typically too late to clearly explain the situation to her and instruct her not to push. Often, the only remaining options are attempts to 'massage away the edema' or to perform a cesarean section. Prompt correction of slow progress, good coaching, and effective pain relief with epidural block should have prevented this problem at a much earlier stage.

Cervical edema should not be confused with "maximal cervical relaxation." The latter condition is characterized by a symmetrically, maximally dilated cervix that hangs loosely in the vagina and on which the high-station head no longer impacts during contractions. This phenomenon is clinical proof of mechanical obstruction (Chapter 22).

> *Cervical edema originates in poor labor attendance and inept labor management, whereas maximal cervical relaxation indicates mechanical birth obstruction.*

21.4 Secondary arrest at full dilatation

Occasionally progress of labor halts for the first time at complete dilatation (Fig. 21.7). This becomes manifest when the fetal head fails to descend and the mother shows no inclination to push despite the achievement of full dilatation. By definition, the active expulsion stage has not yet begun (10.5.2), so the woman should not be encouraged to bear down. It is a disorder of the first stage of labor and should be treated as such: in first labors with oxytocin (Fig. 21.8). Attempts at expulsion, in the absence of the physiological reflex to push, are generally ineffective and a waste of maternal energy.

> *Secondary arrest at full dilatation is a disorder of the first stage of labor and should be treated accordingly: in nulliparous labors with the use of oxytocin.*

It must be noted that epidural analgesia obscures proper diagnosis. With an effective epidural block, active pushing is, therefore, best delayed until the

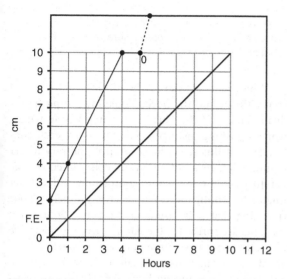

Figure 21.8 Oxytocin for secondary arrest at full dilatation in nulliparous labor.

fetal head reaches the pelvic floor, meaning it is visible when the labia minora are spread.

21.4.1 Mechanistic fallacies

The classic tenet, which marks full dilatation as the onset of the second stage, may have rather unfortunate consequences for women. Too many obstetricians still regard full dilatation as the demarcation line between an abdominal and a vaginal delivery. Whenever there is a need for intervention at this juncture, an instrumental delivery is all too often viewed as a permissible procedure, not to mention a challenge to the obstetrician's manual dexterity. This approach must change. Oxytocin is a much safer alternative (Fig. 21.8). Rotational forceps or vacuum extraction in the passive stage of labor can be genuinely traumatic for both child and mother. Delivery will entail forced traction and a difficult rotation, and although the cervix is fully dilated the vagina and pelvic floor are not. Thus, the maneuver is associated with an unacceptable risk of serious injuries to both mother and child. In such a case, mother and baby would have fared better were full dilatation not achieved at all. Whenever the need for an urgent delivery arises with a fetal head at high station, it should be done by a cesarean.

Attempts at vacuum or forceps delivery late in the first stage of labor are evidence of an archaic mechanistic view of birth. This practice should be renounced.

21.4.2 Expert management

Absence of the pushing reflex at full dilatation is a disorder of the first stage of labor. This problem should, therefore, be handled in a manner identical to that described in 21.3. Nulliparas should receive oxytocin, which can be given with confidence that no harm will befall mother or baby. In most cases, progress is quickly restored (Fig. 21.8). If 2 hours of oxytocin treatment does not effect descent to the level where the pushing reflex is activated (at least 0-station), a cesarean delivery for proven mechanical birth obstruction is the only safe solution. One might start a trial of pushing in the mostly vain hope that the fetal head will yet descend, but the temptation to attempt delivery by traction from 0-station or higher should be resisted. If instrumental delivery of the head should succeed, severe shoulder dystocia will follow in most cases (Chapter 22).

Once again, the fundamental difference between nulliparas and multiparas must be constantly kept in mind: as a rule of thumb, oxytocin in secondary labor arrest is disallowed in multiparas. Cesarean delivery is the only safe option in arrested parous labor.

21.5 Failed expulsion in nulliparas

The natural second stage of labor only begins when the irresistible pushing reflex is activated after the attainment of full dilatation by the impact of the fetal head on the levator ani muscle, rectum, and pelvic floor (10.5.2). At this point, vaginal delivery is virtually assured and – should the need arise – a forceps or vacuum extractor can be used safely. Apart from extremely exceptional women with a selective narrow outlet of the bony pelvis – in whom an otherwise uncomplicated instrumental extraction is no more possible than a spontaneous birth – pelvic dimensions no longer play any obstructive role during expulsion (Chapters 10, 11). Having reached the true expulsion stage, as redefined in Chapter 10, the largest diameter of the head (biparietal plane) has passed well through the pelvic inlet and the entire head is in the pelvis. From this point on, the woman only has to overpower soft-tissue resistance, which, admittedly, requires a lot of force in a first labor. Failure to overcome the soft-tissue resistance is a dynamic problem, not a sign of mechanical obstruction. Slow progress during nulliparous expulsion should be treated with oxytocin.

There is no principal time constraint for the active expulsion stage unless a woman fails to achieve any

Table 21.2 Causes of failing expulsion

1. Maternal exhaustion
2. Pushing too early
3. Ineffective pushing technique
4. Insufficient uterine force

further progress after 1 hour of pushing. Too few birth attendants seem to appreciate that a baby who can be safely born by instrumental traction can also be pushed out, provided the woman has enough reserves of energy. If scrutinized, there are four, primarily iatrogenic, factors involved in failed expulsion (Table 21.2).

21.5.1 Maternal exhaustion

Failure to accomplish expulsion by the woman's own efforts is often related to the antecedent events, because the mother is emotionally drained and physically exhausted after too long a first stage of labor and is now unable or unwilling to push. An operative delivery then seems the only solution, but this problem should have been anticipated and prevented much earlier. In current conventional practice an instrumental or cesarean delivery is performed in 20–30% of all nulliparas who achieve full dilatation (2.2). Execution of the expert birth-plan – provided it is employed in all its components – effectively diminishes this inappropriate operative delivery rate in second-stage labor.

Failing expulsion in first labor is a dynamic birth disorder.

21.5.2 Pushing too early

The prevalent misconception that the expulsion stage begins at full dilatation is a direct cause of many iatrogenic expulsion arrests. All too often women are instructed to push too early and thereby lose too much strength too soon. Impatience on the part of the birth attendants at full dilatation (especially at night) in awaiting the start of the actual pushing reflex to occur, or the vain hope of speeding up the conclusion of the woman's labor, may play a role. In fact, one should have acted much earlier. Pushing before the onset of the natural pushing reflex is generally ineffective and counterproductive in its effect: operative delivery rates rocket sky-high.

Too often energy and resolve are wasted by encouraging women to push before the true reflexive urge to do so has occurred.

When the fetal head reaches the level of the ischial spines (0-station) the irrepressible urge to push gradually arises (10.5). There is nothing wrong with a woman pushing instinctively at the top of each contraction. At this stage, however, it is contrary to her natural instincts and thus wrong policy to encourage her to push for the whole contraction with all her might. Not until the caput reaches the pelvic floor (meaning that it is visible at the pelvic floor when the labia are spread) is the natural, irrepressible urge to push from the beginning of each contraction activated. The woman will not fail to show this herself. The sudden pressure on her pelvic floor is an overwhelming and often cataclysmic sensation that marks the transition from her passive role in the first stage of labor to an active role in the expulsion stage (10.5.3). The wise birth attendant makes the most of this natural process and keeps a close eye on the woman. From this moment forward, all reserves of strength must be gathered. With adequate coaching and expert conduct of first-stage labor, expulsion takes nulliparas about 35 minutes on average and multiparas even substantially less.

It is worth noting that, in vaginal breech deliveries, women are wisely instructed not to give way to their pushing reflex for as long as possible so as to effect deep descent and internal rotation of the breech, after which they can push with all their might. Indeed, the delay in active pushing helps to promote a smooth and safe spontaneous expulsion. Strangely, this physiological fact is often forgotten with cephalic presentations, where women are encouraged to push even before the onset of the physiological reflex to do so.

With expert labor management and adequate coaching, expulsion takes nulliparas only about 35 minutes on average and multiparas even substantially less.

21.5.3 Ineffective pushing techniques

In many places pregnant women are being prepared for labor by independent birth instructors who teach them how to push, for instance in the upright position, sitting on a birthing stool, or squatting supported by a specialized pillow, only to find that such facilities are not available. Similarly, the pre-labor instructions on how to breathe and push often do not correspond with the instructions given by the birth attendants in the delivery room. Confusion resulting from mismatches between training and actual practice strongly undermines the effectiveness of a woman's efforts in delivering her baby. To reiterate: pre-labor education that corresponds with actual practice is critical (18.1), and all birth attendants should be trained in supporting women giving birth in a position of their choice (11.1.3).

Furthermore, faulty pushing techniques are not infrequently the result of thoughtless care providers who allow three or more onlookers, position the woman with her legs in stirrups, and place an intern or student-midwife between her legs facing her vulva closely. Can this be the setting in which caregivers expect women to push best?

Women's natural embarrassment, conditioned prudishness, and their natural desire to maintain personal cleanliness tend to override the pushing reflex. Measures with the declared purpose of stimulating the pushing reflex, such as applying pressure on the rectum using fingers placed in the vagina, as well as stretching the perineum, are painful, woman-unfriendly, and often counterproductive. Additional encouragement including making comparisons to "pooping" (literally heard in many delivery rooms) will not improve a woman's pushing technique either. For didactic sport, every birth attendant should at least once during her/his training strip down (if only to the underpants), put her/his legs in stirrups, and have strangers offer the same "encouraging" words.

> *Faulty maternal pushing techniques are often iatrogenic in origin.*

21.5.4 Insufficient uterine force at expulsion

Despite or because of the management of labor up to the second stage, the expulsive force can be insufficient to effect the cardinal movements of the fetal head and conquer the resistance of the pelvic floor. The assumption that a delayed rotation is the cause of stagnation – which must be manually corrected and/or resolved by rotational forceps or vacuum extraction – is a misconception of the mechanistic perspective (11.2.5). The truth is that flexion, internal rotation, and deflexion of the fetal head originate from force. That is why oxytocin is the first measure in nulliparas and an instrument-assisted delivery should be the last resort. Maximization of uterine force can still bring about the cardinal movements, resulting in a spontaneous delivery. If not, it at least ensures that the caput is as deep as possible and that its attitude is more favorable for facilitating a safe instrumental delivery. The higher the level at which instrumental extraction begins, the greater the risk of fetal and maternal trauma (11.2.3).

21.6 Failing expulsion in multiparas

The overriding proposition that prolonged parous labor originates in fetal obstruction remains valid at all times including the expulsion stage. After a properly managed first stage, failing expulsion is exceedingly rare in multiparas. Less maternal force is required because the soft birth canal has already been stretched at the previous birth. Long parous expulsion mostly results from instructions to push while the true expulsion stage has not yet been reached. If the fetal head is unusually molded with an extensive caput formation (the so-called "pharaoh head"), full engagement might not have taken place even though the head appears to be at 0-station (11.2.4). A decelerative partogram should alert that this might occur. Problematic obstruction should be anticipated. Even when, after secondary delay, the parous woman reaches full dilatation, efforts at expulsion are still likely to fail. In these circumstances, any attempt at vaginal extraction poses inexcusable risks of maternal and fetal injury. If instrumental delivery of the fetal head succeeds, severe shoulder dystocia will almost certainly follow.

In conclusion: instrumental delivery for arrested parous labor must be judged as unsafe and malpractice in most cases. The only exception is a frightened multipara (with a traumatic first experience that should have been avoided) who now hardly dares to push while the fetal head can be easily delivered by outlet forceps or vacuum extractor.

> *The use of forceps or vacuum to resolve second-stage arrest of parous labor is dangerous for both mother and child.*

21.7 The refractory or unresponsive uterus

Ineffective labor is common in nulliparas, and this problem – regardless of when it occurs – can virtually always be resolved with amniotomy and oxytocin, provided treatment is started in a timely fashion and oxytocin is properly dosed. Two clinical conditions wherein the uterus often fails to respond properly to oxytocin should be recognized: induction and the exhausted uterus.

21.7.1 Failed induction

In mainstream practice, induction is the most frequent cause of uterine resistance to oxytocin. The pathophysiology was explained previously (8.8.2). Clinically, induction sets in motion effects that are the exact opposite of those of good care in spontaneous labor (Chapter 23). Moreover, induction hampers proper diagnosis and treatment of all labor disorders described in this chapter. Unsuccessful induction must be recognized as the iatrogenic disorder that it is and should be recorded as "failed induction," not as "dystocia." Exact diagnosis and meticulous audit of all procedures are the key ingredients of quality improvement programs aimed at lowering cesarean rates (Chapters 26 and 27).

21.7.2 Inordinate delay

Picture the legs of a marathon runner who hits the proverbial "wall" and collapses as a result of either lack of strength or muscle cramp. The exhausted myometrium reacts similarly. Over an extended period, lactic acid accumulates and the uterus gradually loses its ability to respond to oxytocin (8.5.4). The exhausted, refractory uterus is a common problem in conventional obstetrics, but is hardly ever seen when the rules of *proactive support* are applied. Incidentally, postpartum hemorrhage also occurs more often in women with a depleted uterus after too long a labor.[13]

When oxytocin treatment is started at too late a stage, the response is also much less safe. The uterus may react as any overburdened muscle loaded with lactic acid: with tetanic spasms (8.5.4). The result is inadequate uterine relaxation between the contractions and consequently fetal distress (8.7.2). The longer the uterus has run ineffectively, the smaller the therapeutic range of oxytocin.

The exhausted, refractory myometrium

An exhausted uterus fails to respond properly to oxytocin or may react with hypertonia in the inter-contraction intervals, leading to fetal distress.

The refractory uterus is a plainly preventable predicament as it results from induction or from unfounded tolerance of long labor. Clinical stalemate, whereby overdue stimulation fails to restore progress or triggers fetal distress, is a frequent indication for cesarean delivery that could have been prevented by timely and far less intrusive measures. The root of the problem – depletion of the uterus – is seldom recognized. It is this lack of understanding as well as the use of too-low doses (17.3.3) that feeds the unfounded skepticism surrounding oxytocin as therapy for dysfunctional labor. Clearly, expert conduct and care of labor prevent this dynamic and iatrogenic problem.

21.8 Hypertonic or uncoordinated dystocia

Most textbooks subdivide dysfunctional labor into two types only: hypotonic and hypertonic inertia. This view is typically coupled with the warning that while oxytocin could be useful in the former, it could be detrimental in the latter. In reality, however, signs of imminent fetal hypoxia are the only contraindication for oxytocin treatment. Hypertonic dystocia is a separate clinical entity altogether (8.5.5) that may occur in nulliparous and multiparous labors alike.

In pathological circumstances, chorioamnionitis, fresh meconium, or free intrauterine blood may randomly excite the myometrium cells to the extent that the electrical orchestration and consequently the efficiency and effectiveness of the contractions are lost (8.5.5). Progress halts, and persistent hypertonia between contractions further compromises fetal oxygenation, setting a dangerous vicious circle in motion. This dual problem characterizes true hypertonic or uncoordinated dystocia.

Hypertonic dystocia

This term is reserved for a singular clinical entity in which meconium, blood, or pus disturbs uterine coordination, leading to a vicious circle of dysfunctional labor and fetal compromise.

Heavy meconium suspension is the most frequent cause. Whether intrauterine infection results from or in dysfunctional labor is a typical chicken-or-egg riddle that cannot be answered in conventional practice where long labors are tolerated. The sequence of events will become evident when the rules of *proactive support* are applied. Clearly, the chance of infection increases with an extended duration of labor as more vaginal examinations are performed and intrauterine catheters are used. This typically happens with poorly managed, out of control labors. A preventable component is then not difficult to identify.

As may happen with all overburdened muscles loaded with lactic acid, an exhausted uterus after too long a labor may also react with spasms (8.5.4). After a long labor, this predicament is difficult if not impossible to distinguish from hypertonic dystocia resulting from beginning infection. This diagnostic problem is circumvented by adherence to the proposed policies because *proactive support* effectively prevents long labor, uterine exhaustion, and intrauterine infection.

Clinical measures should primarily address the underlying problems with amnion-infusion in cases of heavy meconium, and antibiotics (Chapter 24). However, owing to the practical dilemma in which the uterus cannot be stimulated safely but progress remains minimal, a cesarean delivery is often the only feasible solution. Waiting will benefit neither the fetus nor the mother. As always, decisive action is required.

If the fetus does not tolerate the contractions required for normal progress, a cesarean delivery is the only rational and safe option.

21.9 Final diagnosis for effective audit purposes

Dystocia – or equivalent labels such as "failure to progress" or "dysfunctional labor" – is heterogeneous in its causation and manifestation, and the term thus represents a pseudo-diagnosis. These terms should, therefore, no longer be used without further explanation. Instead of simply attributing the indication for operative delivery to "dystocia," the precise nature and causal diagnosis of the birth disorder at hand should be assessed. Cause and effect need to be explored before the conduct and care of labor can be improved with any semblance of a rational basis.

What is more, only detailed and causal diagnoses allow for meaningful audit of all procedures and outcomes (Chapter 26).

Detailed diagnosis is the most important single issue in responsible labor care and critical for meaningful medical audit.

References

1. Cheng YW, Shaffer BL, Bryant AS, Caughey AB. Length of the first stage of labor and associated perinatal outcomes in nulliparous women. J Obstet Gynaecol 2010;**116**:1127–35
2. Gharoro EP, Enabudoso EJ. Labor management: an appraisal of the role of false labor and latent phase on the delivery mode. J Obstet Gynecol 2006;**26**:534–7
3. Maghoma J, Buchmann EJ. Maternal and fetal risks associated with prolonged latent phase of labor. J Obstet Gynaecol 2002;**22**:16–9
4. Bailit JL, Dierker LR, Blanchard MH, Mercer BM. Outcome of women presenting in active versus latent phase of spontaneous labor. Obstet Gynecol 2005;**105**:77–9
5. Jackson DB, Lang JM, Ecker J, Swartz WH, Heeren T. Impact of collaborative management and early admission in labor on method of delivery. J Obstet Gynecol Neonatal Nurs 2003;**32**:147–57
6. Chelmow D, Kilpatrick SJ, Laros RK. Maternal and neonatal outcomes after prolonged latent phase. Obstet Gynecol 1993;**81**:486–91
7. Friedman EA, Neff RK. Labor and Delivery: Impact on Offspring. Littleton, MA: PSG, 1987
8. Malone FD, Geary M, Chelmow D, *et al.* Prolonged labor in nulliparas: lesson from the active management of labor. Obstet Gynecol 1996;**88**:211–15
9. Holmes P, Oppenheimer LW, Wen SW. The relationship between cervical dilatation at initial presentation in labor and subsequent interventions. Br J Obstet Gynaecol 2001;**108**:1120–4
10. Hemminki E, Simukka R. The timing on hospital admission and progress of labor. Eur J Obstet Gynecol Reprod Biol 1986;**22**:85–94
11. O'Driscoll K, Meagher D, Robson M. Active Management of Labour, 4th edn. London: Mosby; 2003
12. Funai EF, Norwitz ER. Persistent anterior cervical lip. In: Management of normal labor and delivery. UpToDate. Accessed November 2014
13. Belfort MA. Overview of postpartum hemorrhage. UpToDate. Accessed November 2014

Chapter 22

Obstructed labor

Assuming the diagnosis of labor to be correct, the onset to be spontaneous, and efficient uterine contractions to be assured, there remains but one reason why labor may continue to stagnate: obstruction. Obstructed labor may be caused either by disparity between the absolute size of the fetal head and the pelvic capacity – generally referred to as "cephalopelvic disproportion" (CPD) – or by its clinical analog: malposition of the fetal head, including occiput posterior, deflexion attitudes, or asynclitism. This chapter discusses CPD and fetal head malposition under one heading, as their clinical picture and clinical approach are virtually identical.

> **Definition**
>
> *The term mechanical dystocia refers to obstruction of the fetal head such as to preclude safe vaginal delivery. Causative factors are fetal size, pelvic functional capacity, and malposition of the fetal head.*

22.1 Diagnosis

Obstructed labor is a clinical diagnosis by exclusion. Adequate forces of labor need to be assured and proven by substantial molding and caput succedaneum formation, before obstruction can be diagnosed with a reasonable degree of certainty. The ratio between the dimensions of the pelvic inlet and those of the fetal head plays a decisive role in the progression of dilatation only during the wedging phase of first-stage labor (10.4.1). Therefore, anatomical (mechanical) obstruction cannot be diagnosed before at least 6 cm dilatation has been attained.

> **Diagnosis of mechanical labor disorder**
>
> *Secondary arrest at 6 cm dilatation or more and failure to descend, despite strong contractions proven by substantial molding and sizable caput formation.*

22.2 Overdiagnosis of CPD

The classic concept of cephalopelvic disproportion originally described obstructed labors occurring as a result of pelvic contracture or deformity, which is a permanent condition. By inference, once CPD was diagnosed, future vaginal birth was deemed impossible. But CPD or contracted pelvis proves to be a very unreliable diagnosis: two-thirds or more of women diagnosed as having this disorder and therefore delivered by cesarean section deliver equally large or even larger babies vaginally with their next pregnancy, if given the chance.[1] Clearly, CPD or its equivalent, "contracted pelvis," is generally overdiagnosed. The main reason is underdiagnosis and undertreatment of dynamic labor disorders (Chapter 21). Although oxytocin is extensively used in many hospitals, it is commonly used too late or in too low a dose (17.3.3).

> **Elusive concept of cephalopelvic disproportion (CPD)**
>
> *CPD or contracted pelvis is a tenuous diagnosis frequently abused as an excuse for a cesarean delivery in women who did not get a fair chance to prove the functional capacity of their pelvis.*

The second reason for overdiagnosis of CPD is the fact that obstructed labor is not associated simply with contracted pelvis or excessive fetal size. Unfavorable position of the fetal head – persistent occiput posterior, asynclitism, deflexion – may similarly obstruct the passage through the birth canal. Obviously, CPD is ill-defined and in most cases the concept of CPD does not cover the accepted clinical significance of contracted pelvis and permanent impossibility of birth. As strict definition and reliable diagnosis are critical for rational and responsible obstetrics, preference should be given to the more neutral and more accurate terms "mechanical birth disorder" or "obstructed labor."

22.2.1 Inaccurate prediction

This terminology also serves to eliminate the widespread but mistaken practice of diagnosing "CPD" even before labor has begun. In reality, reliable selection of a fetal size threshold to predict obstruction remains impossible, despite advanced sonographic fetometry.[2,3] This is because of the inaccuracy of the method and because most cases of diagnosed disproportion occur in fetuses whose weight is well within the range of the general obstetric population. Efforts to predict CPD on the basis of the fetal head circumference have proven equally disappointing, in part because malposition of the fetal head is an additional causative factor. This also explains why sophisticated imaging techniques of the pelvis, including CT and MRI, are unable to predict obstructed labor reliably.[2,3] The only reliable test is labor itself.

> *Neither fetal size estimation nor radiological assessment of pelvic dimensions is particularly accurate in predicting the outcome of labor.*

Although induction is widely practiced for suspected fetal macrosomia ("to prevent the child from growing even bigger"), there is no evidence to support this policy.[4] Rather the reverse is true, because induction mainly induces dynamic labor disorders (Chapter 23). A meta-analysis of studies in women with suspected fetal macrosomia showed similar neonatal outcomes, but cesarean rates were twice as high in women whose labor was induced as in the group with expectant management (16.6% vs. 8.4%).[5] Through circular logic, though, faulty policies tend to create their own justification again. After induction, uterine contractions are often inefficient and thus ineffective. Lack of progress is then wrongly attributed to the anticipated birth obstruction. Such misinterpretations explain the stubborn persistence of wrong policies.

> *"All efforts to anticipate birth obstruction are not only misguided, they result in a rate of intervention grossly in excess of the true prevalence of fetopelvic disparity."[6]*

A floating, non-engaged fetal head in late pregnancy is also not predictive. In black nulliparous women, in whom non-engagement commonly occurs, it is slightly associated with longer labors, but not with operative delivery or increased maternal or fetal morbidity.[7] Not even women with short stature (or small feet) need be regarded with suspicion, since smaller mothers usually give birth to smaller babies. This observation is as important in countries with immigrants from Asia and Africa as it is in the developing world. Western doctors tend to place undue emphasis on short stature without directing equal attention to low birth weight.

In conclusion, a floating fetal head in late pregnancy is no reason for pelvimetry or fetometry. It is imperative, however, to exclude placenta previa or occasionally occurring obstructive cysts and myomas in the lesser pelvis.

> *The only reliable test for disparity between the head and the pelvis is labor itself.*

Occiput posterior before labor has no prognostic significance. At the onset of labor, 15% of fetuses present with occiput posterior.[9] On the basis of old radiographic studies, this position is still construed as a sign of a narrow forepelvis.[10] In reality, however, occiput posterior is predominantly associated with anterior placentation.[9] With adequate driving force, 85–90% of cases will rotate to the anterior position as soon as the occiput reaches or passes the pelvic floor.[11] Labor is not lengthened appreciably in these cases.

> *The majority of cases with initially occiput posterior position undergo spontaneous anterior rotation during expulsion, most often followed by uncomplicated delivery.*

22.3 Expert approach

Clearly, birth obstruction is a diagnosis by experiment, and the appropriate clinical approach is, therefore, purely pragmatic. No consideration whatsoever should be given to the possibility of obstruction in the course of routine antenatal care.

22.3.1 Positive attitude

The pelvic size should never be assessed, either by clinical means or by radiographic pelvimetry or MRI. Fetal weight in the upper league should never be estimated, either by palpation or by sonographic fetometry. All reference to occiput posterior or macrosomia should be either avoided or put into perspective.[12] For a woman carrying an undeniably big baby it is better emphasized that she is built normally and in perfect condition to deliver her child by her own efforts.

Cautionary notes should not be written in the woman's chart by senior staff, because such reservations place an unbearable burden of responsibility on the midwives and junior doctors who actually attend the labor. Pessimistic anticipations tend to self-fulfillment. For similar reasons, the discouraging term "trial of labor" should never be used; a "trial of labor" often fails simply because the outcome is prejudiced beforehand. Induction of labor is contraindicated rather than indicated, so the spontaneous onset of labor is patiently awaited. A positive state of mind is radiated, as "all is well."

> *The greater the emphasis on macrosomia or occiput posterior, the more likely it is that difficulties will follow. Anxious caregivers tend to create their own problems under these headings.*

22.3.2 Clinical diagnosis

The possibility of a mechanical obstruction should be first considered only when initially normal labor ceases to progress secondarily, but such a diagnosis should never be entertained seriously until efficient uterine force has been proven by substantial caput succedaneum formation and molding. In first labors, this usually requires oxytocin that can be administered in the sure knowledge that this treatment does not cause rupture of the nulliparous uterus or trauma to the child. That is certainly not the case in parous labor.

Occiput posterior and asynclitism are usually transient when uterine force is (made) strong.[11] Only if adequate uterine force has been demonstrated by sizable caput formation and molding, or in nulliparous labor progression fails to recover despite 2 hours of judicious stimulation, can a mechanical birth obstruction be diagnosed. A cesarean delivery is then the only rational and safe option.

> *Whenever labor stalls, fetal obstruction should be considered only after efficient uterine contractions have been established. In first labors this usually requires the use of oxytocin.*

Unfounded reservations about oxytocin originate in failure to draw a clear distinction between nulliparous and parous labor. Obstructed nulliparous labor bears no risks; long-term follow-up of 5- to 6-year-old infants delivered after secondarily prolonged labors shows no more neurological abnormalities than matched controls.[13]

Clearly, obstruction of a first birth can be safely diagnosed by assuring optimal uterine force, provided the vertex presents and fetal status is monitored as carefully as in any labor (Chapter 24). An extensive search in Medline/PubMed yields zero counter-evidence for this contention. The power of contractions poses no threat to the mother or the fetus, even in obstructed labor. Uterine rupture is a calamity that only befalls parous women, whereas the nulliparous uterus is virtually rupture-proof. Serious fetal and maternal trauma is associated almost exclusively with forcible traction, regardless of parity.

It is not birth obstruction that carries the dangers for mother and child but mainly the obstetrician who neglects the significance of parity, disregards proper definitions, and misconstrues full dilatation as the deciding demarcation line between abdominal and vaginal operative delivery (21.4.1).

> *Birth obstruction can be safely diagnosed by assuring optimal uterine force through oxytocin therapy. Again, there is one overriding reservation: multiparity.*

22.4 Failing expulsion

Proper understanding of the nature and sequence of cardinal movements of the fetal head during expulsion (11.1) prevents mechanistic misinterpretations in cases of failing expulsion. Since the entire fetal head is in the pelvis when the reflex action is activated, and because isolated constriction of the bony pelvic outlet is extremely rare, the normal capacity of the bony pelvis to allow passage of the fetal head is virtually assured when the true expulsion stage of labor begins. The only physical resistance remaining at this stage of labor comes from the soft pelvic tissues that, admittedly, may require tremendous effort to surmount.

It must be concluded that in almost every case in which expulsion in the true second-stage fails, the predominant cause is dynamic in origin, not mechanical obstruction. When expulsion fails, the composite force of uterine contractions and reflex action of voluntary muscles is evidently not equal to the task. Prevention and treatment of failed expulsion were therefore discussed in more detail under the heading "dynamic labor disorders," where they predominantly belong (Chapter 21).

> *True birth obstruction is a disorder of first-stage labor, not of the second stage. Protraction and arrest of expulsion is a dynamic disorder, not a mechanical disorder.*

22.5 Shoulder dystocia

After delivery of the fetal head, occasionally mechanical problems with the delivery of the fetal shoulders arise resulting from a size discrepancy between the fetal body and the pelvic inlet. The incidence varies between 0.2% and 3% depending on the criteria used for diagnosis.[14] Despite its infrequent occurrence, shoulder dystocia continues to represent a subject of immense importance because the intrusive maneuvers needed to deliver the shoulders are associated with severe fetal trauma, including transient or permanent brachial plexus palsy, bone fractures, hypoxic brain injury, and even perinatal death.[15] Maternal injuries include fourth-degree lacerations extending into the rectum and permanent psychological trauma.

22.5.1 Unpredictability

Maternal risk factors – multiparity, obesity, diabetes – all exert their effects because of the association with increased birth weight.[16] Despite this, a prophylactic cesarean delivery for suspected fetal macrosomia is hardly ever appropriate.[15,17] Such a policy does not eliminate the problem because half of the newborns with shoulder dystocia weigh less than 4000 g, and even if the birth weight of an infant is more than 4000 g, shoulder dystocia complicates only 3% of the deliveries.[15,17] Rouse and Owen argued that a policy of prophylactic cesarean for identified macrosomia involves "a Faustian bargain" because it would require more than 1000 cesarean deliveries and millions of dollars to avert a single permanent brachial plexus injury.[18] In light of the available evidence, preparedness and optimizing the management of shoulder dystocia is the most immediate and tenable approach to the prevention of its related birth traumas.

22.5.2 Intrapartum warning signs

Anticipation implies recognition of pre-existing risk factors (previous shoulder dystocia) and intrapartum harbingers: a secondary protraction disorder and difficult instrumental delivery.[15–17] In those circumstances, the obstetrician on duty should be called into the delivery room in time for stand-by assistance in case shoulder dystocia should occur.

> *Undue attention is given to pre-labor identification of risk factors for shoulder dystocia whereas clearly identifiable warning signs in late labor are often neglected.*

These intrapartum warning signs are the more ominous if occurring in parous labors. The only rational preventive measure is an absolute bar on instrumental deliveries in parous labor for failure to progress. If instrumental traction is needed for the conclusion of protracted parous birth, shoulder dystocia almost certainly follows.

> **Intrapartum predictors**
> 1. *Prolonged wedging phase, in particular in multiparas*
> 2. *Prolonged second stage*
> 3. *Difficult instrument-assisted delivery*

22.5.3 Preparedness

As shoulder dystocia may occur without any prediction, all providers, including those who only attend "low-risk" labors, must be prepared to deal with this obstetric emergency.

Thorough knowledge of the composite actions and maneuvers[14,19] required for the alleviation of shoulder dystocia as atraumatically as possible is important, not only for obstetric residents and attending house staff but also for midwives, nurses, and family practitioners attending home births. Periodic institutional "skills and drills" should be performed, not only to coordinate a teamwork approach to this obstetric emergency, but also to provide an opportunity to practice the proper maneuvers on a regular basis.

22.6 Obstetric rarities

Discussions on the mechanics of birth and related birth disorders are often confused and frustrated by the introduction of exceptional cases. Therefore, a short comment on some obstetric curiosities makes sense here.

22.6.1 Brow presentation

Persistent brow presentation makes birth a mechanical impossibility, unless the fetal head is small (premature infants) or the pelvis is unusually large. However, persistent brow presentation is extremely rare (incidence 1:10 000).[20] Brow presentation in early labor is commonly unstable and often converts to an occiput or a face presentation in the first stage of labor.[21] In both circumstances the fetus can be delivered smoothly through the normal vaginal route. Failure to progress in the wedging phase of labor with a brow presentation is a straightforward indication for cesarean delivery. Obsolete attempts to manipulate the fetus vaginally to occiput or face presentation are dangerous and reminiscent of veterinary interventions. An instrumental delivery of a fetus in persistent brow presentation is, of course, malpractice.

22.6.2 Pelvic deformity

Anatomical deformity of the bony pelvis is equally rare since the elimination of rickets. It usually originates in a limp from early childhood (poliomyelitis) or from injury in a road traffic accident. Fractures of the pubic rami may compromise the birth canal by malunion or callus formation.[22] Identification of women at risk for pelvic deformity presents no problem since they declare themselves by their gait and their medical history.

Only in these exceptional cases is pre-labor assessment of the pelvis warranted. If no pelvic abnormalities are found, a vaginal delivery can be pursued. If a deviant pelvic architecture is manifest, a pre-labor cesarean delivery might be justified.

Exceptional women with pelvic deformity declare themselves by their gait and/or their history of pelvic fracture.

22.7 Final classification for meaningful audit

From the foregoing analyses it is evident that the great majority of dystocia cases that are currently resolved by cesarean delivery actually involve dynamic birth disorders that can be prevented or corrected in a timely manner in most cases. Where a proper labor management protocol is followed and strict definitions are used, birth obstruction occurs far less frequently than generally assumed and recorded in obstetric databases. If properly defined, labor obstruction occurs in only about 1% of all term pregnancies (Chapter 27).

While the evidence and common sense dictate that "dystocia" should not be anticipated ante partum, a detailed diagnosis of each labor disorder is critical for meaningful audit. All operative deliveries for "dystocia" should therefore be formally reviewed at the daily peer review sessions on the basis of all the evidence available (Chapter 26).

First, a differential diagnosis between dynamic and mechanical dystocia should be made (Chapter 21). If, in retrospect, dynamic factors for secondary protraction of labor have been convincingly excluded, a formal decision on the cause of obstruction is made: either malposition of the fetal head or true CPD. This final diagnosis is recorded in the patient's chart because the definitive conclusion may imply consequences for the next pregnancy and route of delivery.

Where rigorous standards of diagnosis are applied, true CPD is exceedingly rare, occurring in less than 0.5% of all pregnancies. Birth obstruction attributable to malposition of the fetal head occurs in another 0.5% of all pregnancies (Chapter 27). Well-defined mechanical obstruction is a relatively rare birth disorder indeed.

References

1. Brill Y, Windrim R. Vaginal birth after cesarean section: review of antenatal predictors of success. J Obstet Gynaecol Can 2003;25:275–86
2. Pattinson RC, Farrel E. Pelvimetry for fetal cephalic presentations at or near term. Cochrane Database Syst Rev 2007
3. Maharaj D. Assessing cephalopelvic disproportion: back to the basics. Obstet Gynecol Surv 2010;65:387–95
4. Orion O, Boulvain M. Induction of labour for suspected fetal macrosomia. Cochrane Database Syst Rev 2011
5. Sanchez-Ramos K, Bernstein S, Kaunitz AM. Expectant management versus labor induction for suspected fetal macrosomia: a systematic review. Obstet Gynecol 2002;100:997–1002
6. O'Driscoll K, Meagher D, Robson M. Active Management of Labour, 4th edn. London: Mosby; 2003

7. Ehsanipoor RM, Satin AJ. Overview of normal labor and protraction and arrest disorders. UpToDate. Accessed November 2014

8. Verhoeven CJ, Mulders LG, Oei SG, Mol BW. Does ultrasonographic foetal head position prior to induction of labour predict the outcome of delivery? Eur J Obstet Gynecol Reprod Biol 2012;**164**:133–7

9. Gardberg M, Laakkonen E, Salevaara M. Intrapartum sonography and persistent occiput posterior position: a study of 408 deliveries. Obstet Gynecol 1998;**91**:746–9

10. Cunningham FG, Leveno KJ, Hauth JC (eds). Normal Labor and Delivery. In: Williams Obstetrics, 22nd edn. New York: McGraw-Hill; 2005:407–41

11. Cruikshank DP, White CA. Obstetric malpresentations: Twenty years' experience. Am J Obstet Gynecol 1973;**116**:1097–104

12. Sadeh-Mestechkin D, Walfisch A, Shachar R, *et al.* Suspected macrosomia? Better not tell. Arch Gynecol Obstet 2008;**278**:225–30

13. Rosen M, Debanne S, Thompson K, Dickinson JC. Abnormal labor and infant brain damage. Obstet Gynecol 1992;**80**:961–5

14. Rodis JF. Shoulder dystocia: Intrapartum diagnosis, management, and outcome. UpToDate. Accessed November 2014

15. ACOG Practice Bulletin 40. Clinical Management Guidelines for Obstetrician-Gynecologists. Obstet Gynecol 2002;**100**:1045–50

16. Øverland EA1, Vatten LJ, Eskild A. Pregnancy week at delivery and the risk of shoulder dystocia: a population study of 2,014,956 deliveries. Br J Obstet Gynaecol 2014;**121**:34–41

17. Rodis JF. Shoulder dystocia: Risk factors and planning delivery of at risk pregnancies. UpToDate. Accessed November 2014

18. Rouse DJ, Owen J. Prophylactic cesarean delivery for fetal macrosomia diagnosed by means of ultrasonography; a Faustian bargain? Am J Obstet Gynecol 1999;**181**:332–8

19. Politi S, D'Emidio L, Cignini P, *et al.* Shoulder dystocia: an Evidence-Based approach. J Prenat Med 2010;**4**:35–42

20. Cruikshank DP, Cruikshank JE. Face and brow presentations: A review. Clin Obstet Gynecol 1981;**24**:333–51

21. Stitely ML, Gherman RB. Labor with abnormal presentation and position. Obstet Gynecol Clin North Am 2005;**32**:165–79

22. Speer DP, Peltier LF. Pelvic fractures and pregnancy. J Trauma 1972;**12**:474–80

23. Riehl JT. Caesarean section rates following pelvic fracture: A systematic review. Injury 2014;**45**:1516–21

Chapter

23

Curtailed use of induction

As documented in nearly all chapters, induction of labor has a profoundly adverse effect on the conduct and care of birth. Induction deteriorates the course and outcome of labor and, consequently, women's experience of childbirth. For this reason, we strongly advise against a liberal use of this intervention. Despite this clear stand, the subject needs to be discussed because the popularity of induction shows that, in addition to direct iatrogenic harm, other disadvantages are seriously underestimated: indirect negative effects on other parturients, educative drawbacks, and detrimental effects on maternity care as a whole. This chapter is meant as an eye-opener to promote self-exploration and reflection by those well-intending colleagues who practice liberal induction policies.

Induction of labor impinges on women's experience of birth and has a profoundly adverse effect on the management of labor and the childbirth service as a whole.

23.1 Overriding biology

Pre-labor biological transformation of both the cervix and the myometrium is essential for a smooth and safe birth (8.1–8.3). Since neither of these two processes has had a chance to achieve completion when labor is induced, every pregnant woman who undergoes this intervention is put at a disadvantage from the outset. The cervix is always more resistant than it would have been if labor had started spontaneously, and the uterus is less efficient at exerting force. Incomplete or absent transformation explains the longer duration of induced labor and associated co-interventions including operative deliveries.

Furthermore, oxytocin is much less safe and much less effective in induced labor than in spontaneous labor. There are few oxytocin receptors present, if any, and the myometrium may lack the connexon-proteins needed to make gap junctions for the activation of effective and safe labor. As a result, oxytocin used for induction may have little effect or may lead to hypertonic uterine dysfunction. Incomplete myometrial transformation is the reason induction does include an artificial latent phase.[1]

Induction leads at best to a longer labor and at worst to a failed induction.

23.1.1 Failed inductions

Apart from false extrapolations from misleading RCTs – heavily criticized in Chapter 6 – virtually all cohort and match-controlled studies on elective induction exploring the consequences came up with the same answers: longer labors, more co-interventions, more need for epidural analgesia, more abdominal and vaginal operative deliveries, and less satisfaction of women with the birth experience.[2-21] Most studies report a 2- to 3-fold increase in the chance of a cesarean delivery following induction of first labors. This trend appears to persist even when the cervix is "favorable" for induction. Yeast *et al.*, for example, found a 70% higher cesarean rate in nulliparas whose labors were induced with a "favorable cervix" as compared with matched spontaneous labors (RR 1.7; 95% CI 1.4–2.0).[13] This finding proves that it takes more than just "cervical ripeness" to ensure a smooth induction, namely myometrial transformation (Chapter 8).

Impact of labor induction

The duration of labor is artificially prolonged, physical and emotional stress soars, the workload of nurses and midwives is increased disproportionately, there is a greater demand for analgesia, and spontaneous vaginal delivery rates plummet.

The negative impact of induction on the course and outcome of labor is most pronounced in nulliparas, though not entirely absent in multiparas.[9,13] In the study of Yeast et al., multiparas whose labor was induced with a favorable cervix were also significantly more often delivered by cesarean section (RR 1.3; 95% CI 1.0–1.7).[13] Recent research re-examined the impact of parity on the outcome of induction.[15] Nulliparas who underwent elective induction were 2.3 times more likely to have a cesarean delivery than electively induced multiparas (26.2% versus 9.0%, $P < 0.05$) while the average Bishop's score did not differ. The risk of instrumental vaginal delivery for nulliparous women was 13.9 times higher than for multiparous women after induction (17% versus 1.5%, $P < 0.01$). In conclusion, nulliparity and unfavorable cervical status are the most important risk factors for a failed induction.

23.2 The cesarean controversy

Recently, confusion about the risks of failed induction has been created by disputable meta-analyses claiming a tempering effect of induction on cesarean rates.[22] In particular, uncritical providers with a narrow idea of EBM – relying exclusively on evidence from (poor) RCTs and disregarding all other forms of research (6.5) – are susceptible to this misguidance. Five analytical obstacles in clinical research fuel the confusion.

23.2.1 Methodological flaws

The first two problems relate to (1) lack of stratification by parity and (2) lack of stratification by cervical status.[23] No-one will deny that rupturing the membranes in a para 3, who is still 2 weeks before her due date, has a soft and ¾-effaced cervix that is accessible for two fingers, and wants her baby to be born, is an entirely different prospect from trying to do the same in a G1P0 who is 3 weeks further on, but has a "wooden" cervix that is 3 cm long. It also ought to be clear that lumping them together in a study, randomized or not, renders distorted information and dangerously underestimates the risks of a failed induction in nulliparas (6.5.9).

The third methodological problem is the composition of the control groups. The non-randomized studies used women in spontaneous labor as controls, whereas most RCTs prospectively allocated women "managed expectantly" in the control groups. From a clinical point of view, the latter is more appropriate, as this is the management choice to be made in practice at a given point in time; the risks of labor induction need to be weighed against the risks of continuing the pregnancy. By implication, RCTs provide evidence for or against a particular policy (induction or expectancy) in specific patient groups, not about the risks of the induction procedure in itself. The observational studies provide more information on causality, and consistently evidenced the increased risk of cesarean delivery after induction. This finding is not surprising as it is in full accordance with the basic scientific understanding of the physiology of parturition (Chapter 8).

> RCTs provide evidence on **what** happens in particular patient groups, but **not why**. The causal relationship between induction and high operative delivery rates has been documented over and over again and is particularly strong in nulliparas.

The fourth analytical challenge relates to the management in the control groups. In RCTs, expectantly managed women may go into spontaneous labor or develop complications that require intervention such as a "medically indicated" induction or cesarean delivery. However, risk assessment varies widely, and policies are heavily doctor-biased. Ergo, these trials provide more evidence on the overall intervention rates in the participating hospitals than on whether induction increases or reduces cesarean rates. Practice variation in the control groups (what is "normal care"?) also hampers clarity; what was compared with what? Apparently, normal labor and delivery skills in many participating hospitals have already plummeted to a level that even induction does not deteriorate the outcomes any further. Unsurprisingly, in most observational studies, the adverse effect of induction (failed inductions) proved to be most pronounced in the hospitals with the lowest baseline cesarean rates. In other words: the better the labor and delivery skills are (controls), the more manifest the negative impact of induction on cesarean rates will be. Accordingly, recent survey studies claiming no or a decreasing effect of induction on cesarean rates were conducted in hospitals with excessive overall cesarean rates.[24–26]

The fifth methodological problem in clinical research is the composition of the study population and the induction methods used. Most RCTs concerned specific patient groups such as post-term pregnancies or pregnancies complicated by IUGR, or hypertension, and so on. Results from these trials cannot and should not be extrapolated to "low-risk" pregnancies. Some RCTs claim to have examined the effects of "elective" inductions, but it remains completely unclear what was meant by "elective."[27,28] Furthermore, various induction methods were used within and amongst the RCTs, disallowing any meaningful conclusions. Yet several meta-analyses lumped all RCTs together (Chapter 6), and claimed to have found "robust evidence" that "elective" induction of labor has no negative effects or even a tempering effect on cesarean delivery rates.[22,29–32]

Clearly, this "evidence" is far from convincing (see also 6.5.9). The meta-analyses certainly do not merit what uncritical bloggers and Tweeters heralded as "dispelling the myth" that induction increases cesarean odds, or what an accompanying editorial referred to as "waking the sleeping dogma."[33] As long as no better evidence is produced, this particular dogma is better left to rest. "When woken up, it may not only bark; it can also have a fearsome bite."[27]

> The overall negative effects of labor induction are seriously underestimated.

23.3 Collateral damage

The procedure of induction of labor cannot and should not be evaluated in isolation. An institutional policy that invokes a high rate of induction not only carries unnecessary risks for the women in question, but also frustrates and disrupts the entire obstetrical service. In addition, liberal use of induction of labor wreaks absolute havoc with obstetrical training and precludes the acquisition of an in-depth understanding of physiological birth.

23.3.1 Effects on others

Inductions make disproportionate claims on the labor ward staff. Facilities, especially in terms of human resources, are dissipated in the care of women who are not in labor and who, therefore, should not be in the delivery unit. The nurses and midwives need to take care of women for prolonged periods who are experiencing the burden of a false or otherwise slow start and women who have an iatrogenic long labor. Induction sparks a cascade of co-interventions that require extra precautions, distracting the nurses from their support role. This medical and nursing attention can only be made available at the expense of personal attention for the other women who started labor spontaneously. The financial costs involved are also considerable.[10]

> The staff resource implications of inductions are staggering. Nurses, midwives, and doctors are occupied with non-laboring patients or iatrogenically long labors to the detriment of the care for all other women who started labor spontaneously.

23.3.2 Educative harm

A normal reaction to the misfortune of others is to trivialize one's own role by looking for external causes. Doctors are very human in this regard. Many a cesarean to resolve a failed induction is performed under pseudo-diagnoses such as "dystocia" or "CPD." The inconvenient truth, however, is that surgery was the only way out of a situation caused by the doctor her- or himself, and often on dubious grounds that in themselves would not have warranted a cesarean section. The turmoil surrounding the surgical conclusion easily conceals the reality that the need for the knife should be attributed to the induction procedure itself. In most cases, it is the procedure of induction that causes the hardship of ineffective labor or uterine hypertonia with fetal distress, not the underlying condition that was used as "indication" for induction. Natural reluctance to acknowledge the plain truth that the problem is doctor-caused is destructive in a training situation where residents are malconditioned by the liberal induction practices of their superiors.

When obstetric training is largely based on experience with inductions, the critical importance of the diagnosis of labor remains completely obscure to aspiring specialists. Even worse, long labors are considered normal and an epidural as an indispensable component of modern obstetrics. Residents and students no longer follow labors from beginning to end, and, owing to fragmented involvement, it has become nearly impossible to gain insight and overview. Personal involvement and commitment are increasingly seen as impossible ideals from times past, before the legal labor act that disallows duty shifts of more than 12 hours was passed. Disastrous vicious circles are the inevitable result (Chapter 6). The fundamental difference between induction and acceleration of spontaneous labor is hardly recognized or not realized at all. Consequently, the possibilities and limitations of oxytocin in these different situations are completely misjudged. After induction, mechanical birth obstruction cannot reliably be discerned from iatrogenic dynamic labor disorders, resulting in a sharp overdiagnosis of CPD (Chapters 21 and 22).

In conclusion: liberal induction practices operate at virtual loggerheads with responsible obstetric training. Certainly, residents and fellows may develop dexterity with forceps, vacuum extractor, and scalpel, but they remain mostly lacking in fundamental insight into the physiology of spontaneous labor and fail to acquire expert labor and delivery skills by which operative deliveries can largely be prevented.

Induction of labor and obstetric training

Nowadays, the acquisition of obstetrical skills and confidence is frequently built on a constant repetition of the same mistakes.

Clearly, the direct and indirect adverse effects of inductions on childbirth as a whole are so wide-reaching that strongly curtailed use of this intervention will undoubtedly instigate significant improvements in the quality of childbirth. Induction of labor is not a trivial intervention and should, therefore, be restricted to a select number of individuals in whom the indication is genuine, and conditions seem to be favorable.

23.4 Indications

Despite the obvious objections, induction rates continue to climb, and rates up to 25% or more of all pregnancies are now common practice.[34-36] A part of these interventions may be employed for serious medical conditions such as pre-eclampsia, but marginally indicated and "elective" inductions undoubtedly account for the bulk.[27,37-39] Many providers easily give in to requests for an induction when women perceive late pregnancy as uncomfortable or desire to arrange a convenient time of delivery. An effective way to reduce these requests is to provide these women with honest information about the prospect of a long and difficult labor with a greater chance of operative delivery, and then ask them to sign an informed consent. Most women will abandon their demand.

Given the direct and indirect adverse effects, induction without a medical indication cannot be defended in any circumstances: "If it ain't broke, don't fix it."

One of the many unfortunate consequences of selective reading, uncritical interpretation, and unjust extrapolation of "randomized evidence" is an almost unbridled expansion of "indications" for induction to encompass, as it seems, almost all births in some hospitals. Although most guidelines dissuade providers from induction in the absence of a medical reason, they leave much leeway in deciding the indication. Boundaries between what is elective and what is selective, what is medically indicated and what is not, and what is maternal request or persuasive coercion, remain as vague as ever.[27,28] Alleged "medical" but dubious indications for induction that deserve special attention include post-term pregnancy at 41 weeks, pregnancy-induced hypertension, and fetal macrosomia.

23.4.1 Post-term pregnancy

The recommendation in guidelines for induction at 41 weeks is predicated on a 2012 Cochrane meta-analysis, claiming: "a policy of labor induction compared with expectant management is associated with fewer perinatal deaths."[30] However, the absolute risk of fetal demise between 41 and 42 weeks is so small that the estimated number needed to treat (number needed to harm) in order to (possibly) prevent one stillbirth is 410 (95% CI 322 to 1492). Most importantly, information on the frequency and methods of fetal assessments in the controls managed expectantly was missing. So, the RCTs and the meta-analysis thereof have neither examined nor determined the optimum policy between 41 and 42 weeks. Induction at 41 weeks on a rule-of-thumb basis does not conform to any critical standards. If there are no complications and the fetus is moving well in a normal amount of amniotic fluid, waiting for spontaneous labor has a much brighter prospect for an individual mother and her baby than induction. In our institution, women who want to wait until 42 weeks visit the antenatal clinic every other day and are given the chance of a spontaneous onset of labor, unless complications arise such as evidence of impaired placental function as shown by a significantly reduced liquor volume, reduced fetal movements, or a non-reassuring CTG.

23.4.2 Hypertension

Hypertension in late pregnancy is another condition in which uncritical application of the laudable principles of EBM has become counterproductive in its effects (6.5). Clinical management is increasingly guided by the results of poorly designed RCTs of which the influential HYPITAT trial is an illustrative example.

This multicenter Dutch study compared induction (n = 377) with expectant management (n = 379) in women with hypertension between 36 and 41 weeks.[40] Although no single case of eclampsia or perinatal death was recorded, the authors recommended induction of labor in all cases of (mild) hypertension because they had found an association of induction with a lower rate of "maternal complications" (i.e. progression of the disease). An amazing recommendation, indeed, as the trial was fatally flawed by the logical fallacy of using hypertension as both an entry and major endpoint criterion in determining whether interruption of pregnancy benefits the mother in ways that matter.[41] Of course, induction will lead to an earlier resolution of most pregnancy-associated problems (e.g. varicose veins), but without any evidence of lessened permanent morbidity.

The most important problem with the HYPITAT trial was the heterogeneity of the study population. The composite measure of maternal morbidity was inadequate; two-thirds of the women did not have pre-eclampsia at randomization. The study designers had ignored the fact that hypertension in late pregnancy is not a diagnosis, but a sign detected by screening asymptomatic women. High blood pressure can indicate pre-eclampsia, indeed, in the minority, but is imperfect in isolation, requiring confirmation by proteinuria.[42] Blood pressure rises physiologically towards term, and the physiology of pregnancy-induced hypertension (PIH) is fundamentally different from that of pre-eclampsia, which is characterized by endotheliopathy with significant alterations in biochemistry and hemodynamics.[42] Certainly, women with pre-eclampsia are at risk for eclampsia, but women with isolated mild hypertension in whom diastolic pressure does not exceed 100 mmHg are not.[42,43] In hypertensive but otherwise well women, producing less severe hypertension alone does not justify a recommendation for induction of labor.

Potential ill effects on the baby were not powered for in the HYPITAT-trial. Nonetheless, induction led to significantly smaller babies (270 g lighter, equivalent to >8% of birth weight).[40] Moreover, iatrogenic late prematurity (36–39 weeks) imposes serious but underestimated risks for babies, including NICU admission and even neonatal death.[44–48] Such unfortunate sequels remain underdetected in a trial of this size.

Clearly, this RCT has not decided optimum management of (mild) hypertension in late pregnancy. Yet this trial is prominently used in guidelines and has a significant impact on clinical practice worldwide. For example, a US study of 5077 patients with gestational hypertension showed a significant increase in delivery interventions after the publication of the HYPITAT trial, but without any improvements in maternal or neonatal outcomes.[49] A Dutch survey study by the HYPITAT researchers themselves identified 43 641 women with hypertensive disease beyond 36 weeks in the National Perinatal Registry and distinguished the period before and after the HYPITAT trial.[50] The induction rate increased from 58.3 to 67.1% ($P < 0.001$), and the prevalence of eclampsia decreased from 0.85 before to 0.19% after the trial ($P < 0.001$). This is a relevant finding indeed with statistical and clinical significance, but not helpful for decision-making in women with mild PIH.

Clearly, the evidence supports the policy to terminate pregnancy in patients with pre-eclampsia, and the HYPITAT trial made an important contribution to the abolishment of the typically Dutch conservative approach to pre-eclampsia. In women with (mild) PIH, however, induction might be much more dangerous than the disease. Instead of adopting a policy of indiscriminate use of induction, childbirth as a whole would be much better served if doctors were to be educated in basic science again, and regain proper skills in differential diagnostics between PIH and pre-eclampsia, and in proper risk assessment.

23.4.3 Fetal macrosomia

Induction of labor is also widely employed for suspected fetal macrosomia "to prevent the baby from getting too big" but again this policy is not supported by quality evidence.[51] On the contrary, the evidence from pooled randomized and observational data suggests that labor induction for suspected macrosomia results in a doubled cesarean delivery rate without improving perinatal outcomes.[52]

> Given the evidence, induction of labor should be restricted to a select number of women in whom the indication is genuine and conditions seem to be favorable.

23.5 Suitability

Cervical status and parity are the most important factors for predicting the likelihood of a successful induction, defined as achieving vaginal delivery. However, assessment of the cervix is highly subjective and even experienced examiners may differ in their appraisal of cervical suitability for induction. So-called pelvic scores – the classic Bishop score is most used – suggest a level of precision that does not exist. Some studies have suggested transvaginal ultrasound for the assessment of "inducibility," but there is no evidence that sonography performs any better than digital examination.[53–55] What is more, all attempts to assess "inducibility" by the assessment of the cervix completely disregard the other biological requirement to enable an effective start of labor, and that is adequate pre-labor transformation of the myometrium. Absence of myometrial connexons and CAPS (8.3) explains cases of a failed induction despite a "favorable" cervix (8.8).

Besides, Bishop based his pelvic score purely on multiparas and wrote specifically: "Owing to the unpredictability in the nullipara, even in the presence of apparently favorable circumstances, induction of labor brings little advantage for either obstetrician or patient." He continued, "Few other advantages can be presented to justify induction of labor during the first pregnancy."[56] Bishop would turn in his grave if he knew that currently tens of thousands of nulliparous women are induced on a daily basis because of a "favorable Bishop score."

23.5.1 Cervical priming

Amniotomy plus oxytocin is the classic method of induction, requiring at least some cervical maturation to the extent that the membranes can be artificially ruptured. Since the clinical introduction of prostaglandins, however, this physical barrier can be circumvented and the state of affairs around induction has become even more confusing. Prostaglandins are claimed to improve the readiness of the cervix for induction. The effect is that prostaglandins are now widely used for pre-induction "priming" or the induction procedure itself. Most patients, though, do not realize the difference, and a disastrous false start is not infrequently the unfortunate result (14.6).

> Cervical priming is by no means a trivial intervention and should be considered as an implicit part of the induction procedure: priming is induction.

The risks involved are not limited to those related to priming itself – false expectations, unrest, uterine irritability, discomfort, and uterine hypertonia with related fetal distress – but include all the risks associated with induction, including excessive cesarean rates. Prysak and Castronova, for example, reported a threefold higher cesarean delivery rate in women who underwent cervical priming compared with case-controls with spontaneous onset of labor (RR 3.06; 95% CI 1.46–6.4).[57]

> The level of indifference toward priming/induction determines the magnitude of the iatrogenic problems created by this intervention in each hospital.

All indirect adverse effects of induction are intensified by the use of prostaglandins. Indeed, it is a strange paradoxical reality in many institutions that women who are being "primed" and not in labor receive more attention from staff and for a longer time than women who are in labor.

The greatest hazard of cervical priming is erosion of its indication. The technical ease of the procedure may tempt providers to prime/induce women with an unripe cervix ("like a carrot"), for whom an induction of labor would not have been contemplated otherwise. In current practice, women with an "unfavorable" cervix are now readily exposed to the procedure of priming, sometimes for several days in a row, without the prospect of any advantage to themselves or their babies. On the other hand, if effective labor is easily achieved, labor was most likely to start spontaneously within a very short period anyhow. The gain? Zero!

An exploratory gift of prostaglandins, "just to see what happens," is frequently undertaken but is utterly imprudent. The allegation that "no harm is done" if labor is not achieved because the membranes are left intact is invalid, since expectations are raised that are difficult to undo. Disappointment, agitation, and a full-blown false start may be the result, or the membranes might rupture without initiating labor. A destructive cascade of events may be induced after a single administration of prostaglandins. Although frequently done, repeated priming for days in a row is an utterly reprehensible practice: it drives women (and nursing staff) nuts.

The greatest hazard of prostaglandins is erosion of the indication for their use.

23.5.2 Methods of labor induction

To date, investigators have concentrated almost exclusively on the evaluation of diverse techniques for labor induction rather than on the far more important question of when an induction is preferable to well-defined watchful expectation. The efforts and financial costs spent on these comparative studies are disproportionate to their value. All induction methods – be it various types, or dosages, or methods of prostaglandin administration, or an intrauterine balloon catheter, or amniotomy plus oxytocin – have their inherent risks. In general, the more effective a method is in inducing uterine contractions, the more complications due to hypertonia will occur. As the renowned and esteemed godfathers of evidence-based obstetrics concluded a good 20 years ago: "The most important decision to be made when considering induction of labor is whether or not the induction is justified, rather than how it is to be achieved... There is too little evidence to allow any judgment about whether prostaglandins are safer for the babies or the mother than amniotomy plus oxytocin or to claim superiority of any of the various prostaglandins or method of administration."[58] Little has changed since.[59]

As the integral policy framework of *proactive support* primarily concerns labor and delivery after spontaneous onset, a detailed evaluation of the diverse induction methods is not relevant here and, hence, not included in this book.

There is little purpose in assessing the relative merits of different ways of achieving elective delivery if there is no need for elective delivery in the first place.

23.6 Weighing the trade-offs

On balance, the direct and indirect drawbacks of priming/induction are so numerous and striking, and the individual advantages in most cases so dubious, that this intervention should be used only with maximum restraint. An induction must be seen as the lesser of two evils. Even with a favorable cervix, induction of labor remains a calculated risk, especially in nulliparous women. This gamble is only justified if the pathological condition for which induction of labor is considered is so serious that a cesarean delivery is a responsible alternative if induction proves to be impossible or unsuccessful. Therefore:

- The entire staff should agree with the indication for priming/induction. Consequently, the indication for each case has to be discussed at the daily plenary staff session. This is the most effective method for reducing inappropriate induction rates (Chapter 26). There are hardly any indications for induction that cannot wait until the next morning.
- To prevent any false expectations and associated confusion, junior staff ought to forbidden even to suggest induction of labor to a complaining woman, without prior approval from the responsible senior staff.
- To impress on all involved that this is not a physiological labor, all inductions should be conducted in a labor room especially assigned for this purpose (the induction room).

Firmness clause

The pathological condition for which priming/induction is considered should be so serious that a cesarean delivery is justified if the procedure proves impossible.

23.7 Continual audit

The frequently heard suggestion that cesarean delivery after induction was inherent in the problem for which labor was being induced is mostly untenable: most conditions regarded as indication for induction do not in themselves constitute causes of labor disorders, except perhaps postmaturity beyond 42 weeks (meconium).

One of the most important boosts to quality improvement in childbirth is continual evaluation of each labor procedure and its outcome by daily, plenary staff review (Chapter 26). The aim of the induction procedure is to effectuate a vaginal delivery. Therefore, each cesarean delivery after priming/ induction should be classified as a "failed induction." This is no accusation that the policy was wrong – that is to presume that the indication for induction was valid – just logic and clarity of thought.

> *Each cesarean delivery after priming/induction should be put on record in the hospital files as a "failed induction."*

If the professional will is there, the institutional induction rate can responsibly be limited to 12% of all term nulliparas and even less in multiparas, without any detriment to fetal outcomes (Chapter 27). It mainly concerns patients (not clients) with more than 24 hours pre-labor rupture of membranes, preeclampsia, and postmaturity at 42 weeks or earlier in case of anhydramnios or other signs of fetal compromise.

23.7.1 Food for thought

It should be noted that most diagnoses of so-called "fetal compromise" are extremely nebulous and ill defined whereas the impaired placental circulation of the truly endangered fetus disallows a safe labor and vaginal delivery in advance. It is astonishing, on consideration, how many supposedly "compromised" fetuses are exposed to the extra hazards of priming-related uterine hypertonia, and often even without continuous fetal surveillance at the antenatal ward. Besides, the fetus that does tolerate the induced contractions without problems has, by definition, an excellent placental circulatory reserve (Chapter 8). So what is or was the need for induction? Current obstetric practice is often incomprehensible. Safe care of the fetus is the subject of the next chapter.

> *For most alleged indications, induction of labor does not save children but does inflict harm on mothers and the childbirth service as a whole.*

References

1. Harper LM, Caughy AB, Odibo AO, *et al.* Normal progress of induced labor. Obstet Gynecol 2012;**96**:671–7

2. Seyb ST, Berka RJ, Socol ML, Dooley SL. Risk of cesarean delivery with elective induction of labor at term in nulliparous women. *Obstet Gynecol* 1999;**94**:600–7

3. Macer JA, Macer CL, Chan LS. Elective induction versus spontaneous labor: a retrospective study of complications and outcome. *Am J Obstet Gynecol* 1992;**166**:1690–6

4. Cammu H, Marten G, Ruyssinck G, Amy JJ. Outcome after elective induction in nulliparous women: a matched cohort study. *Am J Obstet Gynecol* 2002;**186**:240–4

5. Luthy DA, Malmgren JA, Zingheim RW. Increased Cesarean section rates associated with elective induction in nulliparous women; the physician effect. *Am J Obstet Gynecol* 2004;**191**:1511–15

6. Dublin S, Lydon-Rochelle M, Kaplan RC, Watts DH, Critchlow CW. Maternal and neonatal outcomes after induction without an identified indication. *Am J Obstet Gynecol* 2000;**18**:986–94

7. van Gemund N, Hardeman A, Scherjon SA, Kanhai HH. Intervention rates after elective induction of labor compared to labor with a spontaneous onset: a matched cohort study. *Gynecol Obstet Invest* 2003;**56**:133–8

8. Maslow AS, Sweeny AL. Elective induction of labor as a risk factor for cesarean delivery among low-risk women at term. Obstet Gynecol 2000;**95**:917–22

9. Jonsson M, Cnattingius S, Wikström AK. Elective induction of labor and the risk of cesarean section in low-risk parous women: a cohort study. Acta Obstet Gynecol Scand 2013;**92**:198–203

10. Kauffman K, Bailit J, Grobman W. Elective induction: an analysis of economic and health consequences. Am J Obstet Gynecol 2002;**187**:858–63

11. Vahratian A, Zhang J, Troendle JF, *et al.* Labor progression and risk of cesarean delivery in electively induced nulliparas. Obstet Gynecol 2005;**105**:698–704

12. Guerra GV, Cecatti JG, Souza JP, *et al.* WHO Global Survey on Maternal Perinatal Health in Latin America Study Group. Elective induction versus spontaneous labour in Latin America. Bull World Health Organ 2011;**89**:657–65

13. Yeast JD, Jones A, Poskin M. Induction of labor and the relationship to cesarean delivery; a review of 7001 consecutive inductions. *Am J Obstet Gynecol* 1999;**180**:628–33

14. Johnson DP, Davis NR, Brown AJ. Risk of cesarean delivery after induction at term in nulliparous women with an unfavorable cervix. Am J Obstet Gynecol 2003;**188**:1565–72

15. Johnson AM, Bellerose L, Billstrom R, Deckers E, Beller P. Evaluating outcomes of labor inductions beyond 39 weeks of gestation. Obstet Gynecol 2014;**123** Suppl 1:58S

16. Vrouenraets FP, Roumen FJ, Dehing CJ, *et al.* Bishop score and risk of cesarean delivery after induction of labor in nulliparous women. Obstet Gynecol 2005;**105**:690–7

17. Nuutila M, Halmesmäki E, Hiilesmaa V, Ylikorkala O. Women's anticipations of and experiences with induction of labor. Acta Obstet Gynecol Scand 1999;**78**:704–9

18. Bramadat IJ. Induction of labor: an integrated review. Health Care Women Int 1994;**15**:135–48

19. Shetty A, Burt R, Rice P, Templeton A. Women's perceptions, expectations and satisfaction with induced labour—a questionnaire-based study. Eur J Obstet Gynecol Reprod Biol 2005;**123**:56–61

20. Henderson J1, Redshaw M. Women's experience of induction of labor: a mixed methods study. Acta Obstet Gynecol Scand 2013;**92**:1159–67

21. Hildingsson I, Karlström A, Nystedt A. Women's experiences of induction of labour: findings from a Swedish regional study. Aust N Z J Obstet Gynaecol 2011;**51**:151–7

22. Mishanina E, Rogozinska E, Thatthi T, *et al.* Use of labour induction and risk of cesarean delivery: a systematic review and meta-analysis. Can Med Assoc J 2014;**186**:665–73

23. Grobman WA. Elective induction: when? ever? Clin Obstet Gynecol 2007;**50**:537–546

24. Gibson KS, Waters TP, Bailit JL. Maternal and neonatal outcomes in electively induced low-risk term pregnancies. Am J Obstet Gynecol 2014;**211**:249. Epub 2014 Mar 12

25. Stock SJ, Ferguson E, Duffy A, *et al.* Outcomes of elective induction of labor compared with expectant management: population based study. Br Med J 2012;**344**:e2838

26. Darney BG, Snowden JM, Cheng YW, *et al.* Elective induction of labor at term compared with expectant management: maternal and neonatal outcomes. Obstet Gynecol 2013;**122**:761–9

27. Keirse MJ. Elective induction, selective deduction, and cesarean section. Birth 2010;**37**:252–56

28. Berghella V, Blackwell SC, Ramin SM, Sibai BM, Saade GR. Use and misuse of the term "elective" in obstetrics. Obstet Gynecol 2011;**117**:372–6

29. Caughey AB, Sundaram V, Kaimal AJ, *et al.* Systematic review: elective induction of labor versus expectant management of pregnancy. Ann Intern Med 2009;**151**:252–63

30. Gülmezoglu AM, Crowther CA, Middleton P, Heatley E. Induction of labour for improving birth outcomes for women at or beyond term. Cochrane Database Syst Rev 2012

31. Wennerholm UB, Hagberg H, Brorsson B, Bergh C. Induction of labor versus expectant management for post-date pregnancy: Is there sufficient evidence for a change in clinical practice? Acta Obstet Gynecol Scand 2009;**88**:6–17

32. Wood S, Cooper S, Ross S. Does induction of labour increase the risk of caesarean section? A systematic review and meta-analysis of trials in women with intact membranes. Br J Obstet Gynaecol 2014;**121**:674–85; discussion 685

33. Macones GA. Elective induction of labor: Waking the sleeping dogma? Ann Intern Med 2009;**151**:281–2

34. NHS maternity 2010. NHS maternity statistics, 2009–10. NHS Information Centre (http://www.hes online.nhs.uk/Ease/servlet/ContentServer? siteID=1937&categoryID=1475)

35. Martin JA, Hamilton BE, Ventura SJ, Osterman MJK, Mathews TJ. Births: Final data for 2011. Natl Vital Stat Rep 2013;**62**:1–90

36. Goffinet F, Dreyfus M, Carbonne B, Magnin G, Cabrol D. Survey of the practice of cervical ripening and labor induction in France. J Gynecol Obstet Biol Reprod 2003;**32**:638–46 (in French)

37. Wing DA, Lockwood CJ, Barss VA. Induction of labor. UpToDate, Accessed November 2014. www. UpToDate.com

38. ACOG Committee on Practice Bulletins. Induction of labor. ACOG Practice Bulletin no. 107, 2009

39. Leduc D, Biringer A, Lee L, Dy J. Induction of labor. SOGC Clinical practice guideline No 296, September 3013. J Obstet Gynaecol Can 2013;**35**:S1–18

40. Koopmans CM, Bijlenga D, Groen H, *et al.* Induction of labour versus expectant monitoring for gestational hypertension or mild pre-eclampsia after 36 weeks' gestation (HYPITAT): a multicentre, open-label randomised controlled trial. Lancet 2009;**374**:979–88

41. Bewley S, Shennan A. HYPITAT and the fallacy of pregnancy interruption. Lancet 2010;**375**:119

42. North RA. Classification and diagnosis of pre-eclampsia. In: Lyall F, Belfort M, eds. Pre-eclampsia: Etiology and Clinical Practice. Cambridge University Press; 2007

43. National Collaborating Centre for Women's and Children's Health. Commissioned by the National Institute for Health and Clinical Excellence. Hypertension in pregnancy: the management of hypertensive disorders during pregnancy. August 2010 (revised reprint January 2011) www.nice.org.uk (accessed October 2014)

44. Tomashek KM, Shapiro-Mendoza CK, Davidoff MJ, Petrini JR. Differences in mortality between late-preterm and term singleton infants in the United States, 1995–2002. J Pediatr 2007;**151**:450–56

45. Loftin RW, Habli M, Snyder CC, *et al.* Late preterm birth. Rev Obstet Gynecol 2010;**3**:10–9

46. Ramachandrappa A, Jain L. Health issues of the late preterm infant. Pediatr Clin North Am 2009;**56**:565–77

47. Santos IS, Matijasevich A, Domingues MR, *et al.* Late preterm birth is a risk factor for growth faltering in early childhood: a cohort study. BMC Pediatr 2009;**9**: 71. Published online November 16, 2009. doi: 10.1186/ 1471-2431-9-71

48. Bassil KL, Yasseen AS, Walker M, *et al.* The association between obstetrical interventions and late preterm birth. Am J Obstet Gynecol 2014;**210**:538.e1–9

49. Pauli JM, Lauring JR, Stetter CM, *et al.* Management of gestational hypertension: the impact of HYPITAT. J Perinat Med 2013;**41**:415–20

50. van der Tuuk K, Koopmans CM, Groen H, *et al.* Impact of the HYPITAT trial on doctors' behaviour and prevalence of eclampsia in the Netherlands. Br J Obstet Gynaecol 2011;**118**:1658–60

51. Rossi AC, Mullin P, Prefumo F. Prevention, management, and outcomes of macrosomia: a systematic review of literature and meta-analysis. Obstet Gynecol Surv 2013;**68**:702–9

52. Sanchez-Ramos K, Bernstein S, Kaunitz AM. Expectant management versus labor induction for suspected fetal macrosomia: a systematic review. Obstet Gynecol 2002;**100**:997–1002

53. Pereira S, Frick AP, Poon LC, Zamprakou A, Nicolaides KH, *et al.* Successful induction of labor: prediction by preinduction cervical length, angle of progression and cervical elastography. Ultrasound Obstet Gynecol 2014 May 15. doi: 10.1002/uog.13411. [Epub ahead of print]

54. Verhoeven CJ, Opmeer BC, Oei SG, *et al.* Transvaginal sonographic assessment of cervical length and wedging for predicting outcome of labor induction at term: a systematic review and meta-analysis. Ultrasound Obstet Gynecol 2013;**42**:500–8

55. Gokturk U, Cavkaytar S, Danısman N. Prediction of successful labor induction by measuring cervical length, fetal head position and posterior cervical angle can be alternative method to Bishop score? J Matern Fetal Neonatal Med 2014;**15**:1–30. [Epub ahead of print]

56. Bishop EH. Pelvic scoring for elective induction. Obstet Gynecol 1964;**24**:266–8

57. Prysak M, Castronova FC. Elective induction versus spontaneous delivery: a case-control analysis of safety and efficacy. *Obstet Gynecol* 1998;**92**:47–52

58. Enkin M, Keirse MJNC, Neilson J, *et al.* Preparing for the induction of labor. In: *A Guide to Effective Care in Pregnancy and Childbirth*, 3rd edn. Oxford: Oxford University Press; 2000

59. Grobman WA. Predictors of induction success. Semin Perinatol 2012;**36**:344–7

Chapter 24

Safe care of the fetus

Although the great majority of fetuses fare well during labor and delivery, for some babies birth can be a hazardous journey. Risks to the fetus include infection, trauma, and asphyxia (hypoxia leading to acidemia). The chance of perinatal infection is directly related to the length of time from membrane rupture to birth, and proactive steps taken to ensure short labor largely prevent this complication. Trauma is to be avoided at all costs, and trauma is least likely to occur when women deliver their babies by their own efforts. Clearly, both mother and child benefit from short labor and spontaneous delivery as promoted in this book. The present chapter focuses on the prevention, timely detection, and expert treatment of intrapartum fetal hypoxia/acidemia.

Promotion of short labor largely prevents perinatal infection, trauma, and asphyxia.

The desire to prevent fetal hypoxic injury has led to the development and introduction of electronic fetal heart rate monitoring (cardiotocography or CTG). Initially, it was used in high-risk patients, but gradually electronic fetal surveillance came to be used in nearly all hospital births. Its benefits, however, fall short of the initially high expectations that intrapartum CTG could reveal all about fetal condition. In fact, CTG is a good method for screening for fetal hypoxia, but the main drawback is its high false-positive rate. This often results in superfluous operative interventions, rescuing babies from normal physiological events and needlessly inflicting harm on mothers.

24.1 Leading physiological and clinical concepts

Care of the fetus should be aimed at guarding fetal well-being without sliding into medical excess that adds risks to mothers and babies. Safe reduction of operative deliveries for erroneous suspicion of fetal distress requires understanding of the fetus's abilities to cope with the exigencies of physiological birth. Good clinical practice is governed by basic knowledge of fetal physiology and rational patterns of thought and action. Rational care rests on the awareness of the fundamental differences between screening and diagnosis, and takes the possibilities and limitations of various fetal assessment techniques into account. In addition, expert care focuses on the causes of the fetal problems, if they occur, because identification of the causes allows preventive and corrective measures. Basically, intrapartum threats to fetal oxygenation include:

- Insufficient placental reserves (extremely rare at term);
- Umbilical cord compression (very frequent);
- Impaired uteroplacental blood flow (hypotension and hypertonic dystocia).

24.1.1 Placental circulatory competence

Overall intrapartum care is based on the leading premise that the fetus that thrived in pregnancy and enters labor in good condition is equipped by nature with placental reserve capacity to cope with normal labor contractions (8.7.1). If the fetus has been perceptibly active during the past 24 hours and if the amniotic fluid is clear and, most importantly, if the fetal heart rate (FHR) is not affected by contractions in early labor, it can confidently be concluded that the placental circulatory reserve capacity is adequate and that the fetus can withstand normal labor contractions.[1,2] Early labor contractions are *de facto* the ultimate test for fetoplacental competence.

The fetus that tolerates early contractions of labor without problems has adequate placental reserve capacity to sustain it through the pressures and stress of a normal, physiological labor and delivery.

Reassuring findings in early labor, therefore, signify that pre-existing placental failure is virtually excluded as the cause of fetal compromise whenever troubles develop later. The cause of later-occurring oxygenation problems should, therefore, be sought primarily elsewhere, beginning with umbilical cord compression. A less frequent but equally dangerous threat to the normal fetus involves impaired uteroplacental blood flow, mostly due to uterine hypertonia in the intervals between contractions (abnormal labor). Another cause of reduced uteroplacental blood flow is maternal hypotension, which is almost exclusively caused by epidural analgesia (20.1.4).

24.1.2 Physiological labor

Since the basic contention is that normal placental reserves are sufficient to sustain the fetus through "normal" labor, it is necessary to have a clear understanding of what "normal labor" means: spontaneously begun, and over and done with within 12 hours (Chapter 10). If fetoplacental competence has been assessed at the outset, the only remaining risks for the fetus are brought about either by abnormal labor (induction, unnecessarily prolonged labor, infection, presence of meconium) or by accidental cord compression, which can happen in any "normal" labor.

24.1.3 Normal fetal stress and coping ability

Fetal oxygenation is entirely dependent on the free-floating umbilical cord; as a result, blood flow is constantly in jeopardy. Inevitably, most fetuses have experienced brief periods of hypoxemia due to cord compression during pregnancy. The incidence and risks of cord compression are greatest during uterine contractions. The frequency and inevitability of transient cord occlusion have provided the fetus with hemodynamic regulation mechanisms and buffer capacities as a means of coping with brief periods of hypoxia.[1,2] Many characteristics or "abnormalities" of FHR tracings during labor, therefore, reflect physiological responses to stress rather than pathological signs of fetal distress.[3] The challenge is to distinguish normal fetal stress from abnormal fetal distress.[3]

24.1.4 Fetal distress

Hypoxic insults are usually slow in onset and may be transient or persistent over time. The healthy fetus is able to compensate hypoxemia (reduced pO_2) by cardiovascular and homeostatic adaptations, including metabolic adjustments. If no corrective action is taken or the fetal insults persist, fetal compensation mechanisms may progressively fail, leading to hypoxia (reduced oxygen in the tissues) and ultimately to acidosis (increased H^+ within the tissues). Fetal acidemia is the clinically important end-point of hypoxia (genuine "fetal distress"), requiring immediate intervention.

The fetus has adequate survival strategies to cope with the physiological stress of brief periods of hypoxia due to cord compression in physiological labor.

Brief and transient periods of fetal hypoxemia/mild hypoxia are normal during labor and delivery, and the fetus has physiological reserves as a competent strategy for survival. For brain damage to occur, the term fetus must be exposed to much more than brief periods of hypoxemia: it takes profound and prolonged fetal hypoxia with barely sub-lethal metabolic acidosis with pH ≤ 7.00 and base deficit ≥ 12.[4,5] Fortunately, such cases are rare,[6] and fetal hypoxia with beginning acidemia can be detected in time by electronic FHR monitoring supplemented with fetal scalp blood sampling. Severe and dangerous fetal acidosis can be prevented this way in nearly every case.

The fetal heart rate is very sensitive to fetal hypoxemia and hypoxia, but lacks specificity for fetal acidosis, which explains overdiagnosis and overtreatment based on FHR decelerations alone. Assuming "fetal distress" can be defined as hypoxia leading to acidemia, the term is still too broad and too vague to be applied with any precision to FHR readings. Uncertainty about the diagnosis "fetal distress" has led to the use of CTG classification systems[7-9] and descriptions as *reassuring* or *non-reassuring* CTG. These patterns, however, are dynamic during labor in that they can rapidly change from reassuring to non-reassuring and vice versa.[10] Partly because of liability concerns, an operative delivery is commonly performed when the obstetrician loses confidence or cannot assuage doubts about fetal condition. It should be recognized, however, that this clinical judgment, if based purely on the morphology of FHR tracings, is highly subjective and inevitably subject to gross imperfection.[11]

Clearly, sophisticated knowledge of the fetal physiology underlying FHR modulations is required in order to reduce unnecessary operative delivery in non-acidotic fetuses.[3] It is also imperative that a non-reassuring CTG is supplemented with (serial) fetal scalp blood samplings (FBS) to assess fetal pH and buffer reserves.[12] Knowledgeable differential diagnostics of the cause of fetal compromise further offers opportunities for causal treatment and corrective measures.

The clinical diagnosis "fetal distress" based on fetal heart rate tracings needs quantification by fetal blood sampling, and refinement and qualification by differential causal diagnostics.

24.1.5 Umbilical cord compression

Cord compression is the most prevalent and practically the only fetal problem in *"normal"* (i.e. physiological) labor. It can be diagnosed by the typical variable FHR decelerations characterized by transient series of decelerations in FHR that vary in duration, intensity, and relation to uterine contraction.

It should be noted that the umbilical blood vessels of growth-retarded fetuses are more susceptible to compression because cords of dysmature babies contain less Wharton's jelly. This explains the increased rate of variable decelerations in term small-for-date fetuses, often misinterpreted as placental circulatory failure (the latter is detected by congruent, "secondary" or "late" decelerations after each contraction before labor or in early labor in severely compromised and mostly severely preterm pregnancies).

Occasional cord compression can be identified in about 40% of all healthy term fetuses in the retraction phase, increasing to 83% by the end of the wedging phase of first-stage labor.[10,13] This high prevalence attests to the physiological nature of these events. In second-stage labor, FHR decelerations are virtually ubiquitous, and these can be attributed to cord compression and fetal head compression. In fact, more than 98% of all fetuses respond to second-stage labor contractions with heart rate decelerations.[10,13]

In conclusion: virtually no intrapartum FHR tracing is "normal" as judged by antepartum criteria of normalcy. This explains the difficulty in assessing intrapartum fetal well-being on the basis of CTG alone and emphasizes the importance of additional diagnostics.

Umbilical cord compression is the most prevalent threat to fetal well-being that can happen in any labor and delivery.

Although short periods of umbilical cord compression do not pose a real threat to the healthy fetus, serious acidemia can develop during frequent and prolonged interruption of the cord circulation. Whether and how quickly harm is inflicted on a child depends on:

- The frequency and duration of cord occlusion;
- The recovery time between the contractions, which is needed for the supplementation of oxygen and the removal of waste products of anaerobic glycolysis;
- The fetal cardiovascular and metabolic buffer reserves;
- The duration of labor.

Fetal well-being during birth is highly dependent on expert labor management ensuring physiological, short labor.

24.1.6 Abnormal labor

The second threat to fetal oxygenation after cord compression is impaired uteroplacental blood flow. This menace results from insufficient uterine relaxation in the intervals between contractions, which, in turn, results from:

1. Labor induction, or
2. A needlessly exhausted uterus, loaded with lactic acid (refractory uterus), or
3. Disorganized uterine action due to infection, meconium, or intrauterine free blood.

Abnormal labor jeopardizes uteroplacental blood flow.

The proactive steps dictated by the policy-concept of *proactive support of labor* largely eliminate these hazards and leave umbilical cord compression as practically the only unpreventable threat to the healthy fetus during *"normal"* labor and delivery. Vigilant surveillance to detect these cord accidents in time remains mandatory in any labor.

24.1.7 Meconium

Passage of meconium is a separate issue and a complicating factor. It has traditionally been regarded as a warning sign of placental failure and fetal compromise.[14] However, the appearance of meconium during labor does not in itself indicate fetal hypoxia or acidemia, as it is often associated with well-oxygenated fetuses.[15]

Amniotic fluid is contaminated with meconium in about 20% of pregnancies at term, and it is now recognized that meconium indicates a normally maturing gastrointestinal tract in the majority of cases, or that it occurs as the result of vagal stimulation from umbilical cord compression.[15,16] In currently prevailing opinion, passage of meconium during labor in most cases represents a sign of physiological reaction to sensory input, a part of the autonomic stress response rather than a marker of fetal distress.[15] Nevertheless, passage of fresh meconium during labor is always a reason for extra vigilance with continuous CTG monitoring and often for additional diagnostic measures.

> *In most cases, passage of meconium represents a sign of fetal physiological responses rather than a marker of fetal hypoxia.*

The true clinical significance of the passage of fresh meconium is its potentially detrimental impact upon the myometrial efficiency and the fetal airways when inhaled. Meconium contains corrosive bile acids and salts that may spark a chemical inflammation reaction that may severely disorganize myometrial electrical coordination (Chapter 8). This may result in poor efficiency and thus poor effectiveness of the contractions, compounded by inadequate uterine relaxation during the contraction intervals (hypertonic dystocia). A vicious cycle of fetal distress and dysfunctional labor may ensue (21.8).

Even more importantly, fresh meconium constitutes a direct environmental hazard for the fetus. The presence of thick meconium in the fetal nasopharynx or bronchi obstructs the airways at birth, resulting in acute neonatal hypoxia. In addition, deep inhalation of meconium may lead to chemical inflammation of pulmonary tissues. In severe cases, chemical pneumonitis may progress to persistent pulmonary hypertension, other neonatal morbidity, and even death.[17]

It is crucial to emphasize that meconium aspiration may occur before birth as a result of fetal gasping triggered by hypoxia/acidemia.[18–22] Evidently, both intrauterine fetal gasping and inhalation at the first breaths at birth may lead to meconium aspiration syndrome, which is still a major cause of severe long-term neurological morbidity and neonatal mortality in term infants.[18]

> *Fresh thick meconium may lead to a vicious cycle of dysfunctional labor and fetal distress, complicated by intrauterine meconium aspiration due to fetal gasping when hypoxia/acidemia supervenes.*

Not every passage of meconium has the same clinical significance, however. There is a world of difference between a mild discoloration of a normal amount of amniotic fluid and undiluted, thick meconium with the umbilical cord, membranes, and even decidua colored green through the entire depth when exposed subsequently at cesarean section. Therefore, a distinction should be made between three grades of meconium.

> **Meconium grading**
>
> *Grade 1: Normal amount of amniotic fluid, lightly stained with diluted thin meconium.*
>
> *Grade 2: Reasonable amount of fluid with a heavy suspension of fresh meconium.*
>
> *Grade 3: No amniotic fluid and pure meconium that resembles thick pea soup.*

Since the grade of meconium dictates further clinical measures (24.3.3), all cases of meconium and its grade should be reported to the obstetrician who is ultimately responsible for the management and outcome of that labor.

24.2 From screening to diagnosis

Electronic fetal surveillance with CTG has now become widely regarded as the standard of intrapartum fetal care. Its use is credited with the near-elimination of unexpected fetal mortality and reduction of early onset neonatal seizures.[23,24] However, its diagnostic imperfection inevitably leads to many superfluous operative deliveries of non-acidotic babies.[25,26] To take full advantage of intrapartum CTG without introducing unintended maternal risks, a strict distinction must be made between screening for and diagnosis of fetal hypoxia:

- **Screening** requires techniques with as high sensitivity as possible to miss as few as possible cases. By definition, false-positive rates are high. Because the labor progresses over time, screening procedures must be repeated periodically. This is called fetal monitoring.
- **Diagnosis,** on the other hand, requires techniques with high specificity to determine the cases of true fetal hypoxia. Ideally, false-positive rates are low.

24.2.1 Screening/monitoring

FHR monitoring is mandatory in any labor. In "low-risk" labors, FHR can be counted by repetitive auscultation (24.3.2). In most hospitals, however, routine use of intrapartum CTG in all labors is standard practice.

As FHR is highly sensitive for fetal hypoxia, a normal FHR symbolizes fetal well-being, normoxia, normal acid-base status, and a low probability of developing intrapartum fetal asphyxia, virtually barring perinatal catastrophes.[27]

An abnormal FHR pattern, however, inevitably includes a high false-positive rate and, therefore, merely constitutes a warning sign that mandates continuous CTG with knowledgeable interpretation and, if necessary, further diagnostic tests (FBS). Operative interventions should be based on a clear diagnosis instead of a shady screening symptom.

The challenge is to distinguish normal fetal stress from abnormal fetal distress.

24.2.2 Diagnosis

Current training of obstetricians and midwives focuses on the morphological appearances of CTG patterns and their descriptive labels, rather than understanding how the fetus defends itself and compensates for intrapartum ischemic insults. As a result, FHR decelerations are often inexpertly equated with "fetal distress" prompting expeditious delivery. This simplistic interpretation is actually promoted in clinical guidelines and contributes to operative delivery of non-acidotic infants.[3] Guidelines emphasize reference values for baseline FHR, variability, and classification of FHR decelerations into label categories, and de-emphasize an accurate understanding of fetal physiology and how the fetus responds and adapts to (transient) oxygen deprivation. Understandably, there is now a growing lack of confidence, and defensive practices are increasing proportionally.

Lack of physiological knowledge may also lead to a failure to recognize discrete alterations in FHR patterns that reflect progressive loss of fetal hemodynamic and biochemical compensation, resulting in undertreatment and adverse outcomes. Clearly, a more physiological approach to the interpretation of CTGs is a precondition for safe care of the fetus and mother.[3] For an in-depth understanding of intrapartum cardiotocographic patterns, readers are referred to the excellent lessons by Austin Ugwumadu.[1]

Intrapartum CTG is basically a screening method. It can only be used as a diagnostic technique if interpretation is based on a thorough knowledge of fetal physiology.

Whenever – rightly or wrongly – there is any doubt about fetal oxygenation, additional diagnostics is mandatory. Reliable diagnosis of fetal hypoxia/acidemia requires a technique with high specificity. The only objective and direct intrapartum test for fetal hypoxia/acidemia is fetal blood gas analysis by fetal scalp blood sampling (FBS).

Adequate screening/monitoring techniques for fetal hypoxia require high sensitivity (FHR), whereas reliable diagnosis requires a technique with high specificity (FBS).

24.2.3 Causal diagnostics

Clinical action taken for fetal compromise should depend on the cause of the problems and be aimed at elimination of any fetal insult, if possible. Most causes of fetal hypoxemia in labor are accidental and often transient if treated correctly.

Differential causal diagnostics is based on sophisticated interpretation of FHR tracings in combination with intelligent interpretation of the partogram and all other clinical characteristics of that particular labor. A differential diagnosis between umbilical cord compression, maternal hypotension, and interval uterine hypertonia can be made in nearly every case, often allowing causal treatment and corrective measures (see below).

Clinical action taken for fetal hypoxia should be aimed at elimination of the cause of the fetal problems, rather than prompt operative delivery.

24.3 Safe practice: fetal surveillance

Responsible care aimed at safety of both mother and fetus is based on the concepts and considerations discussed above. Like expert care for mothers, safe care of the fetus also requires an overall plan, based on science and knowledgeable clinical mind-lines.

24.3.1 Fetal assessment at labor onset

Since the leading notion is that a healthy fetus can smoothly sustain "normal" labor, it is imperative to assess that the fetus is healthy at admission and that labor is and remains "normal." Expert intrapartum care of the fetus, therefore, begins with:

1. Verification that pregnancy was uneventful;
2. Confirmation that the fetoplacental starting condition in early labor is good;
3. An overall plan to promote "normal" labor.

The first question is answered during the antenatal visits. The second issue must be addressed at the onset of any labor in order to identify cases of fetoplacental compromise that have escaped detection in late pregnancy, before the additional stress of labor causes an already precarious balance to deteriorate abruptly. The necessity of appropriate fetoplacental assessment at the onset of labor dictates:

- Explicit inquiry about recent fetal movements;
- Inspection of amniotic fluid (if membranes are broken);
- A thorough check of FHR in relation to contractions, either by auscultation or CTG.

Reassuring findings attest to adequate placental reserves. A normal FHR pattern also establishes that the fetal neurological and cardiovascular systems are sufficiently intact and able to react and respond to defend the fetus against intrapartum insults if these should occur later on.

Reassuring fetal assessments in early labor signify that pre-existing placental failure is excluded as the cause of fetal compromise if troubles should develop later.

If fetoplacental competence has been established at labor onset, the only remaining risks for the fetus are brought about either by maternal hypotension (epidural), or by abnormal labor (induction, prolonged labor, meconium, infection), or by accidental umbilical cord compression, which can happen in any normal labor. Guarding fetal well-being during labor, therefore, further entails:

4. Ensuring that labor is and remains normal, meaning at least 1 cm/h progression;
5. Vigilant surveillance to detect unforeseeable cord accidents in time.

The basic tools for these assessments include:

- Serial fetal heart rate counts or electronic fetal heart rate monitoring;
- Keeping a partogram from the very onset of labor;
- Artificial rupture of membranes whenever labor is too slow.

24.3.2 Intrapartum fetal heart rate monitoring

FHR is monitored (i.e. repetitive screening) either by intermittent auscultation or by CTG. Both methods are highly sensitive in detecting fetal hypoxia but poorly specific. There is no reliable evidence that has identified either of the two as the superior screening technique in low-risk pregnancies.[28]

Many midwives and laboring women give preference to intermittent auscultation with a handheld Doppler device, because it implies personal bedside-nursing procedures at defined intervals and allows fetal assessments with the woman in any position. There are even waterproof machines for use in baths.

Auscultation should be performed at the end of a contraction. Although there is no evidence to indicate the frequency or duration of fetal heartbeat counts, official bodies recommend auscultation every 15–30 minutes during first-stage labor and every 5–15 minutes in second-stage labor.[29,30] A FHR above 150 or below 110 beats/min for more than 5 minutes and any slowing by more than 15 beats/min after contractions is regarded as an indication for electronic fetal monitoring. Women laboring at home should be transferred to the hospital immediately (Chapter 25).

Despite emphasis on continuous electronic monitoring in most hospitals, other institutions have taken positive steps to promote intermittent auscultation, not only as an option, but also as the most reasonable choice of fetal surveillance in low-risk labors. Indeed, when CTG monitoring is routinely practiced while the nurse is elsewhere, all standards of care slide down a slippery slope (4.3).

Both intermittent auscultation and electronic fetal heart rate monitoring are highly sensitive but poorly specific methods for detecting fetal hypoxia/acidemia.

Routine intrapartum CTG is the most prevalent obstetric procedure without the benefit of scientific validation. Its role in reducing perinatal morbidity – and ultimately improving long-term outcomes – remains to be defined.[27] Moreover, CTG patterns are affected by a variety of physiological mechanisms and interpretation is notoriously subjective. Although specialists can reliably distinguish severely abnormal from normal patterns, this is much more difficult for beginners. They often detect fetal problems where there are none, producing unfounded worries in both provider and parturient and triggering unnecessary medicalization.

Indiscriminate use of electronic fetal monitoring may create more problems than it prevents.

24.3.3 Detection of meconium and clinical consequences

Artificial rupture of membranes to check amniotic fluid for meconium is a poor screening test and should not be performed on a routine basis (17.1.1). Drainage of clear amniotic fluid does not exclude fetal compromise, whereas the passage of meconium does not in itself indicate fetal distress.[31] Amniotomy should be performed selectively for attachment of a fetal scalp electrode when FHR rate is non-reassuring. The membranes should also be ruptured whenever progress of labor is too slow, not in the last place to see whether there is passage of meconium that might explain the dysfunctional labor. If meconium is present, continuous electronic monitoring is mandatory, and the CTG-reading plus the meconium grade should determine clinical management:

- **Grade 1 meconium** still allows for a wide margin of discretion. After careful review of all clinical details, no further action beyond continuous electronic FHR monitoring is needed in most cases. In healthy, well-oxygenated newborns, inhaled thin meconium grade 1 is readily cleared from the lungs by normal physiological mechanisms.
- **Grade 2 meconium** is an indication for FBS to assess fetal oxygenation and buffer reserves, unless the fetus was electronically monitored during the previous hours and had a completely normal CTG.[12] Whenever such reassuring data is not available (intrapartum transfers from home), a fetal blood sample is taken as reference-value for later samples and for medico-legal reasons. The

fetal acid–base status and the progress of labor will dictate further management.[12]

As long as the FHR pattern remains normal, there is no increased likelihood of fetal hypoxia and no risk of intrauterine meconium aspiration. However, presence of abnormal FHR patterns in conjunction with grade 2 meconium is a compelling reason for (serial) FBS.

Fetal hypoxia/beginning acidemia (pH $\leq$ 7.25) is an indication for immediate delivery given the risk of intrauterine meconium aspiration when fetal acidemia (pH $\leq$ 7.20) supervenes. When the fetus is in good condition, poor progress of labor should be accelerated as in all other cases, but when the uterus responds with inter-contraction hypertonia, or whenever the fetus does not tolerate the contractions needed for normal labor progression, operative delivery should be undertaken without delay. Special attention – preferably by an experienced neonatologist – should be paid to proper airway management immediately after birth, and ventilation facilities must be present.

- **Grade 3 meconium** with FHR pattern suggestive of fetal hypoxia is a sufficient indication for immediate cesarean delivery – even if the fetal pH is still normal – unless an easy vaginal delivery is imminent. Meconium grade 3 mostly occurs in early labor as a sign of pre-existing fetal compromise pointing to placental failure. A smooth labor and delivery are exceptional, and the risk of fetal gasping with intrauterine meconium aspiration is maximal. Perinatal mortality is increased seven-fold.[32] Prompt cesarean delivery is, therefore, warranted.

The grade of meconium determines the clinical consequences.

Whenever there is uncertainty how to grade meconium (grade 1 or 2), the classification should be – for reasons of safety – grade 2. Failure to recover any amniotic fluid at artificial rupture of membranes should for similar reasons be approached as meconium grade 2, although clear amniotic fluid frequently appears at a later stage.

24.3.4 Fetal scalp blood sampling (FBS)

Accumulated evidence indicates that in the presence of a non-reassuring CTG, use of FBS can avoid harmful operative delivery of non-acidotic babies.[33–35] The NICE guideline recommends: "Where assisted birth is contemplated because of an abnormal FHR pattern, in cases of suspected fetal acidosis FBS should be undertaken in the absence of technical difficulties or any contraindications."[12] The only exception is clear evidence of acute and severe fetal compromise as manifest, for example, in the case of prolonged deceleration greater than 3 minutes plus complete loss of beat-to-beat variability.

Unfortunately, fetal scalp blood sampling is laborious and may be technically challenging. Many hospitals have, so it seems, permanent technical difficulties as judged by its widespread underuse, particularly in the USA.[27] However, given the otherwise technocratic approach, underuse of FBS more likely reflects diagnostic laxity and a worryingly indifferent attitude toward superfluous operative interventions. Anyhow, the option for FBS is no longer available in many units.[27] A review of 392 publications on emergent cesarean delivery for fetal distress identified only 31 publications that even mentioned the use of scalp pH before surgery, and only three of them provided information on how frequently it was used.[36]

The relative objections of inconvenience and difficulty can be largely circumvented if fetal scalp blood sampling is used for the measurement of fetal lactate instead of pH and base deficit.[37-39] Much less fetal blood is needed (5 μl versus 35 μl), so the procedure for fetal lactate measurement is much easier, faster, and more successful than that for measuring pH and base deficit. Moreover, less dilatation of the cervix and fewer scalp punctures are needed.

> **Fetal scalp blood sampling**
>
> *Micro-sampling methods of measuring fetal lactate are suitable for assessing fetal acid–base buffer reserve in a way that is simpler, cheaper, and more reliable.*

Only fetal hypoxia/acidosis should be accepted as a definitive proof of fetal distress. Therefore, a woman should not be subjected to cesarean section for suspicion of fetal distress without this confirmation by fetal scalp blood sampling. In practice, the indication for FBS arises most frequently in the presence of abnormal heart rate tracings in combination with grade 2 meconium where cesarean section would have to be performed – often unnecessarily – were the test not available. Clearly, in any labor and delivery unit with the slightest pretence of providing high-quality care, facilities for fetal scalp blood sampling should be present and be used.

> *Whenever fetal hypoxia/acidosis is suspected on the basis of CTG, FBS should be performed, unless there is clear evidence of acute and severe fetal acidosis.*

24.3.5 New techniques

The low predictive value of intrapartum CTG for fetal acidemia as well as reluctance to undertake FBS has fueled interest in the development of other fetal assessment techniques. These methods include fetal pulse oximetry and ST-segment analysis of the fetal electrocardiogram (STAN). Unfortunately, history seems to repeat itself through the premature introduction of new technology whose benefits may ultimately be disproved.

Four RCTs (n = 6678) failed to detect evidence that fetal pulse oximetry as an adjunct to intrapartum CTG improves neonatal outcome or reduces cesarean deliveries.[40-43]

> *Fetal pulse oximetry should not be used because the evidence indicates no benefits whatsoever (Evidence level A).*

The software of the STAN device claims to detect fetal hypoxia through recognizing ST-segment depression of the fetal ECG, which is obtained via a fetal scalp electrode. The technique is hampered by the failure rate of 10 to 30% owing to poor signal quality. The STAN-monitor displays "ST-events." A 2014 meta-analysis of five RCTs involving a total of over 15 000 pregnant women evaluated the use of STAN as adjunct to continuous CTG monitoring.[44] In comparison with CTG alone, the adjuvant use of STAN was associated with a reduction in FBS (RR 0.64, 95% CI 0.47–0.88). There were, however, no differences in the rates of cesarean delivery and adverse perinatal outcomes.

> *The potential but limited benefit of STAN is a reduced need for fetal blood sampling.*

Obstetricians applying STAN should be trained and accredited in its use and its interpretation. For now, however, there are insufficient clinical and cost data from a variety of hospital settings to recommend the application in routine practice.[27]

If STAN is to be used, clinicians should be aware of its investigational status, and FBS facilities remain indispensable. The main objection against the use of STAN is that the black box technology may even further prevent doctors from thinking. The fact that, as one of our residents put it, "a fuzzy gnome inside a machine lifts a finger ('ST-event!') telling the doctor to intervene" is perceived as a bad idea by many experienced obstetricians, and rightly so. There is much more to be gained for mothers and babies by new education of doctors in fetal physiological knowledge, and vocational training in intelligent interpretation of intrapartum CTG patterns and FBS results, than by trying to implement a new, entirely opaque fetal assessment technique.

> STAN is not a fully fledged substitute for fetal scalp blood sampling.

24.4 Safe practice: interventions

The appearance of abnormal FHR tracings is not a reason to resort to prompt cesarean delivery, even when mild fetal hypoxia is detected by FBS. It is, however, a compelling reason to decide what may be causing the abnormalities and to attempt to eliminate these problems.[45]

> Appropriate management for significantly variant fetal heart rate patterns consists of correcting any fetal insult, if possible.

24.4.1 Causal treatment

The most frequent problem in normal labor is cord compression, diagnosed by the typical variable decelerations. Although clinicians generally remember to apply oxygen and change maternal position to remove cord compression, they often forget the potential benefits of amnion-infusion and short-acting tocolysis. The Cochrane meta-analysis evidenced that amnion-infusion is associated with a significant reduction in variable heart rate decelerations (RR 0.53, 95% CI 0.38–0.74), cesarean delivery rate (RR = 0.62; 95% CI 0.46–0.83), and meconium below the vocal cords (RR 0.53, 95% CI 0.31–0.92).[46]

> In cases of cord compression – the most frequent cause of fetal compromise in labor – amnion-infusion effectively reduces the need for cesarean delivery (Evidence level A).

Maternal hypotension leading to impaired uteroplacental blood flow is almost invariably related to epidural analgesia, and should be treated with IV fluid loads and vasopressors. In case of uterine tachysystole, oxytocin should be discontinued according to the protocol explained in Chapter 17. It must be emphasized that problematic hyperstimulation leading to fetal distress is mostly iatrogenic since this is particularly related to labor induction or unduly delayed use of oxytocin in spontaneous though slow labor (Chapter 17).

24.4.2 Intrauterine resuscitation

Whatever the cause of fetal compromise, the contractions of labor invariably aggravate the situation. Conversely, uterine relaxation through short-acting tocolysis invariably improves uteroplacental blood flow and alleviates cord compression in nearly all cases.[47] A single bolus of 0.25 mg terbutaline, 0.1 mg fenoterol, or 6.25 mg atosiban effectively inhibits contractions for about 15–20 minutes, restoring adequate fetal gas exchange.

The evidence indicates a significant improvement (RR 0.26, 95% CI: 0.13 to 0.53) of severely abnormal CTG patterns after short-acting tocolysis as compared with no treatment.[48] Although no randomized placebo controlled trials on this subject have been done, it is reasonable to err on the side of fetal safety by using this technique when appropriate.

Intrauterine resuscitation avoids seemingly heroic but superfluous interventions. Fetal resuscitation creates rest and valuable time in which to take a fetal scalp blood sample and to think. Intrauterine resuscitation prevents panicky reactions – especially in less-experienced young doctors who, it must be admitted, attend most labors outside office hours – and gives the obstetrician on duty time to come to the delivery room.

Additional corrective measures often allow labor to continue. If not, (repeated) fetal resuscitation creates time to prepare the operating theater. Pre-cesarean tocolysis diminishes the need to rush and permits meticulous and thus safer surgery. In second-stage labor, intrauterine resuscitation provides the time to place an outlet forceps carefully or to apply vacuum to the ventouse slowly, facilitating an atraumatic instrumental delivery. In conclusion: short-acting tocolysis is an effective and useful temporizing maneuver in the management of intrapartum fetal distress.

Despite the evidence and unequivocal recommendations for intrauterine resuscitation by ACOG, RCOG, and other authoritative institutions, overall compliance with the official guidelines is very poor. A review of approximately 400 publications on cesarean delivery for fetal distress found that only three papers reported the use of tocolytics before commencing the surgery, and in these studies tocolytics were used in only 16% of the potential candidates.[36] Clearly, there is still much room for improving fetal and maternal outcomes if intrauterine resuscitation is used on a more regular basis.

Intrauterine resuscitation with short-acting tocolytics is a very effective but widely undervalued and underused method to (temporarily) restore fetal oxygenation.

24.4.3 Operative delivery

Whenever fetal reserves – estimated by fetal scalp blood sampling – are judged to be insufficient to withstand further labor, and when the abnormal FHR pattern persists despite conservative management and intrauterine resuscitation, delivery should be expedited. In first-stage labor, cesarean delivery is now justified. In (true) second-stage labor, vacuum or forceps delivery is the best option. To permit meaningful audit, the umbilical cord should be doubly clamped at delivery, and an arterial blood sample obtained to determine the neonatal acid–base status.

24.5 Prevention of litigation

Confidential enquiries in several nations on perinatal death and hypoxic-ischemic encephalopathy indicate that roughly half of the labor-related cases could not reasonably be avoided by state-of-the-art intrapartum care.[49–60] To avoid unjust claims and to permit an objective medico-legal judgment, the results of all fetal and maternal assessments as well as all uncommon events and interventions during labor should be well documented. The clinical note should clearly mention the frequency and results of auscultation, the time of onset and type of non-reassuring CTG, the fetal scalp blood gases, the corrective and resuscitative measures undertaken along with the response, and the time of decision for cesarean delivery and the time of incision. CTG tracings should be kept for second opinion. The best way to counteract unjustly incriminating statements by

self-proclaimed CTG experts in court is to provide hard data on fetal scalp blood pH or lactate during labor as well as umbilical artery blood gases immediately after birth.

The enquiries also revealed clearly preventable elements in 20–70% of catastrophic labor outcomes. The five leading areas of clinical error are in decreasing rank order:

- CTG misinterpretation and underuse of FBS;
- Underestimation of risk during labor;
- Management of labor;
- Assessment of risk factors before labor;
- Management of delivery.

Evidently, the best way to prevent malpractice litigation is avoidance of errors. We trust this book might help.

References

1. Ugwumadu A. Understanding cardiotocographic patterns associated with intrapartum fetal hypoxia and neurologic injury. *Best Practice Res Clin Obst Gynaecol* 2013;**27**:509–36

2. Tucker Blackburn S. *Maternal, Fetal and Neonatal Physiology: A Clinical Perspective*, 3rd revised edition. Saunders; 2007

3. Ugwumadu A. Are we (mis)guided by current guidelines on intrapartum fetal heart rate monitoring? Case for a more physiological approach to interpretation. *Br J Obstet Gynaecol* 2014;**121**:1063–70

4. Hankins GD, Speer M. Defining the pathogenesis and pathophysiology of neonatal encephalopathy and cerebral palsy. *Obstet Gynecol* 2003;**102**:628–36

5. ACOG Committee Opinion no. 348, November 2006: Umbilical cord gas and acid–base analysis. *Obstet Gynecol* 2006;**108**:1319–22

6. Hankins GD, MacLennan AH, Speer ME, Strunk A, Nelson K. Obstetric litigation is asphyxiating our maternity services. *Obstet Gynecol* 2006;**107**:1382–5

7. Macones GA, Hankins GD, Spong CY, Hauth J, Moore T. The 2008 National Institute of Child Health and Human Development workshop report on electronic fetal monitoring: update on definitions, interpretation, and research guidelines. *Obstet Gynecol* 2008;**112**:661–6

8. National Institute of Clinical Excellence. Intrapartum Care: Care of Healthy Women and Their Babies During Labour. NICE Clinical Guideline No. 55. *National Collaborating Centre for Women's and Children's Health* London, UK: RCOG Press, 2007

9. American College of Obstetricians and Gynecologists. Practice bulletin no. 116: management of intrapartum fetal heart rate tracings. *Obstet Gynecol* 2010;**116**:1232–40

10. Jackson M, Holmgren CM, Esplin MS, Henry E, Varner MW. Frequency of fetal heart rate categories and short-term neonatal outcome. *Obstet Gynecol* 2011;**118**:803–8

11. Blackwell SC, Grobman WA, Antoniewicz L, Hutchinson M, Gyamfi Bannerman C. Interobserver and intraobserver reliability of the NICHD 3-Tier Fetal Heart Rate Interpretation System. *Am J Obstet Gynecol* 2011;**205**:378.e1–5. Epub 2011 June 29.

12. NICE Guidelines. *Intrapartum care: care of healthy women and their babies during childbirth*. RCOG Press; 2007. Updated 2010 www.nice.org.uk/guidance/cg55

13. Melchior J, Bernhard N. Incidence and pattern of fetal heart rate alterations during labor. In Kunzel W, ed. *Fetal Heart Rate Monitoring: Clinical Practice and Pathophysiology*. Berlin: Springer; 1985:73.

14. Walker J. Foetal anoxia. *J Obstet Gynaecol Br Commonw* 1953;**61**:162–80

15. Ahanya SN, Lakshmanan J, Morgan BL, Ross MG. Meconium passage in utero: mechanisms, consequences, and management. *Obstet Gynecol Surv* 2005;**60**:45–56

16. Nathan L, Leveno KJ, Carmody TJ, Kelly MA, Sherman LM. Meconium: a 1990s perspective on an old obstetric hazard. *Obstet Gynecol* 1994;**83**:329–32.

17. Ramin KD, Leveno KJ, Kelly MA, Carmody TJ. Amniotic fluid meconium: a fetal environmental hazard. *Obstet Gynecol* 1996;**87**:181–4

18. Garcia-Prats JA. Clinical features and diagnosis of meconium aspiration syndrome. UpToDate. Accessed November 2014

19. Ghidini A, Spong CY. Severe meconium aspiration syndrome is not caused by aspiration of meconium. *Am J Obstet Gynecol* 2001;**185**:931–8

20. Blackwell SC, Moldenhauer J, Hassan SS, *et al.* Meconium aspiration syndrome in term neonates with normal acid-base status at delivery: is it different? *Am J Obstet Gynecol* 2001;**184**:1422–5; discussion 1425–6

21. Dollberg S, Livny S, Mordecheyev N, Mimouni FB. Nucleated red blood cells in meconium aspiration syndrome. *Obstet Gynecol* 2001;**97**:593–6

22. Jazayeri A, Politz L, Tsibris JC, Queen T, Spellacy WN. Fetal erythropoietin levels in pregnancies complicated by meconium passage: does meconium suggest fetal hypoxia? *Am J Obstet Gynecol* 2000;**183**:188–90

23. Vintzileos AM, Nochimson DJ, Guzman ER, *et al.* Intrapartum electronic fetal heart rate monitoring versus intermittent auscultation: a meta-analysis. *Obstet Gynecol* 1995;**85**:149–55

24. Thacker SB, Stroup DF, Peterson HB. Efficacy and safety of intrapartum electronic fetal monitoring: an update. *Obstet Gynecol* 1995;**86**:613–20

25. Nelson KB, Dambrosia JM, Ting TY, Grether JK. Uncertain value of electronic fetal monitoring in predicting cerebral palsy. *N Engl J Med* 1996;**334**:613–18

26. Parer JT, King T. Fetal heart rate monitoring: is it salvageable? *Am J Obstet Gynecol* 2000;**182**:982–7

27. Young BK. Intrapartum fetal heart rate assessment. UpToDate. Accessed November 2014

28. Devane D, Lalor JG, Daly S, McGuire W, Smith V. Cardiotocography versus intermittent auscultation of fetal heart on admission to labour ward for assessment of fetal wellbeing. Cochrane Database Syst Rev 2012

29. American College of Obstetricians and Gynecologists. Fetal Heart Rate Patterns: Monitoring, Interpretations, and Management. Technical Bulletin No. 207. July 1995

30. Royal College of Obstetricians and Gynaecologists. *The Use of Electronic Fetal Monitoring: The Use and Interpretation of Cardiotocography in Intrapartum Surveillance*. London: Royal College of Obstetricians and Gynaecologists; 2001

31. Greenwood C, Lalchandini S, MacQuillan K, *et al.* Meconium passed in labor: How reassuring is clear amniotic fluid? *Obstet Gynecol* 2003;**102**:89–93

32. Grant A. Monitoring the fetus during labour. In: Chalmers I, Keirse MJNC, Enkin M, eds. *Effective Care in Pregnancy and Childbirth*, **Vol 2**. Oxford: Oxford University Press; 1989

33. Jørgensen JS, Weber T. Fetal scalp blood sampling in labor: a review. *Acta Obstet Gynecol Scand* 2014;**93**:548–55

34. Reif P, Haas J, Schöll W, Lang U. [Foetal scalp blood sampling: impact on the incidence of Caesarean section and assisted vaginal deliveries for non-reassuring foetal heart rate and its use according to gestational age]. *Z Geburtshilfe Neonatol* 2011;**215**:194–8

35. Alfirevic Z, Devane D, Gyte GM. Continuous cardiotocography (CTG) as a form of electronic fetal monitoring (EFM) for fetal assessment during labour. Cochrane Database Syst Rev 2013

36. Chauhan SP, Magann EF, Scott JR, *et al.* Emergency cesarean delivery for nonreassuring fetal heart rate tracings: compliance with ACOG guidelines. *J Reprod Med* 2003;**48**:975–81

37. Westgren M, Kruger K, Ek S, *et al.* Lactate compared with pH analysis at fetal scalp blood sampling: a prospective randomized study. *Br J Obstet Gynaecol* 1998;**105**:29–33

38. Kruger K, Hallberg B, Blennow M, Kublickas M, Westgren M. Predictive value of fetal scalp blood lactate concentration and pH as markers of neurologic disability. *Am J Obstet Gynecol* 1999;**181**:1072–8

39. East CE, Leader LR, Sheehan P, Henshall NE, Colditz PB. Intrapartum fetal scalp lactate sampling for fetal assessment in the presence of a non-reassuring fetal heart rate trace. Cochrane Database Syst Rev 2010

40. Garite TJ, Dildy GA, McNamara H, *et al*. A multicenter controlled trial of fetal pulse oximetry in the intrapartum management of nonreassuring fetal heart rate patterns. *Am J Obstet Gynecol* 2000;**183**:1049–58

41. Klauser CK, Christensen EE, Chauhan SP, *et al*. Use of fetal pulse oximetry among high-risk women in labor: a randomized clinical trial. *Am J Obstet Gynecol* 2005;**192**:1810–7

42. East CE, Brennecke SP, King JF, *et al*. The effect of intrapartum fetal pulse oximetry, in the presence of a nonreassuring fetal heart rate pattern, on operative delivery rates: a multicenter, randomized, controlled trial (the FOREMOST trial). *Am J Obstet Gynecol* 2006;**194**:606.e1–16

43. Bloom SL, Spong CY, Thom E, *et al*. (National Institute of Child Health and Human Development Maternal-Fetal Medicine Units Network). Fetal pulse oximetry and cesarean delivery. *N Engl J Med* 2006;**355**:2195–202

44. Olofsson P, Ayres-de-Campos D, Kessler J, *et al*. A critical appraisal of the evidence for using cardiotocography plus ECG ST interval analysis for fetal surveillance in labor. Part II: the meta-analyses. *Acta Obstet Gynecol Scand* 2014;**93**:571–86

45. Macones G. Management of intrapartum category I, II, and III fetal heart rate tracings. UpToDate. Accessed November 2014.

46. Hofmeyr GJ, Lawrie TA. Amnioinfusion for potential or suspected umbilical cord compression in labour. Cochrane Database Syst Rev 2012

47. Hendrix NW, Chauhan SP. Cesarean delivery for nonreassuring fetal heart rate tracing. *Obstet Gynecol Clin N Am* 2005; **32**: 273–86.

48. Kulier R, Hofmeyr JG. Tocolytics for suspected intrapartum fetal distress. Cochrane Database Syst Rev 2006

49. Draper ES, Kurinczuk JJ, Lamming CR, *et al*. A confidential enquiry into cases of neonatal encephalopathy. *Arch Dis Child Fetal Neonatal Ed* 2002;**87**(3):176–80

50. Dupont C, Touzet S, Rudigoz RC, *et al*. Critical events in obstetrics: a confidential enquiry in four high-level maternities of the AURORE perinatal network. *Journal of Evaluation in Clinical Practice* 2008;**14**:165–68

51. Papworth S, Cartlidge P. Learning from adverse events – the role of confidential enquiries. *Semin Fetal Neonatal Med* 2005;**10**:39–43

52. Liston R, Crane J, Hamilton E, *et al*. Fetal health surveillance in labour. *J Obstet Gynaecol Can* 2002;**24**:250–76

53. Rosser J. Confidential Enquiry into Stillbirths and Deaths in Infancy (CESDI). Highlights of the 6th annual report. *Pract Midwife* 1999;**2**:8–19

54. Maternal and Child Health Research Consortium. *8th Annual Report. Confidential enquiry into stillbirths and deaths in infancy*. London: Elsevier; 2001

55. Young P, Hamilton R, Hodgett S, *et al*. Reducing risk by improving standards of intrapartum fetal care. *J R Soc Med* 2001;**94**:226–31

56. O'Mahony F, Settatree R, Platt C, Johanson R. Review of singleton fetal and neonatal deaths associated with cranial trauma and cephalic delivery during a national intrapartum-related confidential enquiry. *Br J Obstet Gynaecol* 2005;**112**:619–26

57. Tan KH, Wyldes MP, Settatree R, Mitchell T. Confidential regional enquiry into mature stillbirths and neonatal deaths: a multi-disciplinary peer panel perspective of the perinatal care of 238 deaths. *Singapore Med J* 1999;**40**:251–5

58. Liston R, Sawchuck D, Young D; Society of Obstetrics and Gynaecologists of Canada; British Columbia Perinatal Health Program. Fetal health surveillance: antepartum and intrapartum consensus guideline. *J Obstet Gynaecol Can* 2007;**29**: S3–56

59. Maternal and Child Health Research Consortium. Confidential enquiry into stillbirths and deaths in infancy: 4th Annual Report, 1 January–31 December 1995

60. RCOG. *Confidential enquiry into maternal and child health maternity services in 2002 for women with type 1 and type 2 diabetes*. London: RCOG Press; 2004

Organizational reforms

Chapter 25

Proactive support of labor is an integral concept of childbirth consisting of five strongly interdependent components: pre-labor education, psychological support, prevention of long labor, constant peer review, and sound organization. It would be naive to expect that full implementation of the system could be achieved overnight. As with all major reforms in healthcare and beyond, organization makes all the difference between success and failure. Unlike the situation today, wherein the organization directs the content of offered care, the demands of high-quality care should direct the organization. Most importantly, frontline birth professionals rather than managers must take the lead in the much-needed changes.[1,2] Sound organization needs to be considered at three levels:

1. The labor and delivery ward;
2. Cooperation between doctors, midwives, and nurses;
3. Replacement of provider-centered care by woman-centered care.

25.1 The labor and delivery ward

Many delivery units are so disorganized – unable to cope with additional pressures even though overstaffed for much of the time – that there is no possibility of providing efficient and high-quality care.[3] Nursing services often function in a largely fragmentary manner, usually heavily concentrated in daylight hours. Several doctors come and go, leaving capricious or even contradictory instructions. Residents, midwives, and nurses are frequently placed in the invidious position of having to apply different methods of care – in exactly the same clinical circumstances – for no reason other than that the names of the obstetricians printed on the chart are different. "The sheer irrationality of this situation is a constant affront to the intelligence of labor room staff."[3] As a result, nurses, midwives, and doctors fail to cooperate

closely, and some even work in open conflict. Inevitably, poor corporate spirit and poor organizational standards sustain substandard care.

> In terms of care, many labor wards border on the chaotic, because an agreed central plan and proper organization are missing.

25.1.1 Staff consensus

Clearly, a delivery unit cannot begin to function properly unless all care providers agree on a common goal and strategy of care, obstetricians, midwives, and nurses alike. This book may serve as the evidence-based blueprint for such a plan.

Obstetricians are in a prime position to improve the standards of care in labor, simply by agreeing on a central policy plan. They should provide the tools and back-up needed for the nurses and midwives to execute their pivotal tasks. A group of motivated obstetricians with recognized authority and supported by hospital management should take the lead.[1,2] "All colleagues cooperating within the confines of a delivery unit should be called together and each obstetrician must be prepared to surrender a small portion of his or her jealously guarded independence for the sake of the common good."[3] This is the litmus test of goodwill on the part of the obstetricians.

The next step is to redefine the working relations between regulated midwives and doctors in a mutually satisfactory manner. The common plan should put an end to the silly animosity that all too often exists between these professional groups. Institutional commitment to high-quality care and low operative intervention rates is a corporate undertaking, requiring determination and team spirit.

> Staff consensus on a common goal and strategy is the prerequisite of high-quality care in labor.

Consensus should be reached about a system that is based on nursing and midwifery services with constant medical back-up. Once *proactive support of labor* has been introduced, the nurses and midwives convert most standards into practice, greatly improving care and enhancing the job satisfaction for everybody. With their pivotal roles clearly defined, they will further guard, extend, promote, and carry the system. It is particularly the midwives and nurses in our institution who unremittingly explain the methods and procedures to the ever-rotating undergraduates, residents, and student-midwives who, in turn, profit immensely from the clarity now offered. In our experience, these student-midwives and residents spread the system in their future careers and working environments.

25.1.2 Equal service around the clock

All pregnant women – without exception – are entitled to the same high level of safe care and expertise during labor and delivery, regardless of the hour of the day or the day of the week when birth happens to occur. This fundamental human right implies that the same complement of labor room staff – of equal status – should operate day and night; so-called daylight obstetrics is bad obstetrics (Chapter 23).

Furthermore, the labor and delivery unit should be designated an area of intensive nursing support, exclusively for women in labor. Staff attention should not be distracted by other tasks. The labor and delivery ward is not meant to serve as a gynecological first-aid facility, nor for antenatal assessments, external cephalic version of breech, or intensive surveillance of severely ill pregnant women or post-operative patients, etc. A labor and delivery ward should be used exclusively for labor and delivery; patients/clients who are not in labor do not belong there.

The delivery ward is an intensive care unit, intended exclusively for women in labor and evenly staffed around the clock, seven days a week.

25.1.3 Scale

Adequate scale is an obvious advantage in eliminating peaks and troughs in the number of deliveries at different hours of the day and on different days of the week. A volume of 2000 deliveries permits a nucleus of highly skilled personnel – nurses, midwives, and doctors – to be employed on a whole-time commitment to the delivery unit. They should not be required to divide their attention and responsibility simultaneously with antenatal clinics, antenatal wards, or postnatal care. In smaller delivery units, adequate nursing services might be achieved by a flexible system with on-call nurses, on standby to complement the on-site nurses if needed. Regardless of the scale, one-on-one nursing support extended to all women is a compulsory quality demand. However, cost-efficiency must co-exist, and in the final analysis many small hospitals will need to face the reality that an obstetric unit is not in the best interests of either the parturient or the hospital.

The welfare of pregnant women should not be influenced by the time at which birth happens to occur.

25.1.4 Central direction

A delivery unit catering for low-, medium-, and high-risk deliveries cannot be directed under a committee system and, therefore, a chain of command must be clearly defined. There should be one obstetrician only in charge at any given time. There is no more room for divided direction in a busy delivery unit than there is in the cockpit of an airplane. So, all nurses, midwives, and residents should be subject to the immediate authority of the obstetrician in charge.[3] Obviously, this obstetrician should have no other obligations and activities during his/her labor ward shift. He/she should review every woman and unborn child in the delivery unit, in the company of the attending midwife or resident, at regular intervals. As soon as all attending obstetricians have committed themselves to the common guidelines, policies should be consistent around the clock. Any departure from standard policy should always be explicitly approved by the obstetrician in charge and documented.

One obstetrician only should be in charge of the delivery unit at any given time.

25.2 Professional cooperation

With a common strategy of care, the professional roles and responsibilities of nurses, midwives, and doctors can finally be defined. One-on-one nursing is the backbone of the system and, equally importantly, there is no longer place for rivalry or competition between well-trained and legally certified midwives and doctors. Their roles are fully complementary: the midwife's expertise lies in the supervision of health and the prevention and detection of disease whereas the specialty of the obstetrician is the treatment of disease and the restoration of health. These professional groups should recognize and value their complementary skills and work together for the common good.

> *Optimal care can only be provided when nurses, midwives, and obstetricians acknowledge their specific roles and their complementary skills.*

25.2.1 Nursing services

Good nursing service does not mean a group of nurses caring for an equivalent number of parturients on a collective basis. Hard clinical evidence shows that a woman's childbirth experience largely depends on the quality of the relationship established with the nurse assigned to her personally.[4] The attention of each nurse should, therefore, be confined to one woman in labor only. In contrast to common perception, larger scale favors personal attention and human compassion, provided that the full system of *proactive support* is adopted *in all its components*.

> *Key to high-quality and safe care is supportive nursing attention on a one-on-one basis extended to all women in labor.*

The skills required for supportive nursing care in labor are completely different from nursing skills needed on the antenatal or postnatal ward. Therefore, these groups should not be interchanged for economic efficiency reasons. Quality demands must lead. Labor room nurses are specifically selected for their supportive skills and their ability to cope with the extremely variable reactions of women in labor. It goes without saying that they must be able to function in emergency situations. Although their priorities are the supportive role and the bedside monitoring of maternal and fetal health, all nurses should also be trained and authorized to site IV lines, administer IV medication on the request of midwives and doctors, and so on. Nurses do not perform vaginal examinations or deliveries. In medical terms, they are subject to the authority of the

midwives and doctors. However, in terms of labor support and women's satisfaction, nurses play the most important and most difficult part. Doctors and midwives should openly acknowledge this and show the much-needed respect for what the labor room nurses do.

25.2.2 Midwifery services

A risk assessment should be made in the antenatal clinics and again at admission (Chapter 24), formally assigning the care of each woman either to the midwifery service or to the medical-specialist team. In more than 75% of all women the pregnancy proceeds uneventfully, and the supervision of childbirth can be safely assigned to the midwives, who now supervise all labors according to the principles and guidelines of *proactive support*. There is no place any longer for unfounded midwifery philosophies of wait and see. The midwife is officially authorized to admit the woman on the basis of a strict diagnosis of labor (Chapter 14), and she guards and ensures progression (Chapter 15).

As most complications of labor arise in initially normal cases that are not proactively supervised, the midwives must be vested with the authority and the tools required to conduct labor properly, including correction of slow labor according to protocol (17.3). As long as no other problems occur, midwives can and should take full professional responsibility for (corrected) physiological labor and delivery. To reiterate: *proactive support of labor* does not medicalize birth. Rather, it ensures normality of the birth process, and this is the focus of midwifery care. Ideally, the availability of home-like delivery rooms devoid of redundant technical equipment should emphasize this midwifery assignment. Essential provisions and allowances for women-friendly labor rooms were summarized previously (16.3.3 and 19.3).

> *Midwives play the pivotal role in the supervision and preservation of physiological labor, including acceleration of abnormally slow labor if needed.*

25.2.3 The role of the obstetrician

The obstetrician in charge focuses primarily on the high-risk patients who are not an issue in this book. However, in terms of absolute numbers most problems in labor appear in completely normal women initially assigned to the midwives. The obstetrician, therefore, no longer remains off-stage, "awaiting the occasional summons to perform an emergency operation in a belated attempt to retrieve a situation that could have been anticipated at a much earlier stage."[3] Instead, he or she is continually present and tries to help the midwives and residents prevent such emergencies by regular review of all parturients, regardless of prior risk assessment. It is the obstetrician in charge who will be held accountable for the outcome at the daily peer review (Chapter 26). All obstetricians should be at pains to ensure that policies are executed through constant education on the spot of new residents, midwives, and nurses.

The obstetrician in charge must be instantly available on the premises at all times.

25.2.4 Responsibilities and liability

For an individual client/patient, there exists no such thing as shared responsibility. "A bland institutional declaration to the general effect is meaningless both in medical and legal terms."[3] Therefore, each woman in labor must know exactly who is directly responsible for her welfare. Although low-risk care may be (partly) delegated to student-midwives and high-risk labors to residents, the attending midwife and the supervising obstetrician, respectively, bear ultimate responsibility and liability and must be known to the laboring woman by name and face.

Whenever the midwife judges that the boundaries of her authority are reached, the obstetrician takes over responsibility. There is no place for equivocation on this issue. If the consulted obstetrician decides to further delegate the supervision of the compromised labor to the midwife or a resident, it goes without saying that the obstetrician remains ultimately accountable whenever a mishap might occur. Apart from liability concerns, experience shows that all professionals and clients/patients benefit greatly from intensive cooperation between midwives and doctors based on mutual confidence and respect. Such a congenial working environment can only exist when a common birth-plan is adopted and when specific tasks and responsibilities are clearly defined.

Full responsibility for low-risk labors can and should be assigned to well trained, certified midwives.

25.2.5 Sound economics

The system favors efficient use of the expensive labor and delivery unit because virtually all women now give birth within 12 hours. Investment in one-on-one nursing is cost-effective since the reduction in surgical deliveries greatly reduces overall hospital expenditure. It equally reduces post-operative care, freeing nurses from the postnatal ward to be employed on the labor ward. The costs of time-consuming damage control, liability claims, and insurances will undoubtedly decrease as mistakes diminish, and medical negligence actions will belong to the past. Sound organization not only improves all standards of care but also enhances job satisfaction of staff, reducing the all too common high rates of sick leave and extremely costly burnout. There is no doubt that the system pays for itself.

Expert childbirth practice corresponds with good working conditions for staff and sound economics. All three issues make good sense and are interrelated.

25.3 Grassroots system reforms

The proposals touch the very heart of obstetric services as they segregate the persons who perform antenatal care from those who provide intrapartum care, a trend seen in most institutions in recent decades. The advantages in quality of care should outweigh the potential offsets for both mothers-to-be and their caregivers. In particular, concerns about the inherent disruption of patient–practitioner relationships must be discussed. Doctors, midwives, and women with child will have to adapt to many changes. Fortunately, recent socio-cultural developments lead and pave the way.

Organizational reforms require the courage to make decisions that will benefit the next generation's laboring women and caregivers alike.

25.3.1 Traditional patient–doctor relationships

Traditionally, the doctor or midwife who provides mothers with prenatal care also delivers the baby. For doctors, this provider-centered practice model combines an office practice and hospital practice.

That system locks obstetricians into an unending cycle of office visits, hospital rounds, surgeries, deliveries, more office visits, evening rounds, late-night telephone calls, and more deliveries in the middle of the night. The obstetrician ends up driving across town several times a day to see women at different hospitals, leaving other patients waiting at the office while he or she frequently cannot make it to the labor room in time to deliver the baby. Continuity in patient–doctor relationships is cherished in name, but continuous and personal care in labor is actually non-existent. Even worse, the combination of grueling working hours and demands of personal involvement encourages obstetricians to induce labor for no reason other than doctor's convenience and will equally lower the threshold for cesarean deliveries. These practices inevitably harm their patients' health. Women should realize that the provider-centered system was never designed for and is not aimed at their best interests, nor does it help obstetricians for that matter; both sides suffer greatly under this system.

Poor organization is the rock on which good intentions usually founder.

25.3.2 Current crisis in obstetrics

Hectic and unpredictable working hours, topped by the stifling legal climate, are increasingly causing gynecologists to retire or cut back on obstetric services.[5–8] Job dissatisfaction is not anecdotal but structural; evidence exists for a marked increase in fatigue, substance abuse, poor personal relationships, and burnout.[8–14] Clearly, this is of no service to any pregnant woman.

Little wonder that the number of medical graduates choosing a career in obstetrics has recently dropped markedly.[15–18] Medical students rotating through obstetrics mainly observe stressed or demotivated doctors and understandably decide that there must be better ways to make a living. Future work capacity is jeopardized, and the dwindling workforce recruitment aggravates all problems even further, completing the vicious circle. Clearly, the need for grassroots reforms of the obstetric system is acute.

As it goes now, both access to and the quality of obstetrical care are in real jeopardy. The current provider-centered system should, therefore, be replaced by a new system that is women-centered in design.

25.3.3 Societal changes

Fortunately, major socio-cultural reforms have occurred throughout all western societies in the past decades, including a gradual gender transformation of academic professionals. This trend did not pass by the domain of obstetrics and gynecology; today, more than 75% of all residents are female. Undoubtedly, the greatest benefit to accrue from this change is a heightened sensitivity to "women's issues" in the training programs and practice of medicine, such as the need to balance the demands of work and to raise a family. This has triggered permanent changes.

No longer are doctors – of either gender – willing to work 70–80 hours a week while personal and family life suffer.[14–19] The new lifestyle demands exclude a practice with 24/7 availability and continuous personal commitment. Solo practices are becoming increasingly unpopular, and most obstetricians now practice in groups that provide their members with reasonable call schedules and duty hours. Even part-time practice has now become possible. The new function of OB-hospitalist or laborist-obstetrician, whose job is restricted to working in the labor and delivery ward, is becoming increasingly popular and benefits both doctors and birthing women.[20–23] Certainly, most women in labor prefer the personal attention and time of a dedicated obstetrician who is constantly there, above their "own" doctor, who is there only occasionally and always in a rush. The new breed of obstetrician-laborist fits perfectly in the ideal organization of the delivery unit.

Physicians and midwives want a reasonable work/ family balance, just like all other people, including women who happen to be pregnant. Today the majority of expectant women accept this as a matter of course.

By now, patients/clients are used to seeing different practitioners and understand the inevitability thereof.[24] They only disapprove when reorganization is primarily aimed at making things better for doctors rather than for patients/clients. Dissatisfaction does not result from doctors' discontinuity but frustrating inconsistencies in information by different practitioners and annoying discrepancies between information and actions. The problem is not a group practice, but non-cooperating egos who refuse to adapt to commonly established policies. The opportunity for major breakthroughs is often missed, for it is exactly the joint practice that finally opens possibilities for genuine improvement of all standards of care including personal attention and women's satisfaction. To this end, of course, the prerequisites of a common strategy of care, meaningful cooperation, and consistent client/patient information must be met.

> Women's dissatisfaction with large practices does not result from disruption of doctors' continuity but inconsistencies in information and disappointing mismatches between expectations and practice.

25.3.4 Refocusing obstetric practice

The final logical step is to refocus the specialty of obstetrics on what the discipline originally was meant for, i.e. the pathology of pregnancy and childbirth. In contrast, care during normal pregnancy and childbirth is the specialty of well-trained and legally certified midwives. The evidence shows that it is inherently unwise and often even unsafe for healthy women with normal pregnancies to be cared for by obstetric specialists, even if the required staffing is available (Chapters 2–4). Besides, obstetricians – caring for women with both normal and abnormal pregnancies – have to make an impossible choice because of time constraints: to neglect the normal pregnancies in order to concentrate their care on those with pathology, or to spend most of their time supervising biologically normal processes. In that case, they rapidly lose their specialist expertise. We had better refocus our identity as medical specialists rather than as primary care providers. The benefit will be the re-emergence of the specialty we all chose and love to practice: a technical and surgical profession. The challenge is to restrict the application of these operative skills to those who really need it.

> Obstetricians should refocus on their primary task: the care and treatment of pathological pregnancy, and of labor and delivery disorders.

25.3.5 Integrated primary care

Yet it is still the doctors who provide almost all antenatal care and who deliver more than 90% of all babies in the USA.[25] In the majority of other countries, most babies are delivered by hospital midwives, but it is no secret that cooperation with the obstetricians is often far from ideal, mainly because an integrated and mutually agreed concept of childbirth is lacking. In those institutions, too, there is ample room for improvement.

Every childbearing woman wants personal attention for "rosy issues", which consumes much time, something most medical specialists do not have. The more reason to leave primary care for uneventful pregnancies to the experts in this field – the midwives – provided, of course, they wholeheartedly keep to the principles of *proactive support*, just as medical-specialist staff should do. That implies that midwives and obstetricians must work closely together both at the antenatal clinics and in the delivery ward, ideally in one collective enterprise.

A joint practice guarantees instant consultation and a seamless care continuum if complications arise. Strict division into two independently operating care echelons simply does not work, as the system in the Netherlands clearly shows (Chapter 5). Clients'/patients' preferences and needs are much more complex and contain many elements of both midwifery and medical styles of care, both of which should be honored at all times.[26–31] A systematic review of the international literature on the efficiency and effectiveness of integrated perinatal care confirms the crucial importance of organizing modalities that aim to support woman-centered care and cooperative clinical practice.[32]

> Primary care is preferably provided by midwives who are fully integrated into the system, who know the boundaries of their expertise, and who have instant access to help from cooperating obstetricians.

Reorganization cannot neglect more earthy issues; the collective of obstetricians and midwives should make new financial arrangements with the health insurers, eliminating improper incentives to direct care. In fact, the much more demanding efforts to promote spontaneous delivery should be better paid than the resolution of preventable labor problems by a quick but unnecessary cesarean delivery. Reforms should, therefore, be neutral or positive to the incomes of all participating obstetricians and midwives. A guaranteed and fair income ultimately enhances the quality of care and reduces consequent overall costs. In our experience, most health insurers are glad to cooperate.

25.3.6 Place of birth and emotions

A final issue that needs to be addressed is the place of birth, an endless source of conflict and strong emotions (Chapter 5). Women's preference for a primary midwife-led birth center or a home birth originates in socio-cultural values or reflects fear of hospitals and opposition to overmedicalized hospital birth. As it is now, rejection of hospital birth by women's health groups and home birth activists is all too well founded on women's adverse hospital experiences. Views are particularly polarized in the USA, with reactionary activists on the barricades for home births and hospitals denying independent midwives access when problems occur at home, so that they are forced to smuggle their patients into the ER and leave. Many US hospitals even deny midwives a job when they are also involved with home births.[33] Clearly, there is a lot of rancor there.

> Experiences with overmedicalized, impersonal, and technocratic hospital care will continue to arouse reactionary calls for home births, sometimes even in chancy circumstances. Who is to blame?

In essence, disputes between obstetricians and radical midwives are about who is in charge rather than the place of birth (Chapter 5). Both biomedical obstetrics and the women's health movement's critique of it share a belief in the ability to lead childbirth to a positive and rewarding outcome. However, this emphasis on happy endings – whether believed to be the result of medical intervention or women's natural inborn powers to give birth – exacerbates the adverse experiences of those women whose happy expectations do not come true.[34]

Obstetricians' emphasis on risks may surely disempower women, but home birth activists' emphasis on the "dream delivery" and the importance of women being in control of their own bodies equally contributes to disappointment and women's self-blame when delivery is not completed at home or in the "homelike" birth center.[31,36] Clearly, both attitudes should be abandoned.

> Honoring women's choices means that there should be no pressure for or against planning birth at home or in a midwife-led birth center, provided that it concerns a low-risk labor and instant access to the hospital is guaranteed.

Despite decades of political and academic debate, the relative merits of home versus hospital birth remain unproven.[37,38] This is likely to remain so, as comparisons that are sufficiently unbiased and large enough to address crucial safety issues are unlikely to be forthcoming.[37,39] Be that as it may, women will continue to choose to give birth at home for a variety of reasons, and these women and their babies are equally entitled to effective hospital back-up whenever problems arise. It is, therefore, much wiser to listen to women's wishes, to elaborate and agree on strict selection criteria and safeguards for home births, to define mutual responsibilities, and to monitor results. Entrenched positions, by either party, only make women suffer.

25.4 Women-centered care model

Broadening women's options involves moving from the preconceived biomedical or midwifery notions of appropriate care into a women-based and multi-option setting. This reorientation holds for all aspects of in-hospital as well as out-of-hospital care.

25.4.1 Shared practice

The most logical and ideal answer to the socio-cultural pressures is to integrate both services into one collective system, based on a common, women-centered plan. A joint practice of obstetricians and midwives can offer the possibility of safe home births in selected cases, attended by the midwives who also work in the birth center integrated with the hospital delivery ward. The united practice guarantees consistent policies, a continuum in care, instant access to the hospital, seamless transfer if needed, and a good collaborative relationship between the midwives and the hospital. The joint electronic dossier guarantees that all relevant information is available at all times.

Mutual trust is a matter of fundamental importance on which all else ultimately depends, and this requires mutual respect and undivided adherence to all components of a central plan, both in the hospital and at home. In a collective initiative, there is no place for competition. Like all other professionals, independently operating midwives will have to sacrifice (a part of) their autonomy for the sake of the general good, join the collective practice, adopt its policies, share its profits, and subject themselves to peer review. This is the acid test of goodwill on the part of midwives.

Women's preferences and needs contain many elements of both midwifery and medical styles of care. Integrating out-of-hospital and in-hospital care reconciles these wishes.

The authors work in a highly developed western country where midwifery and home birth are still valued as a cultural heritage (Chapter 5). Recently, we concluded the challenging process of merging some of the formerly independent midwifery practices into a collective system with our hospital, called the integrated birth center "Livive."[40]

25.4.2 Personalized care

Our system combines the best of midwifery and medical care. The first antenatal visit of all women – regardless of any "risk factor" – is between the 8th and 10th week with one of the midwives. She takes a thorough medical and social history and arranges an early ultrasound and routine blood tests. All intakes are discussed with the consultant-obstetrician, and a tailored antenatal "care path" is defined for each woman. The "care path" includes frequency of antenatal visits, additional blood tests and ultrasounds, consultation of other specialists or the social worker, and so on.

In the absence of any relevant medical or obstetrical history, women are scheduled for routine antenatal care with the midwives, either in the hospital/birth center or in one of the midwife offices in the women's approximate neighborhood. All women under the midwives' care visit the obstetrician once – routinely between 32 and 36 weeks – to get acquainted with the medical profession, just in case. This visit emphasizes the integrated nature of the care model. A tailored birth-plan – including the place of birth – is discussed. Practice shows that all women appreciate this visit to the obstetrician, mostly perceived as a welcome reassurance that all is well and medical back-up is instantly available 24/7 should the need arise.

An integrated practice allows a personally tailored antenatal "care path."

Women with relevant pre-existing morbidity are directly assigned to the obstetrician for further medical antenatal care. However, most women with a risk factor remain under the care of the midwives who

comply with the well defined "care path" including extra ultrasound examinations or additional laboratory tests. The timing of the antenatal visit to the obstetrician depends on the nature of the risk factor, the scheduled test results, and the course of the pregnancy.

All women visit the birth-educator between 34 and 36 weeks in order to go into labor well prepared (Chapter 18). After an uneventful pregnancy and in the absence of recognized risk factors, women are given the choice where to give birth. The best practice is to provide pregnant women with data-driven information (Chapter 27), replacing anecdotal horror stories of "what might happen" at home or in the hospital. Only constant and unbiased evaluation (Chapter 26) allows for meaningful bilateral cooperation.

25.4.3 Case selection for home birth

The midwives of our integrated unit now deliver babies both in the hospital/birth center and at the women's homes. Home birth is no longer considered as a goal per se but as a responsible option in strictly selected cases. We have agreed on the following:

1. Home births remain restricted to uneventful, singleton pregnancies with a normal fetus in the cephalic presentation and a gestational age between 37 and 42 weeks.
2. VBACs are not allowed at home. If the cesarean section and the post-operative recovery have been uneventful, VBAC is accepted in the hospital.
3. Stripping of membranes at 41-plus weeks, to induce a home birth before the 42-week limit is passed, should no longer be practiced (14.6.4).
4. The transfer-time to the hospital in case of complications should never exceed 30 minutes, taking into account the usual traffic conditions. Women who live further away deliver in the hospital/birth center under the midwife's supervision.
5. The midwife attending home birth takes full responsibility. The hospital guarantees instant medical back-up.
6. The midwife at home keeps the obligatory partogram. She ruptures the membranes whenever indicated, even at 1 cm dilatation if needed. Whenever progress remains unsatisfactory, the mother is transferred to the hospital in time to allow effective corrective action. The midwife continues attendance in the

hospital and remains responsible for the accelerated labor.

7. The midwife stays at the home from the very onset of labor. In the case of any abnormality in fetal heartbeat counts or passage of meconium, the woman is immediately transferred to the hospital, and the obstetrician takes over responsibility.

Constant and meticulous audit (Chapters 26 and 27) does not reveal any adverse perinatal outcomes that could have been prevented had the mothers been in the hospital from the onset of labor. When strict selection criteria are met, and the policies of *proactive support* carefully followed, the integrated facility of home births proves to be safe.

An integrated in- and out-of-hospital practice can responsibly provide facilities for safe home births in strictly selected cases.

Despite access to all options and neutral counseling, the great majority of "low-risk" women in our region now prove to give preference to the birth center as the place of birth. The main reasons nulliparas report are a feeling of safety should problems arise, the high intrapartum transfer odds, and instant availability of adequate pain relief. Parous women choose the hospital/birth center for similar reasons and because of their satisfaction with the first birth experience there. By now, only 3% of all nulliparas and 10% of multiparas deliver at home attended by one of our midwives. Given the women's preferences, the midwives no longer regard home as the ideal place of birth for nulliparas. Freedom from adverse effects on their income and constant evaluation of results made them discover this by themselves, which is the only way that works.

Home birth should not be an escape from the overmedicalized childbirth services that exist in many hospitals. Home delivery should be the optional bonus for parous women who experienced high-quality integrated care throughout their first childbirth and gained the ultimate prize of a safe and rewarding vaginal first delivery.

25.4.4 Benefits for all

The organizational reforms prove to be a threefold win situation, for women, midwives, and doctors alike, without any objective disadvantages. All women – ranging from the lowest to the highest risks – now profit from complementary midwifery and medical expertise and attention. The only variable is the intensity and frequency of medical involvement. The midwife's antenatal and intrapartum care has been substantially extended, and the medical staff predominantly operates on a consultative basis.

Efficiency and job satisfaction of both professional groups are enhanced markedly. The obstetricians now concentrate on their medical expertise and the midwives, who love to extend their chances for conducting the birth process properly, have regained the pivotal role in the supervision of "normal" pregnancy and childbirth.

Most importantly, women's satisfaction has increased markedly as continuous personal attention is now guaranteed, and long labor is effectively prevented. With the overall birth-plan, all women finally get the maximal chance to deliver their baby safely by their own efforts (Chapter 27).

The integrated childbirth system effectively restores the balance between natural and medicalized childbirth.

References

1. Likosky DS. Clinical microsystems: a critical framework for crossing the quality chasm. *J Extra Corpor Technol* 2014;**46**:33–7

2. Nelson EC, Batalden PB, Godfrey MM. *Quality Design: A Clinical Microsystems Approach*. New York: Wiley; 2006

3. O'Driscoll K, Meagher D, Robson M. *Active Management of Labour*, 4th edn. London: Mosby; 2003

4. Hodnett ED. Pain and women's satisfaction with the experience of childbirth: a systematic review. *Am J Obstet Gynecol* 2002;**186**:S160–72

5. Farrow VA, Leddy MA, Lawrence H, Schulkin J. Ethical concerns and career satisfaction in obstetrics and gynecology: a review of recent findings from the Collaborative Ambulatory Research Network. *Obstet Gynecol Surv* 2011;**66**:572–9

6. Anderson BL, Hale RW, Salsberg E, Schulkin J. Outlook for the future of the obstetrician-gynecologist workforce. *Am J Obstet Gynecol* 2008;**199**:e1–e8

7. Bettes BA, Chalas E, Coleman VH, Schulkin J. Heavier workload, less personal control: impact of delivery on obstetrician/gynecologists' career satisfaction. *Am J Obstet Gynecol* 2004;**190**:851–57

8. Bettes BA, Strunk AL, Coleman VH, Schulkin J. Professional liability and other career pressures: impact on obstetrician-gynecologists' career satisfaction. *Obstet Gynecol* 2004;**103**:967–973

9. Spickard A, Gabbe SG, Christensen JF. Mid-career burnout in generalists and specialist physicians. *JAMA* 2002;**288**:1447–50

10. Defoe DM, Power ML, Holzman GB, Carpentieri A, Schulkin J. Long hours and little sleep: work schedules of residents in obstetrics and gynecology. *Obstet Gynecol* 2001;**97**:1015–8

11. Storr CI, Trinkoff AM, Anthony JC. Job strain and non-medical drug use. *Drug Alcohol Depend* 1999;**55**:45–51

12. Myers MF. Don't let your practice kill your marriage. *Med Econ* 1998;**9**:78–87

13. Maulen B. Depression, divorce, malpractice, bankruptcy: why do so many physicians commit suicide? *MMW Fortschr Med* 2002;**144**:4–8

14. Kravitz RL, Leigh JP, Samuels SJ, Schembri M, Gilbert WM. Tracking career satisfaction and perceptions of quality among US obstetricians and gynecologists. *Obstet Gynecol* 2003;**102**:463–70

15. Queenan JT. The future of obstetrics and gynecology. *Obstet Gynecol* 2003;**102**:441–2

16. Gibbons JM. Springtime for obstetrics and gynecology: will the specialty continue to blossom? *Obstet Gynecol* 2003;**102**:443–5

17. Pearse WH, Haffner WHJ, Primack A. Effect of gender on the obstetric-gynecologic work force. *Obstet Gynecol* 2001;**97**:794–7

18. Frigoletto FD, Greene MF. Is there a sea change ahead for obstetrics and gynecology? *Obstet Gynecol* 2002;**100**:1342–3

19. Fang YM, Egan JF, Rombro T, Morris B, Zelop CM. A comparison of reasons for choosing obstetrician/ gynecologist subspecialty training. *Conn Med* 2009;**73**:165–70

20. Weinstein L. The laborist: a new focus of practice for the obstetrician. *Am J Obstet Gynecol* 2003;**188**:310–12

21. Funk C, Anderson BL, Schulkin J, Weinstein L. Survey of obstetric and gynecologic hospitalists and laborists. *Am J Obstet Gynecol* 2010;**203**:177.e1–4 Epub 2010 June 26

22. Feldman DS, Bollman DL, Korst LM, *et al.* The laborist: what is the frequency of this model of care and how is it being used in California? *Obstet Gynecol* 2014;**123** Suppl 1:144S

23. Olson R, Garite TJ, Fishman A, Andress IF. Obstetrician/gynecologist hospitalists: can we improve safety and outcomes for patients and hospitals and improve lifestyle for physicians? *Am J Obstet Gynecol* 2012;**207**:81–6. Epub 2012 June 23

24. McNeil DA, Vekved M, Dolan SM, *et al.* A qualitative study of the experience of CenteringPregnancy group prenatal care for physicians. *BMC Pregnancy Childbirth* 2013;13 Suppl 1:S1-6. Epub 2013 January 31

25. Martin JA, Hamilton BE, Ventura SJ, *et al.* Births: final data for 2009. *Natl Vital Stat Rep* 2011;**60**:1–70

26. Pitchforth E, Watson V, Ryan M, *et al.* Models of intrapartum care and women's trade-offs in remote and rural Scotland: a mixed-methods study. *Br J Obstet Gynaecol* 2008;**115**:560–9

27. Huntley V, Ryan M, Graham W. Assessing women's preferences for intrapartum care. *Birth* 2001;**28**:254–63

28. Spurgeon P, Hicks C, Barwell F. Antenatal, delivery and postnatal comparisons of maternal satisfaction with two pilot Changing Childbirth schemes compared with a traditional model of care. *Midwifery* 2001;**17**:123–32

29. Hundley V, Ryan M. Are women's expectations and preferences for intrapartum care affected by the model of care on offer? *Br J Obstet Gynaecol* 2004;**111**:550–60

30. Lyon DS, Mokhtarian PL, Reever MM. Predicting style-of-care preferences of obstetric patients: medical vs midwifery model. *J Reprod Med* 1999;**44**:101–6

31. de Jonge A, Stuijt R, Eijke I, Westerman MJ. Continuity of care: what matters to women when they are referred from primary to secondary care during labour? A qualitative interview study in the Netherlands. *BMC Pregnancy Childbirth* 2014;**14**:103. doi: 10.1186/1471-2393-14-103

32. Rodriguez C, des Rivières-Pigeon C. A literature review on integrated perinatal care. *Int J Integrated Care* 2007;**7**:1–15

33. Declercq ER, Sakala C, Corry MP, Applebaum S. *Listening to mothers: report of the first national US survey of women's childbirth experiences.* New York: Maternity Center Association; 2002

34. Laynne LL. Unhappy endings: a feminist reappraisal of the women's health movement from the vantage of pregnancy loss. *Soc Sci Med* 2003;**56**:1881–91

35. Christiaens W, Gouwy A, Bracke P. Does a referral from home to hospital affect satisfaction with childbirth? A cross-national comparison. *BMC Health Services Res* 2007;**7**:109–17

36. Rijnders M, Baston H, Schönbeck Y, *et al.* Perinatal factors related to negative or positive recall of birth experience in women 3 years postpartum in The Netherlands. *Birth* 2008;**35**:107–16

37. Olsen O, Clausen J. Planned hospital birth versus planned home birth. Cochrane Database Syst Rev 2012

38. Catling-Paull C, Coddington RL, Foureur MJ, Homer CS. Birthplace in Australia Study; National Publicly-funded Homebirth Consortium. Publicly funded homebirth in Australia: a review of maternal and neonatal outcomes over 6 years. *Med J Aust* 2013;**198**:616–20

39. Hendrix M, Van Horck M, Moreta D, *et al.* Why women do not accept randomisation for place of birth: Feasibility of a RCT in The Netherlands. *Br J Obstet Gynaecol* 2009;**116**:537–42

40. Website of the integrated midwifery-obstetrical birth center "Livive" at the St. Elisabeth hospital in Tilburg, the Netherlands. http://www.Livive.nl

Implementation and ongoing audit cycle

Promoting women's satisfaction with childbirth is as much about caregivers' re-education as about changing behaviors, and neither can be accomplished in a haphazard manner. Altering the mind-set and practice patterns of highly educated professionals is not an easy task. Successful implementation of *proactive support of labor*, therefore, requires clinical leadership, careful planning, determination, and constant maintenance.

26.1 Initiative

The first step is to identify the most sensitive areas of care and to standardize the general outline of procedures.[1] These matters have been addressed in the previous chapters under the headings diagnosis of labor, prevention of long labor, curtailed use of inductions, pre-labor educational service, continuous labor support, and organization. A continual cycle of audit should then be introduced, leading to step-by-step improvements in labor supervision, labor support, and overall care.

26.1.1 Leadership and peer pressure

Strong clinical leadership is critical. Many quality improvement initiatives in healthcare have failed in the past because of a lack of authoritative direction.[2] As childbirth management decisions are "local", activities to bring about practice change have to be driven locally, and such initiatives are destined to fail in the absence of committed leadership. Authority should not rest on status, gender, or age, but on example, in-depth knowledge, and the ability to inspire and motivate all co-workers. Although a system with a formal "head of department" or "Master" may greatly facilitate decision-making for practice change, the collective senior staff must support the reforms and maintain constant "peer pressure" as well. Doctor and midwife habits and inveterate practice patterns are unlikely to change in the absence

of recognition, praise, public accord, and private admonishments by committed senior staff.

> *Initiatives for altering practice patterns require committed clinical leadership and constant peer pressure of expert staff.*

26.2 Close peer review on a daily basis

Reduction of practice variation is one of the major hallmarks of quality improvement.[3] Key to achieving enduring success is an ongoing system of close peer review within the unit, weaving all medical and non-medical components of *proactive support* into an overall pattern of practice. The main platform for an effective audit cycle is the daily morning report, attended by all obstetricians, residents, midwives, and nurses.

> **The morning report**
> *Daily evaluation of all the medical and non-medical processes involved is the most important contributor to establishing and maintaining expert care in childbirth.*

26.2.1 Internal audit for educational purposes

Instead of the usual team meeting rushing through last night's problems and briefly summarizing the operative deliveries, each woman operatively delivered during the past 24 hours is now made the object of scrutiny. Insistence on the precise use of well-defined terms and strict diagnoses is a matter of prime importance. Vague observations such as "dystocia" and "indiscriminate" or "non-reassuring CTG" should no longer be accepted. Instead, exact diagnoses – as defined in the previous chapters – and the underlying cause of each problem should be assessed, and the timing and nature of corrective actions analyzed. Cause and effect need to be explored if progress is to be made.

Although there will always be some subjective elements in clinical diagnosis, a collective judgment on the appropriateness of diagnosis and treatment can be reached in almost every case, provided the details of each labor have been carefully documented. Omissions in relevant information should, therefore, be exposed. An honest review looks at what could have been done differently in the timing of intervention (*prompt*), the amount of labor support (*sufficient*), and the type of corrective measures or treatment (*appropriate*).

> To promote new standards of care, peer review must be detailed, inspiring, and high-profile, and a positive and safe atmosphere must be carefully guarded at all times.

Initially, providers may feel threatened by these rigorous reviews ("comply or explain"), but experience shows that their job satisfaction and prestige improve markedly with their growing understanding of labor and the quality of care. Peer review should not be directed to assigning blame to individuals or to deflecting criticism from others. Critique should be focused on medical and/or non-medical care aspects, never on individual care providers; public *ad hominem* attacks are counterproductive. Inspiring peer review is aimed at enhancement of the general fund of knowledge – both scientifically and clinically – and promotion of new standards and expectations.

26.2.2 Staff commitment to low intervention rates

Reported indications for operative deliveries should be reviewed, distinguishing between fetal reasons and dystocia and the respective causal diagnoses. Through these daily plenary sessions, the whole staff, including all consultants, become actively involved in the regular review of labor as never before, and the morning reports gain enormously in substance, relevance, educational value, appreciation, and fun.

> Exact causal diagnoses and close analysis of the corrective measures taken are critical for meaningful audit and ongoing education.

Every decision to terminate pregnancy – be it by induction of labor or a pre-labor cesarean delivery – should be discussed at the plenary morning report. Just the strict peer review will reduce the rates of these interventions and related iatrogenic complications. Since the aim of labor induction is to effectuate a vaginal delivery, each cesarean birth after priming or induction should be classified as "failed induction" (23.7). This very assessment proves to be an eye-opener to many doctors, and will help to further reduce the institutional induction rate.

> Each proposal for priming/induction and pre-labor cesarean should be reviewed at the plenary morning report. The same goes for the maternal and fetal outcomes.

26.2.3 Resetting the mind

Daily review of procedures and outcomes identifies gaps between the ideal and practice and guides improvements. This is a continual process, especially in teaching hospitals where constant turnover of young registrars, residents, student-nurse/midwives, and interns strains compliance with the system. It takes time for new team members to break habits they have learned elsewhere, inevitably making mistakes along the way. While the medical protocols are the easiest to teach, it is far more difficult to instill the positive attitude, redirecting attention from the exclusive focus on risks to the promotion of comfort, reassurance, and a positive birth experience. It takes a while for new team members to reset their minds and put trust in this new approach. One of the most important learning objectives is the avoidance of planting psychological "black worms" (4.2) that inevitably trigger unnecessary inductions of worried though otherwise well women. In this respect, many women need to be re-educated as well, and that is, in fact, the greatest challenge of all. However, the more the system is adopted and spread, the easier this will be.

> Quality improvement requires a mind reset in both providers and clients/patients.

26.3 Regular perinatal audit

Changing practice patterns serves no useful purpose if the reduction of interventions is achieved at the expense of perinatal outcomes. Therefore, formal feedback from the pediatricians must be provided at least every week. In these multidisciplinary meetings, the obstetric and neonatal details of every case with suboptimal perinatal outcome should again be subjected to scrutiny. In our experience, following low-risk pregnancies, adverse outcomes such as perinatal infection, trauma, and asphyxia are virtually the exclusive result of protocol violations.

Ongoing audit of interventions linked to maternal and perinatal outcomes is the very foundation of proactive support of labor.

26.4 Mother debriefing and personal feedback

Standard debriefing 6 weeks after delivery by the childbirth educator (18.6) evaluates women's satisfaction with their childbirth experience. These structured interviews on the basis of validated questionnaires provide indispensable information – both positive and negative – for meaningful feedback to individual nurses, midwives, and doctors. In fact, intensive use of all mothers' feedback is the most effective tool to improve bedside manners on the personal level. All staff members – ranging from nurses to consultants – should be provided with the aggregated feedback data (Chapter 27). Complaints about an individual caregiver should be discussed in private, and a plan for improvements should be made. The motto is: don't talk about people; talk with people.

26.4.1 Regular nursing audit

The labor ward nurses and midwives play the pivotal role in high-quality childbirth. That is why they should be encouraged to hold regular meetings to discuss the art, skill, and science of labor support on the basis of mutual experiences, nursing studies, and the structured feedback from all women subjected to their care.

A continuous, multidisciplinary audit system ensures that every important aspect of birth care is kept under constant review.

26.5 Meaningful year reports

A current account of interventions and outcomes must be maintained on a regular basis, and the overall year results should be discussed in plenary. It is difficult to address what "a good induction rate" or "a good cesarean birth rate" is for a given hospital, since not every maternity center is dealt the same cards. Socio-cultural and medical characteristics of the population may vary widely between hospitals. What is obligatory, though, for any institution, is to know their population and the level of interventions, and to have an opinion on whether or not they are appropriate.[4] A meaningful hospital year report enables learning from trends over time and from comparisons with other centers, both nationally and internationally. That is the subject of the final chapter.

Effective audit cycle

"Quality is related to outcome, and outcome will guide processes." [4]

References

1. Nelson EC, Batalden PB, Godfrey MM. Quality Design: A Clinical Microsystems Approach. New York: Wiley; 2006

2. Lukas CV, Holmes SK, Cohen AB, *et al.* Transformational change in health care systems: an organizational model. Health Care Manage Rev 2007;**32**:309–20

3. Wennberg JE. Dealing with medical practice variations: a proposal for action. Health Affairs 1984;**3**:6–32

4. Robson M, Hartigan L, Murphy M. Methods of achieving and maintaining an appropriate caesarean section rate. Best Practice Res Clin Obstet Gynaecol 2013;**27**:297–308

Chapter 27

External audit of procedures and outcomes

Every woman deserves high-quality care during pregnancy and childbirth. While no one is likely to question this basic human right, there may be marked disagreement about what quality of care is. This issue must be resolved by defining simple and replicable quality indicators that allow fair comparisons to be made for meaningful external audit. The most relevant quality benchmarks are maternal satisfaction with the childbirth experience and intervention rates in relation to maternal and neonatal outcomes.

27.1 Women's satisfaction

Although mothers' satisfaction should be considered as the principal measure of quality, few obstetricians and midwives evaluate this outcome in their own practice on a systematic basis. Consequently, their impressions of women's attitudes to labor may be colored by reactions of (prejudiced) women with strong views, or complainants who may not be representative. General ideas about women's desires – whether these be a general preference for "all natural birth" or a cesarean section without any medical indication – are often biased and reinforced by self-selection. Generalizations are then readily made, and strong opinions defended without any serious attempt at systematic verification with their patients/clients after delivery.

> *Women's satisfaction with the childbirth experience is the predominant quality indicator that needs to be monitored constantly.*

27.1.1 Constant monitoring

All women who gave birth in our integrated obstetrical/midwifery birth center are interviewed 6 weeks after delivery by the childbirth educator (Chapter 18) or sent a questionnaire for structured feedback. The response rate is 70 to 80%. Validated questions explore their

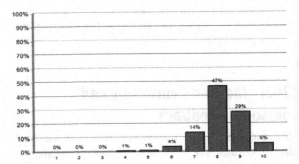

Figure 27.1 Satisfaction with the childbirth experience of the women under the care of the in- and out-of-hospital integrated birth center "Livive" of the St. Elisabeth hospital in Tilburg, the Netherlands (2011–2013; *n* = 3107).

appreciation of the antenatal care, the pre-labor information, the labor experience, the postpartum care, the attitudes of the caregivers, the organization, and the in- and out-of-hospital facilities. The mothers score their overall appreciation on a 0 to 10 scale (Figure 27.1). The overall satisfaction scores are available to the public on the birth center's website and updated every 6 months.[1]

This feedback invariably confirms women's appreciation of the integrated organization with complementary roles of midwives and obstetricians, closely working together and placing the pregnant woman first. Mothers also appreciate the well-informed birth-plan and emphasize the importance of pre-labor information that corresponds with actual practice. Very few women complain afterward of the birth-plan, as long as the policies were fully executed, the promises about labor support were kept, and the reasons for any intervention or deviation from protocol were clearly explained. Of course, 100% satisfaction will never be reached, but women's dissatisfaction, if critically analyzed, nearly always proves to originate in disappointing mismatches between expectations and practice. This emphasizes the necessity of strict adherence to the agreed birth-plan.

27.2 Benchmarking intervention rates

There is a lack of standardized information allowing meaningful comparisons of intervention rates between hospitals or nations. Annual reports vary widely in patient stratification, reporting parity-based or mixed-parity data and subdivisions into varying gestational age groups as well as arbitrarily defined subsets of low-risk, medium-risk, and high-risk pregnancies, to name just a few confounders. Furthermore, intervention rates may be affected by several demographic, fetal, and obstetric factors, such as the profile of the index population and the ratio between nulliparas and multiparas. No less confusing is a substantial though unknown number of midwife-led (low-risk) deliveries outside the hospital leading to underestimation of the numerator and overestimation of the intervention rates for some hospitals, particularly in the Netherlands. The missing values cannot be traced reliably because independent midwives move between various hospitals. Most of the above-mentioned factors are beyond the control of obstetricians. That is why the "raw" cesarean birth rate of a given institution is unsuitable for assessing the labor and delivery skills of its providers. Several suggestions for risk-adjusted algorithms have been made to facilitate inter-unit comparisons, but so far none of these complex concepts has gained wide acceptance.[2–11] What is more, the incidence of "dystocia" and "fetal distress" currently reported in hospital year reports are merely statements of the number of operative deliveries included under those headings on an arbitrary basis. The same holds true for national databases. Such data relay nothing about the quality of the care processes involved.

> *Blunt comparison of overall operative delivery rates between hospitals is meaningless. Cause and effect need to be determined if safe changes are to be made.*

27.2.1 The ten groups classification

To solve these problems, Robson introduced a classification system recognizing labor induction and cesarean delivery as the two dominant factors that determine the quality of care. Quality control is based on the analysis of ten groups (Table 27.1) that are totally inclusive and mutually exclusive, meaning that all deliveries ranging from "low risk" to "high risk" are included and a woman can be classified in one single group only.[13]

The "ten groups" classification avoids debates on arbitrary definitions of "risks" and distinguishes between the main obstetric factors that determine operative intervention rates: parity, spontaneous labor onset or induction, previous cesarean section, fetal presentation, and gestational age. The ten groups are objective, clinically relevant and withstand close scrutiny.[14] The system assesses the quality of a given birth center in a standardized way, and year reports based on the ten groups allow fair comparison of intervention rates between units nationally and internationally as well as monitoring trends over time.

The ten-group system helps to understand the care processes per group, the related interventions, and their consequences in terms of benefits and costs. The way the sizes of the groups relate to each other (Table 27.2) and the intervention rate per group (Tables 27.3–27.5) are strong indicators for the quality of the policies in a particular institution and the labor and delivery skills of its professionals. Careful interpretation of the results will guide practice changes, and the ten-group system allows monitoring improvements.

Table 27.1 The ten groups classification (Robson) for internal and external audit purposes

1	Nulliparas, single cephalic, ≥37 weeks, spontaneous labor onset
2	Nulliparas, single cephalic, ≥37 weeks, induced or pre-labor cesarean section (CS). 2A: primed/induced; 2B: pre-labor CS
3	Multiparas (excluding previous CS), single cephalic, ≥37 wks, in spontaneous labor
4	Multiparas (excl. prev. CS), single cephalic, ≥37 wks, induced or pre-labor CS. 4A: primed/induced; 4B: cesarean delivery before labor
5	Multiparas with previous CS, single cephalic, ≥37 weeks
6	All nulliparous breeches
7	All multiparous breeches (including previous CS)
8	All multiple pregnancies (including previous CS)
9	All abnormal lies (including previous CS)
10	All single cephalic deliveries, <37 weeks (including previous CS)

Table 27.2 The contribution that each group makes to the overall population

Total	1	2A	2B	3	4A	4B	5	6	7	8	9	10
4059	1245	471	27	1056	336	33	345	108	71	102	10	255
100%	31%	12%	0.7%	26%	8%	0.8%	8.5%	2.7%	1.7%	2.5%	0.2%	6.3%

Table 27.3 The contribution that each group makes to the overall cesarean rate

Overall 19% (772/4059)	1	2	3	4	5	6	7	8	9	10
$n = 772$	88	164	12	20	185	99	47	46	10	91
100%	11%	21%	1.6%	2.6%	24%	13%	7.4%	6.0%	1.3%	12%

Quality relates to maternal and fetal outcomes, and these should be scrutinized per group so that the processes involved can be modified in a tailor-made and safe fashion.

27.2.2 Population characteristics

The tables that follow show the data pooled over a 3-year period (2011–2013) from the integrated midwifery-obstetrical birth center "Livive" as described previously (25.4.1). The women represent an average western European pregnant population: roughly 20% is first- or second-generation non-Europeans. The institution is a regional teaching hospital. Intrapartum transfers ($n = 1043$) from independent, non-affiliated midwives have been excluded from the analysis because policies until transfer were undefined and not always compliant with those advocated in this book. Moreover, if those patients had been included, it would have affected the data in an unknown fashion as the number of non-transferred home deliveries by these independent midwives is unknown.

The data presented here are fully representative for *proactive support of labor* as practiced in our integrated midwifery/obstetrical birth center. The intervention rates should be eligible for comparison with those of any other regional teaching hospital catering for the entire pregnant population.

27.2.3 Inter-group distributions

The relative size of the groups 1 to 5 reveals relevant information. In general, nulliparous women are scheduled for an induction or pre-labor cesarean section (group 2A + B) because of worries about something that might happen. So, the ratio between group 1 and group 2 (A + B) is indicative of risk assessment and coaching skills to encourage low-risk nulliparous women to wait for spontaneous labor. Although this ratio compares favorably to many other units, there is still room for improvement (26.2.3).

The size of group 3 (spontaneous parous labors) relates to the quality of care provided the first time around: the better women's experiences in their first labor, the fewer worries, and the larger becomes group 3 relative to group 4 and 5. Parous women are generally subjected to induction or a pre-labor (repeat) cesarean section (groups 4A + B and group 5) because of worries instigated by something that did happen during the previous pregnancy or birth. The size of groups 6–10 is beyond the control of providers.

The relative size of groups 1 to 5 reveals important information about institutional policies, and labor and delivery skills of its professionals.

27.2.4 Cesarean rates per group

The overall cesarean rate (19%) compares favorably with that of most institutions, both nationally and internationally. Groups 1, 2, and 5 contribute 57% to the overall cesarean delivery rate (Table 27.3), and the main contributors are group 2 (nulliparous inductions) and group 5 (repeat cesareans).

An international comparative study indicates that 98% of the marked inter-institutional variation in overall cesarean delivery rates can be attributed to cesarean deliveries in groups 1 and 2 alone.[15] It is exactly these groups that are amenable to the policies advocated in this book. The data clearly illustrate the tempering effect of *proactive support* on cesarean delivery rates. Evidently, expert care with relatively few cesarean deliveries in groups 1 and 2 keeps the size of group 5 (cesarean scar) to an acceptably low level (8.5%, Table 27.2), thereby effectively reducing overall cesarean rates (Table 27.3).

"Quality is related to outcome, and outcome will guide processes."[13] Therefore, the institutional results should be discussed comprehensively (Chapter 26). Perhaps the most effective initiative to rekindle everyone's desire to promote spontaneous delivery is the provision of each doctor on a regular basis with her/his individual induction and operative delivery rates in term first pregnancies (group 1 and 2).

> The best way to safely reduce overall cesarean rates is to avoid a cesarean delivery first time around by improving the conduct and care in first labors and restrictive use of induction in first pregnancies.

27.2.5 Nulliparous deliveries at term

Proactive support is specifically designed for the supervision of first labors with a single, term fetus in the cephalic presentation. Therefore, the quality of the system is best judged by the intervention and outcome data of groups 1 and 2 (Table 27.4).

Group 1: In 77% of these term spontaneous nulliparous labors, women gave birth spontaneously, 5% ($n = 61$) of them at home. The moderate operative delivery rates illustrate the benefits of the integral approach and the well-defined birth-plan, including diagnosis of labor, early correction of dystocia, and one-to-one supportive care. The relatively high oxytocin treatment rate in this group pays off with a low

cesarean delivery rate (7.1%) and a low instrumental vaginal delivery rate (16%). About 50% of women delivered in 6 hours or less, 98% within 12 hours, and 100% within 14 hours. In 0.9% of group 1 women, obstructed labor was diagnosed and resolved by cesarean delivery: 0.5% cephalic malpresentation and 0.4% CPD. The indications for the other cesareans were oxytocin resistant dynamic dystocia and/or fetal intolerance/distress.

Group 2A: The high operative delivery rates in this group reconfirm the negative effects of priming/induction on the course and outcome of first labors. This finding is consistent with data from all international studies using the ten-group analysis.[15–22] The need for epidural analgesia is more than twice as high as in spontaneous labors, and only 45% deliver spontaneously. The cesarean rate increases fourfold (29%), and the instrument-assisted vaginal delivery rate (26%) is also markedly higher than that after spontaneous labor onset (16%). The conclusion is clear: reduction of labor inductions in first pregnancies is important to reduce overall operative delivery rates.

Group 2B: This group included five cesareans on request without any somatically medical indication (5/1245 = 0.4%). The other 22 pre-labor cesarean sections in term, first, single cephalic pregnancies (22/1245 = 1.8%) were performed for strictly medical reasons.

27.2.6 Multiparous deliveries at term

Table 27.5 shows a completely different picture and clearly illustrates that parous labors are not comparable in any way to first labors (Chapter 13).

Group 3: Dystocia and the need for oxytocin in spontaneous parous labor are rare indeed, and the demand for epidurals is low. Evidently, a safe and rewarding first birth results in low intervention rates

Table 27.4 Interventions and mode of delivery in groups 1 and 2

Nulliparas, single, cephalic, ≥37 weeks (2011–2013)	Number 1743	Oxytocin	Epidural	Cesarean delivery	Vacuum/ forceps	Spontaneous delivery
Group 1: Spontaneous labor	1245 100%	594 48%	386 31%	88 7.1%	196 16%	961 77%
Group 2A: Priming/ induction	471 100%	381 81%	325 69%	137 29%	123 26%	211 45%
Group 2B: Pre-labor C-section	27 100%			27 100%		

Table 27.5 Interventions and mode of delivery in multiparas

Multiparas, single, cephalic, ≥37 weeks (2011–2013)	Number 1762	Oxytocin	Epidural	Cesarean delivery	Vacuum/ forceps	Spontaneous delivery
Group 3: Spontaneous labor	1046 (100%)	39 3.7%	86 8.1%	12 1.1%	9 0.9%	1035 98%
Group 4A: Priming/ induction	336 (100%)	141 42%	155 46%	20 5.9%	10 2.9%	407 91%
Group 4B: Pre-labor CS	33 (100%)			33 100%		
Group 5: With cesarean scar	347 (100%)	6 1.7%	80 23%	185 53%	45 13%	117 34%

Table 27.6 Adverse perinatal outcomes of term, singleton, cephalic pregnancies (*lethal congenital malformation)

	Group 1 $n = 1245$	Group 2 $n = 498$	Group 3 $n = 1056$	Group 4 $n = 369$	Group 5 $n = 345$
Stillbirth	0	0	0	0	1
Intrapartum death	0	0	0	0	0
Umbilical artery pH ≤ 7.00	2	5	1	2	1
NICU admission	4	5	1	2	3
Neonatal death (≤46 days)	1*	0	0	0	1*

in next pregnancies. Roughly 3 out of 4 of the 1.1% intrapartum cesarean deliveries were performed for obstructed labor and the other quarter for fetal compromise. The few instrumental vaginal deliveries (<1%) were performed to expedite delivery for fetal reasons, not failed expulsion.

Group 4: In multiparas too, priming/induction is associated with relatively high cesarean odds. Nearly 6% of parous inductions ends with a cesarean delivery (failed induction).

Group 5: While cesarean rates in this group approach 100% in many centers, VBAC is accepted in our hospital under strict precautions. Induction is avoided or, if necessary, limited to amniotomy alone rather than using pharmacological treatment. The use of oxytocin (if used at all) is limited to the retraction phase of first-stage labor. The repeat cesarean rate is 53% (19% ante partum and 34% intrapartum), and the instrumental delivery rate is 13%.

Remaining groups: As groups 6 to 10 (which include both nulliparous and parous women) do not relate to the policies of *proactive support of labor*, the intervention data are not further analyzed. It should

be noted, though, that, because pre-labor transfers from independent midwives were included in the 4095 pregnancies analyzed, there might be a slight over-representation of these and other "medium- and high-risk" patients in our population.

27.3 Safety

In groups 1 to 5, there was just one stillbirth (at 37+1 weeks) in a woman with a cesarean scar (feto-maternal hemorrhage). There were no other perinatal losses in term, singleton pregnancies of cephalic babies without congenital malformations (Table 27.6). Corrected perinatal mortality only occurred in groups 6 to 10.

In addition to the regular internal audit of perinatal outcomes (Chapter 26), independent multidisciplinary experts from outside the hospital subjected all perinatal deaths and neonatal intensive care admissions to scrutiny as part of the National Perinatal Audit program.[23] None of the adverse perinatal outcomes in groups 1 to 5 could be attributed to the restrictive induction policies, and there has not been a single cause to question fetal safety of the protocols specific for *proactive support of labor.*

> *The protocols of proactive support of labor prove to be safe for babies and mothers.*

Both the intervention and the outcome data compare favorably with those of most other centers catering for pregnancies ranging from "low-risk" to "high-risk".[2–22] The composite outcomes illustrate the safety of the policies for both mothers and their babies.

27.4 Sense of proportion

Institutional cesarean delivery rates should not be judged in isolation from other results and epidemiological features. Operative intervention rates in term pregnancies are only one of many factors that determine the quality of care. The key question is not whether the operative delivery rate of a particular birth center is high or low, but rather whether it is defendable in light of the results, after considering all the relevant information.[13] The ten-group analysis will help to understand cause and effect at the hospital level, and the outcomes will guide structural reforms in the care processes.

Women will always choose the place of birth and the type of delivery that they think is safest for their baby and themselves. To make the right decision, women need to have access to the data of the institution in which they will give birth, not vague epidemiological information from the literature aggregated from completely different settings and contexts (6.5). Professionals should recognize this and be obliged to provide all relevant information of institutional procedures and outcomes per group.[13]

> *The combined data illustrate the balance that has been struck between maternal and neonatal outcomes, resulting in high levels of maternal satisfaction.*

There is no plausible reason why these results could not be reproduced in other institutions. It all depends on rediscovery of basic science, positive psychology, personal attention, strict diagnoses, clearly defined labor and delivery procedures, and – most importantly – constant high-profile audit of all procedures and outcomes. Because the evidence suggests that the spiraling operative delivery rates in term

pregnancies in other institutions are ineffective if not downright harmful (Chapter 2), the ball is in their court to provide good evidence to justify the continuation of their practice.

27.4.1 Sum of the parts

It bears repetition that *proactive support of labor* is an all-embracing concept, and that all medical and non-medical aspects of care discussed in this book must be closely addressed if real quality improvements are to be made. It is the sum of all parts that makes it a highly sophisticated form of maternity care, marked by safety, simplicity, and high quality.

Importantly, the policy framework is not designed with the sole intention of reducing cesarean delivery rates but rather to reset the mind to promote a safe, spontaneous, and relatively easy birth. Significant improvement of women's satisfaction with their childbirth experience is, in fact, the most beneficial and most rewarding outcome.

In conclusion: the approach presented here is of great benefit to all pregnant women, their babies, and the providers who care for both of them. The principles and clear policies of *proactive support of labor* will remain as relevant in the future as they are today. Offering safe and really supportive help at the beginning of life is both a challenge and a privilege.

References

1. Website of the integrated midwifery-obstetrical birth center "Livive" at the St. Elisabeth hospital, in Tilburg, the Netherlands. http://www.Livive.nl

2. Cleary R, Beard RW, Chapple J. The standard primipara as a basis for inter-unit comparisons of maternity care. Br J Obstet Gynaecol 1996;**103**:223–9

3. Main EK. Reducing cesarean births rates with data-driven quality improvement activities. Pediatrics 1999;**103**:374–83

4. Elliott JP, Russell MM, Dickason LA. The labor adjusted cesarean section rate: a more informative method than cesarean section "rate" for assessing a practitioner's labor and delivery skills. Am J Obstet Gynecol 1997;**177**:139–43

5. Lieberman E, Lang JM, Heffner LJ. Assessing the role of case mix in cesarean delivery rates. Obstet Gynecol 1998;**92**:1–7

6. Elferink-Stinkens PM, Van Hemel OJ, Hermans MP. Obstetric characteristics profiles as quality assessment of obstetric care. Eur J Obstet Gynecol Reprod Biol 1993;**51**:85–90

7. Stivanello E, Rucci P, Carretta E, *et al*. Risk adjustment for inter-hospital comparison of caesarean delivery rates in low-risk deliveries. PLoS One 2011;**6**: e28060

8. Chaillet N, Dumont A. Evidence-based strategies for reducing cesarean section rates: a meta-analysis. Birth 2007;**34**:53–64

9. Turcot L, Marcoux S, Fraser WD. Canadian Early Amniotomy Study Group. Multivariate analysis of risk factors for operative delivery in nulliparous women. Am J Obstet Gynecol 1997;**176**:395–402

10. Thomas J, Callwood A, Broklehurst P, Walker J. The National Sentinel Caesarean Section Audit. Br J Obstet Gynaecol 2000;**107**:579–80

11. Wilkes PT, Wolf DM, Kronbach DW, Kunze M, Gibbs RS. Risk factors for cesarean delivery at presentation of nulliparous patients in labor. Obstet Gynecol 2003;**102**:1352–7

12. Robson MS. Classification of cesarean sections. Fetal Maternal Med Rev 2001;**12**:23–39

13. Robson M, Hartigan L, Murphy M. Methods of achieving and maintaining an appropriate caesarean section rate. Best Pract Res Clin Obstet and Gynaecol 2013;**27**:297–308

14. Torloni MR, Betran AP, Souza JP, *et al*. Classifications for cesarean section: a systematic review. PLoS ONE 2011;**6**:e14566

15. Brennan DJ, Robson MS, Murphy M, O'Herlihy C. Comparative analysis of international cesarean delivery rates using 10-group classification identifies significant variation in spontaneous labor. Am J Obstet Gynecol 2009;**201**:308.e1–8

16. Brennan DJ, Murphy M, Robson MS, O'Herlihy C. The singleton, cephalic, nulliparous woman after 36 weeks of gestation: contribution to overall cesarean delivery rates. Obstet Gynecol 2011;**117**:273–9

17. Stivanello E, Rucci P, Carretta E, *et al*. Risk adjustment for inter-hospital comparison of caesarean delivery rates in low-risk deliveries. PLoS One 2011;**6**:e28060

18. Kelly S, Sprague A, Fell DB, *et al*. Examining caesarean section rates in Canada using the Robson classification system. J Obstet Gynaecol Can 2013;**35**:206–14

19. Costa ML, Cecatti JG, Souza JP, *et al*. Using a Caesarean Section Classification System based on characteristics of the population as a way of monitoring obstetric practice. Reprod Health 2010;**7**:13

20. Colais P, Fantini MP, Fusco D, *et al*. Risk adjustment models for interhospital comparison of CS rates using Robson's ten group classification system and other socio-demographic and clinical variables. BMC Pregnancy Childbirth 2012;**12**:54

21. Mueller M, Kolly L, Bauman M, Imboden S, Surbek D. Analysis of caesarean section rates over time in a single Swiss centre using a ten-group classification system. Swiss Med Wkly 2014;**144**:1–11

22. Lee YY, Roberts CL, Patterson JA, *et al*. Unexplained variation in hospital caesarean section rates. Med J Aus 2013;**199**:348–53 doi:10.5694/mja13.10279

23. Website of Dutch National Perinatal Audit Program. http://www.perinataleaudit.nl

Index

Printed in the United States
By Bookmasters